THE HEALTH OF HORSES

LONGMAN VETERINARY HEALTH SERIES

Forthcoming titles

Livestock Health and Welfare:
Edited by Roy Moss

The Health of Poultry:
Edited by Mark Pattison

Small Ruminant Health:
Edited by Tony J Wilsmore & Peter J Goddard

Animal Breeding and Infertility:
Edited by Michael C Meredith:

The Health of Dairy Cattle:
Edited by David G White

The Health of Pigs:
Edited by John R Hill & David W B Sainsbury

Food Hygiene:
Edited by Jeremy Hall

Nutrition and Animal Health:
Edited by John T Abrams

The Health of Horses

Edited by
David G Powell
and
Stephen G Jackson

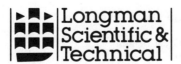
Longman
Scientific &
Technical

Longman Scientific & Technical,
Longman Group UK Ltd,
Longman House, Burnt Mill, Harlow,
Essex CM20 2JE, England
and Associated Companies throughout the world.

First published 1992

ISBN 0-582-08346-X

British Library Cataloguing in Publication Data
A catalogue record for this book is available from the British Library

Set by 3MM in 10/12½pt Plantin roman.

Printed and Bound in Great Britain
at the Bath Press, Avon

CONTENTS

Chapter 4   Pasture Management

Chapter 5   Housing and Ventilation

LIST OF CONTRIBUTORS

Stephen G Jackson, PhD
Vice President Research and Marketing, Kentucky Equine
Research Inc.

Charles T Dougherty, BSc, MS, PhD
Professor of Agronomy, University of Kentucky

John F Leech, MA
Director of the Livingston County Cooperative Extension
Service, Michigan State University

Walter W Zent, DVM
Veterinarian and partner, Hagyard-Davidson-McGee
Associates, Lexington

Eugene T Lyons, PhD
Professor of Veterinary Science, University of Kentucky

J Harold Drudge, DVM, ScD
Emeritus Professor, University of Kentucky

David G Powell, BVSc, FRCVS
Equine Epidemiologist, University of Kentucky

Roberta M Dwyer, DVM, MS
Assistant Professor, University of Kentucky

LIST OF COLOUR PLATES (pp 192–3)

Figure 7.2 Infective larvae of strongyles present in droplets of water on blades of grass awaiting ingestion.

Figure 7.3 Aneurysm of the anterior mesenteric artery caused by migrating larvae of *Strongylus vulgaris*, showing large thrombus in the lumen of the enlarged artery.

Figure 7.4 Mature, blood-engorged large strongyles attached to the mucosa of the large intestine.

Figure 7.5 (a) Larvae of small strongyles embedded in the mucosa of the caecum and colon. Gross view showing range of sizes between large red signet-ring forms and the small black specks.

Figure 7.5 (b) Photomicrograph of small strongyle larvae embedded in mucosa revealing the form of the specks in Figure 5 (a).

Figure 7.6 Mucosa of dorsal colon featuring a darkened crater-like lesion caused by a small strongyle (*Triodontophorus*).

Figure 7.7 Masses of immature (left) and mature (right) ascarids (*Parascaris equorum*) near a rupture of the wall of the small intestine of a foal.

Figure 7.8 Typical clusters of the red-coloured common bot (*Gasterophilus intestinalis*) and the yellow-coloured throat bot (*G. nasalis*) attached to walls of stomach and duodenum, respectively.

Figure 7.9 Tailhead of horse with loss of hair and roughened appearance due to rubbing induced by pinworm infection (*Oxyuris equi*).

FOREWORD

George Bernard Shaw when invited to write a preface for a book replied to the author, 'after reading my preface, who would read your book'. There is no such problem with *The Health of Horses*—read this excellent book and do not waste time reading the preface.

The layout of this book is simple and practical. Take the sub-heading 'colic' as an example. This common and often fatal condition in horses is described in about four hundred words. All the salient points and the digestive upsets, which are part of the problem, are mentioned and the reader is advised to seek further information.

To the busy farm manager or teacher this book should be an invaluable source of basic information. The chapter on pasture management shows how to provide good pasture for horses. The prevention of disease is the basic theme throughout the book—vaccination programme, parasite control, nutritional disorders are all dealt with in different chapters with solid recommendations. Housing and ventilation are dealt with in a cost effective way with good photographs and a very useful building checklist (Appendix 5.1).

Sitting in my library surrounded by countless books on horses, I ask the question—if instant information in easy to read form is required what book would I recommend? *The Health of Horses* is the answer. The topics covered are pertinent to the horse breeding industry and the authors, who are experts of world renown, have the ability to put scientific information in concise form which is easy to understand. The diagrams, charts and photographs throughout are very effective and informative, while the tables of scientific information are well set out. For these reasons, *The Health of Horses* should become a standard reference book for every horse farm manager. Finally, the sections on nutrition are the simple answer to the frequent question, 'how should I feed my horse?'

Michael Osborne
Kildangan Stud
April 1991

PREFACE

The Health of Horses provides information on the basic principles of management and husbandry to ensure the well-being and welfare of the horse. A positive attempt has been made to avoid complex scientific terminology so the reader with a basic knowledge of biology can understand and apply the information provided. The information will be of considerable value to horseowners throughout the world even though queries may arise when terminology differs from one continent to another. This is most apparent in the chapter dealing with housing where reference is made to barns and stalls which are the accepted description of accommodation for horses in North America. Stables is the term used in Europe and they differ in design from North American barns. In recent years, however, the design of American barns has been utilized extensively to build equine housing in Europe. The basic requirements for materials and ventilation are the same whether they are incorporated in barns or stables.

The initial chapters discuss the dietary requirements of the horse during different phases of activity. It should be remembered that the horse evolved as a grazing animal and its digestive system is adapted to cope with a large amount of roughage. Many disease problems which are discussed in the early chapters are associated with the inclusion of grain and extra protein sources in the diet. At present there is a distinct tendency to overfeed the horse, providing an excess of energy and protein to the detriment of roughage available as pasture or hay.

The chapter on housing outlines the minimum requirements

necessary to provide an environment which is safe and hygienic for horses as well as providing conditions which are acceptable to those who look after them in summer and winter. Considerable scientific advances have been made in recent years to improve fertility within the equine population. Many of these procedures are associated with enhancing fertility in the mare including the use of ultrasound to diagnose pregnancy and hormone therapy to synchronize oestrus. However, the traditional management tools of teasing and accurate record-keeping should not be ignored in an efficient breeding operation. An aspect of equine medicine that currently receives less attention because its efficacy is frequently taken for granted is the role of anthelmintics in the control of intestinal parasites. Historically intestinal parasitism was associated with horses in poor condition and showing signs of colic. With the advent of the latest generation of extremely effective anthelmintics intestinal parasitism should be considered a historical event providing horses are treated regularly in the recommended manner.

The introduction over the last 30 years of equine vaccines to control a variety of infectious diseases has resulted in the control but not the eradication of many disease problems. No vaccine can guarantee 100% protection but providing the schedule of vaccination is faithfully followed the risk of clinical disease is significantly reduced. The advice of the farm veterinarian with regard to the most suitable worming and vaccination schedule will ensure an effective programme at the lowest cost. The extensive range of biological and pharmaceutical products to treat and prevent disease in the equine population has tended to diminish the attention given to hygiene and disinfection. The value of both is discussed in the chapter on foal management with special reference to the appropriate selection of disinfectants to minimize outbreaks of contagious disease especially in the foaling unit. The final chapter discusses the procedures necessary to care for the horse's foot and a discussion of some of the more common hoof problems.

While reading this book it is anticipated that readers will develop a better understanding of how to care for their horses and prevent many of the more common disease problems. By doing so they will ensure that their horses perform consistently and provide a considerable amount of pleasure and enjoyment.

David G. Powell, Stephen G. Jackson
June 1991

ACKNOWLEDGEMENTS

The illustrations in the chapters were obtained from a variety of sources. Linda Blake Caddel supplied the photograph of the horse on the weighing scale in Chapter 2. The majority of photographs illustrating aspects of barn design and construction in Chapter 5 were provided by the Blood Horse Magazine and we are especially grateful to their photo librarian Betsy Burroughs for her assistance. Anne Eberhardt, photographer with the Blood Horse Magazine kindly supplied photographs for Figures 5.2, 5.5b and 5.6 in the same chapter. The Keeneland Association provided the photograph of the interlocking paving blocks in Figure 5.10. Many of the illustrations in Chapters 6 and 8 were taken by Dr Charles Issel and the ultrasound photographs in Chapter 6 were provided by Dr Norman Rantanen. Dr Ben Baker supplied the photograph of the mare 'in season' illustrated in Figure 6.1a. Copies of the farm record sheets were provided by Tom Stewart of Stoner Creek Farm. Dr Doug Leach supplied drawings illustrated in Figures 10.1, 10.2 and 10.3.

The time-consuming preparation of the manuscript was undertaken with considerable patience and attention to detail by Diane Haughey, staff assistant in the Department of Veterinary Science of the Gluck Equine Research Center. Without her active participation the book would not have been completed.

The staff of Longman Group UK Ltd. were encouraging, helpful and patient. Dr David Sainsbury was the instigator of our endeavours and a helpful critic.

We are grateful to the following for permission to reproduce copyright figures and tables:
American Association of Equine Practitioners for Fig. 8.3; National Academy Press for Tables 1.3 & 1.5.

1 BASIC PRINCIPLES OF EQUINE NUTRITION
STEPHEN G. JACKSON, PhD

Summary
The digestive system
Nutrients and their uses
Sources of nutrients in equine diets
Feed storage
Further reading

Summary

The horse evolved as a wandering herbivore, equipped with a functional caecum which permits utilization of fibrous feeds to meet a significant proportion of nutrient requirements. Utilization of cellulose and other fibrous fractions of the diet is made possible by the microbial flora in the hind gut. A significant portion of the energy and vitamin needs of the horse are met as a result of microbial digestion. Any management or feeding regime that alters the homeostasis of the hind gut will result in problems, so an understanding of gut function and the dynamics of the intestinal tract is essential to maintaining an effective feed management programme.

Like all species of livestock the horse has a daily requirement for protein, energy, vitamins, minerals and water. Protein should be of high quality such that essential amino acid requirements are met and special emphasis given to availability of the amino acid lysine in the young growing horse. Energy intake, derived from the carbohydrate, fibrous, fat and protein fraction of the diet should be adjusted to maintain growth and body condition. The macro and micro mineral requirements of the horse are met using a combination of organic (contained in feedstuffs) and inorganic sources. The primary macro minerals are calcium, phosphorus, potassium, magnesium, sodium and chlorine. Micro or trace minerals include selenium, copper, zinc, iron, iodine and manganese with others added as local conditions require. Fat-soluble vitamins, which include A, D, E and K, are present in a variety of feeds and are stored in the body. Water-soluble vitamins are not stored and must be synthesized in the intestinal tract by the horse daily or be present in the feed.

Nutrients commonly used to supplement forage in the horse's diet include cereal grains and plant protein. Sources of energy include maize, oats, barley and wheat by-products. Protein sources include soyabean, linseed, and to a lesser extent rape seed and distillers' dried grains. The grain mix should provide major nutrients, including protein, energy, minerals and vitamins, when forage intake is inadequate to meet requirements. The overall ration should be formulated to supplement forages, not replace them.

Forages should form the predominant part of the horse's ration. High-quality cool or warm season grasses maintained in an appropriate manner are capable of meeting the majority of the nutrient needs of most classes of horses. Soil fertility, forage availability and stocking rates should all be considered in assessing the contribution of forage towards meeting the horse's nutrient needs.

Processing such as crimping, rolling, flaking and pelleting is designed to enhance the digestibility and increase the homogeneity of feed. The increase in digestibility may not be worth the cost of processing, especially for mature horses with sound teeth. There are, however, grains such as barley and sorghum that should be processed prior to feeding. Pelleting is advantageous when there are several finely textured ingredients included in the formulation. Regardless of the means used to process or mix feed, proper storage is essential to maintaining feed quality. Even the highest quality feed is of no value if it is allowed to become mouldy or rancid.

Understanding the basic principles of equine nutrition is essential to producing a sound and healthy horse. There is probably no other area of equine management that is so influenced by 'old wives' tales', inaccurate information and superstition. It is illogical to accept progress in other areas of equine science and management but still cling to archaic and misguided methods for meeting the horse's nutrient requirements. The intention of the first three chapters is to present information concerning nutrient requirements and how they are utilized, what factors influence the variation seen in requirements between classes of horses and the impact that the physical form of feed has on its utilization.

The digestive system

The horse evolved as a wandering continuous grazing herbivore and is selective in what it eats, preferring certain species of plants to others. The digestive system evolved in this natural pursuit of a forage diet but the modern horse is asked to perform physical activities which have necessitated a major change in the natural diet.

The mature horse has 18 upper and 18 lower teeth consisting of six upper and lower incisors and 12 upper and lower molars. The function of teeth is prehension (gathering) and chewing and they participate in the digestive process by reducing the particle size of ingested food. Chewing stimulates the flow of saliva, which aids in digestion and swallowing. Hereditary dental problems such as parrot mouth (over-shot) and monkey jaw (under-shot) seriously impair the ability of the horse to gather and utilize food. The horse has fewer dental problems compared to humans, but when they occur horses lose weight and waste feed so annual dental examinations should be part of a horse management programme. As horses age, wearing of the teeth occurs, as a result of which sharp edges may develop on the outside of the upper teeth and inside of the lower teeth. This results in irritation to the cheeks and tongue causing ulcers and lacerations. When this occurs it is necessary to 'rasp' or 'float' the teeth using a file-like instrument to remove the offending sharp edges. After the teeth have been rasped a considerable improvement occurs and the horse no longer wastes food, is a more efficient food converter, gains weight, readily accepts the bit and is more amenable to training.

The oesophagus is a long muscular organ which moves food from the mouth to the stomach by peristaltic waves or muscular contractions. Saliva, produced by secretory glands in the mouth, helps lubricate the passage of food; consequently choking and obstruction within the oesophagus are rare.

The stomach of the horse is similar to that of the pig only larger and has a capacity of about 16 litres. The capacity compared to the rest of the gastrointestinal tract is small and has contributed to the horse being a continuous grazer able to handle many small meals rather than several large ones. It is therefore advantageous to split large amounts of feed into small portions rather than providing too much feed at one time; this decreases the incidddence of digestive problems associated with colic and enterotoxaemia. Digestion in the stomach is facilitated by the secretion of hydrochloric acid and enzymes, which include pepsin and trypsin. Because of the small capacity of the stomach it empties quickly so that food eaten at the beginning of a meal is already in the small intestine before feeding is completed.

The small intestine is a tubular structure approximately 21 m long, holds about 56 litres of ingesta and is composed of three segments, the duodenum, the jejunum and the ileum. The small intestine is the major area for absorption of protein, fat, carbohydrates and some minerals and vitamins. Enzymatic digestion which began in the stomach continues in the small intestine with enzymes secreted by the pancreas and intestinal mucosa.

The caecum of the horse performs the same function as the rumen of the cow and sheep and is the major area of microbial digestion. Microorganisms present in the caecum are capable of digesting fibrous feeds producing a major energy source, the volatile fatty acids. The B-complex vitamins, vitamin K and microbial proteins are synthesized by caecal microflora. The caecum may hold as much as 34 litres of ingesta and feed is held for a longer period compared to previous parts of the digestive system to allow fermentation to take place.

After ingesta passes from the caecum it enters the large intestine, specifically the large colon. The large colon has a capacity of about 68 litres and is composed of seven segments: the right ventral colon, the sternal flexure of the left ventral colon, the left ventral colon, the pelvic flexure of the left ventral colon, the left dorsal colon, the diaphragmatic flexure of the right dorsal colon and the right dorsal colon. Microbial fermentation, which began in the caecum, continues in the large intestine. The absorption of the products of microbial fermentation and minerals occurs in the large intestine as well as the resorption of water. After leaving the right dorsal colon, ingesta enters the small or descending colon. The small colon is about 3.5 m long and empties into the rectum. Faeces are voided via the anus, the posterior opening of the digestive tract.

From a practical standpoint the following should be borne in mind relative to the digestive system. The limit of voluntary dry matter consumption is 3–4% of body weight per day and to maintain normal gut function the horse should receive a minimum of 1% of its body weight per day as long stem hay or pasture. Horses receiving a large amount of feed per day should have it split into several smaller feeds.

Nutrients and their uses

The major classes of nutrients are water, energy, protein, vitamins and minerals. Horses require each of these nutrients in varying amounts for maintenance, growth, reproduction, lactation, work and in some cases fattening. The concentration (%) and amount of each nutrient required depends on several factors including age, use and condition of the horse.

Water

It is absolutely essential that the horse has access to fresh, clean water at all times, bearing in mind that the body of the horse consists of 70–80% water. There is an inverse relationship between body water and fat such that older fatter horses have a lower per cent body water than young horses. The minimum daily water requirement is the sum of water lost via sweat, urine and the respiratory tract plus water required for milk and muscle protein production. In a cool environment a horse requires 42–50 ml of water/kg of body weight per day. Work increases the horse's requirement for water up to 300% depending on the amount, duration and intensity. Elevated environmental temperatures, stress and disease also increase the requirement for water by as much as 50%. The heavy milking mare secretes as much as 13–18 kg of water per day in milk and the lactating mare's requirement is increased by over 200%. The largest single determinant of water intake is the amount of dry matter consumed, the horse consuming 2–4 litres of water for every kilogram of dry matter intake.

Water should always be fresh and clean and as safe as that consumed by humans. Sources listed in order of desirability are: fresh city water, well water, running creeks or rivers, lakes and small stock ponds. The optimum temperature of water for consumption is 7–18 °C.

Protein

Commercial horse feeds are sold on the basis of their protein concentration and are formulated around protein percentages to meet the requirement for various classes of horses. The age and use of the horse are the most important factors to be considered in respect of protein nutrition. Protein is a predominant component of muscles, organs and other tissues in the body and is a critical part of the diet throughout life. It is composed of chains of subunits called amino acids and the amount of the various amino acids available depends on the protein source. There are 25 amino acids of which the 10 listed in Table 1.1 are considered essential in the diet for the horse, including lysine which is considered the most important for growth. The other 15 amino acids are synthesized by the horse.

Table 1.1 Dietary essential amino acids

Phenylalanine	Alanine
Valine	Tryptophan
Threonine	Histidine
Methionine	Isoleucine
Leucine	Lysine

The protein content of feeds is expressed as per cent crude protein, which is determined by analysing the nitrogen content and multiplying the result by 6.25. It is not the most accurate method of expressing the value of protein but will suffice for commonly used protein sources. Of greater value than crude protein is digestible protein, which indicates the protein absorbed. However, basic feed analysis allows only predictions of digestibility not its actual quantitation.

Protein provides a source of amino acids for the synthesis of muscle, enzymes, hormones, bones and other tissues and may serve as a source of energy although this is not a major function. For protein to be used as energy, amino acids must be deaminated, meaning the amine or ammonium component is removed allowing the remaining carbon chain to be used for energy. This happens when excess protein is fed or if the horse is in a negative energy balance or starving. There is an inverse relationship between protein requirement and age. The young horse synthesizes muscle protein and other protein-requiring tissues, so has the greatest demand for protein. Specific protein requirements for the various classes of horses will be discussed in Chapter 2 but the following basic principles should be kept in mind. Protein is the most expensive ingredient in feeds and should not be considered as an energy source. Feeding excess protein will not cause a horse to grow faster. A barn containing horses that smells strongly of ammonia is a sign that protein is being overfed. Strenuous exercise does not significantly increase the horse's requirement for protein.

Protein deficiency rarely exists as more horses are overfed than underfed protein. Signs of protein deficiency in young horses include depressed growth, poor appetite, a rough haircoat and abnormal skeletal development. For older horses, protein deficiency is difficult to assess but in lactating mares a decrease in milk production is likely to occur. Non-protein nitrogen (NPN) includes urea and biuret commonly used in the diet of ruminant animals. Horses are not able to use significant amounts of urea to synthesize protein in the caecum. Urea and other non-protein nitrogen compounds, in elevated levels, may be toxic to the horse, and should not be used in horse rations.

Energy

Energy is provided by carbohydrates, fats and, to a lesser extent, protein. The predominant source of energy is carbohydrate, stored in plants primarily as starch, which is digested in the stomach and small intestine and absorbed as simple sugars. Cellulose, a plant structural carbohydrate, is another source and is digested by bacteria-derived cellulase in the caecum and absorbed as the volatile fatty acids—acetate, propionate and butyrate. In the analysis of feedstuffs, the carbohydrate fraction is represented as crude fibre (CF) and nitrogen free extract (NFE). Readily digested soluble carbohydrates, such as starch, are included in NFE; less digestible fibrous components, such as cellulose, are part of the CF. The more grain mix that is fed, the higher the NFE and the lower the CF; for instance, corn (maize) grain is 70.3% NFE and 2% CF, whereas timothy hay is 45.4% NFE and 32% CF. It follows that the higher the fibre content of the ration, the lower the digestibility and energy value of the ration. Thus cereal grains are used when the energy density of the diet needs to be increased.

Fat or lipids also supply a significant amount of energy to the horse. Fat is 2.25 times higher in energy value per unit weight than carbohydrate and is readily digested by the horse. The fat content of most rations averages 2–3% and is represented in analyses of feedstuffs by the ether extract. The use of supplemental fat in equine diets in the form of corn or maize oil, soyabean oil, blended vegetable fats or animal fat, such as tallow or lard, has received a great deal of attention. Fat has a high energy density, is highly digestible and fairly palatable. The addition of fat to the rations of horses with very high energy requirements may have considerable merit. Maize oil (50–60 g) added to the feed is used to improve the condition of the haircoat of sale horses. Fat as high as 15% of the diet has little effect on the palatability of the ration.

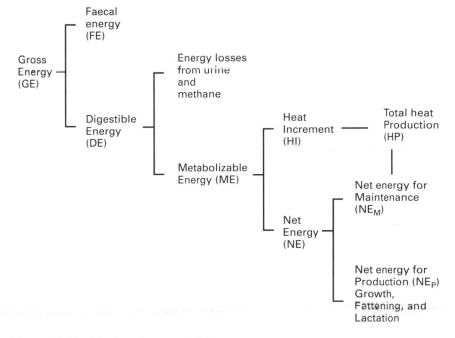

Figure 1.1 Partitioning of energy in feeds.

Figure 1.1 shows the way energy is partitioned in the body. Even though the unit of most importance in understanding the energy value of a feed is net energy (NE), most horse rations are discussed using digestible energy (DE) or more frequently total digestible nutrients (TDN). Digestible energy is expressed in kcal (kilocalories) or Mcal (megacalories or MJ (megajoules). One Mcal is equivalent to 1000 Kcal and 4.187 MJ is equivalent to 1 Mcal. To convert Mcal/kg to MJ/kg multiply by 4.187. The digestible energy value of maize is 3.4 Mcal/kg, whereas timothy hay is 1.98 Mcal/kg. Net energy values are more descriptive of the energy actually available to the horse for maintenance or productive functions. However, the lack of adequate NE values for horse feeds necessitates the use of DE values until such time as adequate research provides meaningful metabolizable and net energy values.

The other method of expressing the energy value of feeds is total digestible nutrients (TDN).

$$TDN = \% \ DCF + \% \ DCP + \% \ DNFE + (\% \ DEE \times 2.25)$$

where % DCF = % digestible crude fibre

% DCP = % digestible crude protein

% DNFE = % digestible nitrogen free extract

% DEE = % digestible ether extract (multiply by 2.25 because fat is 2.25 times as high in energy as carbohydrates)

For comparison purposes:

1 kg of TDN = 4.4 Mcal of DE or 1 lb of TDN = 2 Mcal DE

Minerals

A list of macro and micro or trace minerals required by the horse is shown in Table 1.2. Also, typical mineral levels found in more commonly fed horse feeds are shown in Table 1.3.

Table 1.2 Minerals required in the diets of horses

Macrominerals	Microminerals
Calcium (Ca)	Copper (Cu)
Phosphorus (P)	Zinc (Zn)
Magnesium (Mg)	Iron (Fe)
Potassium (K)	Molybdenum (Mo)
Sodium (Na)	Manganese (Mn)
Chloride (Cl)	Iodine (I)
Sulphur (S)	Selenium (Se)
	Chromium (Cr)
	Cobalt (Co)

Calcium

Calcium is the most abundant mineral within the body and is a major component of bones and teeth. During skeletal development, the cartilage of the skeleton is replaced by calcium in a process known as ossification and adequate dietary calcium is necessary to allow this transformation to occur. In addition to its role in skeletal development, calcium is required for muscle contraction, clotting of blood and maintenance of the acid–base balance. Calcium is present in higher concentrations in forages compared to grains. Rations containing large amounts of grain are supplemented with dicalcium phosphate or ground limestone to meet the horse's requirement for calcium. Deficiency of calcium results in rickets or poor bone mineralization amongst young horses and osteo-malacia or osteoporosis amongst older horses. Although the effect of excess calcium intake in the horse is not well established, it is apparent that high levels of calcium interfere with the absorption of trace minerals, including iron, zinc and copper. Excess calcium intake may be a possible contributing cause of developmental orthopaedic disorders (DOD) including osteochondro-sis (OCD) and epiphysitis.

Phosphorus

Phosphorus has a similar role to calcium and is an important component of bone. Eighty per cent of phosphorus in the body is found in the skeleton as crystalline hydroxyapatite, the major bone mineral. In addition to its role in bone metabolism, phosphorus performs a vital role in energy metabolism as a component of compounds such as adenosine triphosphate (ATP), creatine phosphate (CP) and inosine monophosphate (IMP). Organic or plant sources of phosphorus are not as readily absorbed as the inorganic sources dicalcium phosphate and monosodium phosphate. The amount of fluorine present in rock sources of phosphate may be too high and consequently the fluorine concentration of feeds should be monitored if inorganic phosphorus is used. Deficiencies of phosphorus result in improper bone mineralization, leading to skeletal problems. Inadequate phosphorus intake, especially in conjunction with high levels of calcium, may be one of the more important causes of epiphysitis in young horses. High intakes of phosphorus, along with low calcium, may predispose to symptoms of nutritional secondary hyperpara-thyroidism.

Calcium:phosphorus ratio

Because of the interrelated functions of calcium and phosphorus, the ratio as well as their absolute intake is important. The total ration should never contain more phosphorus than calcium. Ideally, the ratio of the total ration should be 1.2–1.7 calcium to 1.0 phosphorus. This ratio is especially critical at marginal levels of intake, but less so at higher intakes of calcium and phosphorus. Provided phosphorus requirements are met or exceeded, the horse can tolerate higher ratios than mentioned above. High ratios frequently occur when legume

Table 1.3 Vitamin and mineral values for feeds in Horse Diets[1]

Feed	Per cent in feed							I.U. per kg	
	Dry matter	Ca	P	Mg	K	Na	S	Vitamin A equivalent[2]	Vitamin E
Alfalfa (lucerne)									
Hay, sun-cured, early bloom	90.5	1.28	0.19	0.31	2.32	0.14	0.27	50608	23.5
Meal, dehydrated, 17% protein	91.8	1.38	0.23	0.29	2.40	0.10	0.22	29787	81.9
Barley									
Grain	88.6	0.05	0.34	0.13	0.44	0.03	0.15	817	23.2
Hay, sun-cured	88.4	0.21	0.25	0.14	1.30	0.12	0.15	18571	–
Beet pulp	91.0	0.62	0.09	0.26	0.20	0.18	0.20	88	–
Bermudagrass, coastal									
Hay	93.0	0.30	0.19	0.11	1.58	–	–	–	–
Brome, smooth hay, sun-cured, mid-bloom	87.6	0.25	0.25	0.09	1.74	0.01	–	–	–
Canarygrass, reed hay, sun-cured	89.3	0.32	0.21	0.19	2.60	0.01	0.12	6762	–
Canola									
Seed meal, solvent-extracted	90.8	0.63	1.18	0.55	1.22	0.01	1.23	–	–
Clover, Ladino									
Hay, sun-cured	89.1	1.20	0.30	0.42	2.17	0.12	0.19	57475	–
Clover, Red									
Hay, sun-cured	88.4	1.22	0.22	0.34	1.60	0.16	0.15	9727	–
Corn, Dent, Yellow									
Grain	88.0	0.05	0.27	0.11	0.32	0.03	0.11	2162	20.9
Distille's grains	92.0	0.10	0.41	0.06	0.17	0.09	0.42	1104	–
Cottonseed meal	91.0	0.17	1.11	0.54	1.30	0.04	0.26	–	–
Fescue, Kentucky									
Hay, sun-cured	91.9	0.37	0.27	0.14	1.76	0.02	–	–	–
Linseed meal	90.2	0.39	0.80	0.60	1.38	0.14	0.39	–	–
Lespedeza, Kobe									
Hay, sun-cured, mid-bloom	93.9	1.11	0.32	0.27	0.89	–	–	–	–
Milk									
Skimmed, dehydrated	94.1	1.28	1.02	0.12	1.60	0.51	0.32	–	9.1
Millet, Pearl									
Hay, sun-cured	87.4	–	–	–	–	–	–	–	–
Molasses									
Beet	77.9	0.12	0.02	0.23	4.72	1.16	0.46	–	4.0
Sugarcane, dehydrated	99.4	1.03	0.14	0.44	3.39	0.19	0.43	–	5.2
Sugarcane	74.3	0.74	0.08	0.31	2.98	0.16	0.35	–	5.4
Oats									
Grain	89.2	0.08	0.34	0.14	0.40	0.05	0.21	44	15.0
Groats	89.6	0.08	0.42	0.11	0.36	0.03	0.20		14.8
Hay, sun-cured	90.7	0.29	0.23	0.26	1.35	0.17	0.21	10792	–

Table 1.3 (*continued*)

Feed	Dry matter	Ca	P	Mg	K	Na	S	Vitamin A equivalent[2]	Vitamin E
								I.U. per kg	
Orchardgrass									
Hay, sun-cured	89.1	0.24	0.30	0.10	2.59	0.01	0.23	13 366	–
Pangolagrass									
Hay, sun-cured	91.0	0.42	0.21	0.14	1.27	–	–	–	–
Rice									
Bran with germ	90.5	0.09	1.57	0.88	1.71	0.03	0.18	–	85.3
Grain, ground	89.0	0.07	0.32	0.13	0.44	0.06	0.04	–	14.0
Mill run	91.6	0.15	0.46	0.10	0.52	–	0.18	–	5.3
Rye									
Grain	87.5	0.06	0.32	0.11	0.45	0.02	0.15	35	14.5
Ryegrass, Italian									
Hay, sun-cured, late vegetative	85.6	0.53	0.29	–	1.34	–	–	99 287	–
Sorghum, grain	90.1	0.04	0.32	0.15	0.37	0.01	0.13	468	10.0
Soyabean									
Seed meal, solvent-extracted, 44% protein	89.1	0.35	0.63	0.27	1.98	0.03	0.41	–	3.0
Seed meal without hulls, solvent-extracted	89.9	0.26	0.64	0.29	2.12	0.01	0.44	–	3.3
Sunflower									
Seed meal	92.5	0.42	0.94	0.65	1.17	0.02	0.31	–	11.1
Timothy									
Hay, sun-cured, early bloom	89.1	0.45	0.25	0.11	2.14	0.01	0.12	18 719	11.6
Wheat									
Bran	89.0	0.13	1.13	0.56	1.22	0.05	0.21	1048	14.3
Grain, hard, red winter	88.9	0.04	0.38	0.13	0.43	0.02	0.13	–	11.1
Grain, soft, red winter	88.4	0.03	0.36	0.12	0.35	0.01	0.13	–	15.6
Hay, sun-cured	88.7	0.13	0.18	0.11	0.88	0.19	0.19	30 304	–
Mill run, less than 9.5% fibre	89.9	0.10	1.02	0.47	1.20	0.22	0.17	–	31.9
Whey									
Dehydrated (cattle)	93.2	0.85	0.76	0.13	1.16	0.62	1.04	48.8	0.2
Yeast, Brewer's									
Dehydrated	93.1	0.14	1.36	0.24	1.68	0.07	0.44	–	2.1

[1] Adapted from 1989 NRC report *Nutrient Requirement of Horses*.
[2] The vitamin A equivalent was calculated as carotene × 400 except for value for dehydrated whey, which represents actual amounts of vitamin A.

Ca = calcium; P = phosphorus; Mg = magnesium; K = potassium; Na = sodium and S = sulphur.

hays such as alfalfa (lucerne) high in calcium are fed as the major roughage source. Rations with a calcium/phosphorus ratios as high as 3:1 have been fed to young horses and as high as 6:1 to mature horses without detrimental effects. It is when the ratio falls below 1:1 that problems occur.

Sodium and chloride

Salt (sodium chloride) should be freely available at all times and is added to commercial feeds at a level of 0.5–1% of the ration. Sodium and chloride are involved in many metabolic functions including secretion of hydrochloric acid in the stomach, maintenance of body fluid balance, control of pH, nerve conductivity and muscle contraction. Most feedstuffs are deficient in sodium and/or chlorine and so salt must be added. Salt is provided as a mineral salt block or included in the grain mix. Although the latter should provide adequate amounts of salt when the horse is consuming large amounts of feed, it is preferable to provide an additional method of salt supplementation. Even though horses are efficient in conserving salt during hot weather and in heavy training they are at risk of becoming deficient if it is not provided.

Magnesium

Magnesium serves as a cofactor for numerous enzymes and in metabolic pathways. It is involved in carbohydrate metabolism and is critical to the proper function of the nervous system. Most commonly fed rations contain adequate magnesium to meet the horse's requirement, and magnesium deficiency is not of practical significance. Horses appear to be more tolerant of magnesium deficiency than cattle and pastures which result in grass tetany among cattle rarely cause the condition in horses. Should hypomagnesium tetany be a problem, it is possible to supplement the ration with magnesium or add magnesium oxide to the salt mix. The magnesium level generally found in commercial feeds is around 0.25% and is adequate to meet the needs of all types of horses.

Potassium

Potassium is abundant in most forages and if horses are consuming hay in large amounts or are at pasture, potassium inadequacy is not of concern. Potassium is involved in the maintenance of osmotic balance, acid–base balance and digestive secretions. Hays and forages are high in potassium but grains are relatively low. Horses at high work intensity consuming a large amount of grain should be supplemented with potassium chloride. Situations which predispose a horse to loss of potassium include profuse sweating, diarrhoea and anorexia, at which time potassium supplementation is necessary.

Iron

Iron is probably the most abused mineral in horse rations. Iron is a component of red blood cells and functions as haem-iron in the oxygen-carrying pigment of blood, haemoglobin. Estimates of the iron requirement of the horse indicate that 40 ppm in the total diet is sufficient. Many horses receive in excess of 300 ppm iron via 'blood builders', 'iron tonics' and other supplemental sources of iron. The horse is efficient in the conservation and recycling of iron so that it is used repeatedly in haemoglobin synthesis. The only instance when iron deficiency is a problem is following severe blood loss, during heavy parasite infestation or following surgery. Premature foals benefit from iron supplementation as milk is not a good source and iron stored in the premature foal is minimal.

Selenium

The selenium status of the horse should be considered on a geographical basis as there are areas where deficiencies exist and others where toxicities are a problem. Although selenium is an essential nutrient for the horse, the requirement is low, 0.1 ppm, and the toxic level is also low, 4 ppm. It should never be used randomly or 'top dressed' over the feed. Selenium may be involved in the 'tying up' syndrome, which several investigators have reported will respond to selenium therapy. It has also been implicated as a cause of poor reproductive performance in mares causing a prolonged re-breeding interval, abortion, retained placenta and early embryonic death. Blood levels of 0.08–0.1 ppm selenium are considered adequate and horses with levels in this range or above do not benefit from supplemental selenium. If supplementation is necessary, it is commonly provided as sodium selenite.

Copper and zinc

Copper and zinc have received a great deal of attention in recent times due to their possible involvement in metabolic bone disease, including epiphysitis, osteochondrosis and wobbler disease. According to the National Research Council's (NRC) *Nutrient Requirements of Horses*, published in 1989, the minimum requirements for copper and zinc are 8 and 20 ppm respectively, or expressed another way, 8 and 20 mg/kg of dietary intake. The association between the two minerals and metabolic bone disease has not been fully elucidated. Copper deficiency results in impaired haemoglobin formation, muscular incoordination and abnormal bone metabolism. It is the latter which lends credence to the argument that horses develop bone problems due to inadequate copper.

The amount of copper in the diet may be adequate, but due to the presence of antagonists, such as zinc, inadequate absorption from the gut may occur. Copper is easily supplemented in the form of copper sulphate and the horse is more tolerant of high levels compared to ruminants. On a note of caution, it should be mentioned that it is often the practice to randomly, and without justification, supplement the horse's ration with high levels of trace minerals. Such additions should be made only if there is a real need for doing so and recognizing that toxicity problems may occur. There are many interactions involving trace minerals and by adding excess of one mineral a deficiency of another can easily occur. Cases of epiphysitis have been reported to respond to supplemental copper and it has become standard practice to formulate grain mixes for young horses containing 30–40 ppm copper.

Zinc promotes growth, wound healing and serves as a coenzyme or cofactor in many metabolic pathways. Although zinc deficiencies in horses fed conventional diets may occur they are usually the result of the inclusion of high levels of calcium. In other species zinc deficiency results in slow growth, poor hair development, parakeratosis and poor wound healing. Zinc toxicities have been reported in the horse, when excess zinc in the ration interferes with copper and calcium metabolism and results in an interactive deficiency of copper leading to severe bone problems. The NRC's recommendation for zinc is 20 ppm; however, most commercial rations contain 60–80 ppm zinc. If high zinc levels are present, the copper level should be increased.

Iodine

The NRC recommendation is that horses need 0.1 ppm of iodine in the total diet. The iodine requirement is met by allowing access to a mineralized salt block containing iodine or by including trace mineralized salt in the grain mix at 0.5% of the ration. Iodine is involved in the production of thyroxine by the thyroid gland and a deficiency stimulates production of thyroid-stimulating hormone by the pituitary gland causing enlargement of the thyroid gland. Many commercial mineral supplements contain iodine and care must be taken to prevent the inadvertent feeding of toxic levels of iodine, above 5 ppm.

Molybdenum

Most commonly fed feedstuffs contain adequate molybdenum to meet the horse's needs. A far more important problem than molybdenum deficiency is excess molybdenum. Although it has not been shown in the horse, molybdenum ties up copper resulting in copper deficiency among ruminants. There is no need to supplement horse rations with molybdenum.

Sulphur

One of the most important functions of sulphur is as a constituent of the sulphur-containing amino acids, methionine, cystine and cysteine. If adequate protein is being fed, sulphur supplementation is not thought to be necessary and excess may cause an antagonistic deficiency of minerals such as copper.

Cobalt

Cobalt is part of the vitamin cyanocobalamin (B_{12}) synthesized by bacteria in the caecum. Cobalt deficiency is not a problem as horses are more tolerant to low cobalt levels than cattle or sheep.

Vitamins

A vitamin is defined as an organic substance required in small amounts for regulating various metabolic processes in the body. Vitamins are classified as fat- or water-soluble; the fat-soluble vitamins include A, D, E and K, the water-soluble vitamins B and C. Fat-soluble vitamins are stored in the body to a much larger extent than water-soluble vitamins. The water-soluble vitamins are not stored to any appreciable extent and must be provided in the daily diet or synthesized. Most horses receive an excess amount of each vitamin in their diet. With the exception of vitamin A, horses at pasture do not require supplementation. But for horses in heavy work, rapidly growing young horses and foaling mares it may be necessary to add vitamins to the rations. Levels of vitamins A and E in some of the more commonly used horse feed ingredients are shown in Table 1.3.

Vitamin A

When evaluating the vitamin requirements of the horse, vitamin A should receive primary attention. Vitamin A is involved in night vision, maintenance of the epithelium of the respiratory and urogenital tract and bone metabolism, to name but a few of its functions. Fresh forage contains adequate beta-carotene, a precursor of vitamin A, to meet requirements of the horse. Hay made from forage has a lower carotene content and storage over an extended time decreases the amount present. Hays that are properly cured, retaining their green colour, have a higher carotene content than over-cured hay, hay cut in late stages of maturity and hay that was rained on or excessively weathered. Because of the ability to store large quantities of vitamin A, a horse allowed to graze fresh forage will retain an adequate vitamin A status. Horses grazing pasture for a period of a month will store sufficient vitamin A to last 5–6 months. Vitamin A is added to most equine rations due to the variability in vitamin A content of natural sources and storage instability. Also horses are not particularly efficient in the conversion of beta carotene to the active form of the vitamin.

Vitamin D

Vitamin D is required for the absorption and metabolism of calcium and phosphorus. It is also involved in the absorption of zinc, iron, cobalt and magnesium and influences the deposition of these minerals in bone. Rickets in young horses and osteomalacia in older horses may be caused by a deficiency of vitamin D. Natural sources of vitamin D include sun-cured hays and cod-liver oil. The major source of vitamin D is obtained through conversion of precursors present in the skin. The conversion requires exposure to sunlight and horses kept outside will meet their vitamin D requirements in this manner. Vitamin D toxicity can be a problem and massive doses result in calcification of soft tissue, most notably cardiac and skeletal muscle. Vitamin D supplementation in grain mixes is generally 10% of the level of vitamin A.

Vitamin E

Vitamin E, also known as alpha-tocopherol, is involved with many of the functions associated with selenium. The interrelationship between selenium and vitamin E in the horse is not clearly understood, but conditions such as 'tying-up syndrome' (azoturia) do respond to selenium-vitamin E therapy. Vitamin E is a biological and dietary antioxidant and is necessary to maintain cell membrane integrity, including that of red blood cells. Although conclusive experimental data are not available, vitamin E may enhance reproductive efficiency. Vitamin E deficiency and toxicity have not been reported in the horse; however, it is not unusual to supplement equine diets with vitamin E.

Horses prone to tying up syndrome may benefit from a series of vitamin E-selenium injections.

Vitamin K

Vitamin K is involved in the clotting of blood. Since vitamin K is produced in adequate quantities by bacteria in the caecum, supplementation with vitamin K is not warranted. One instance when supplementation may be necessary is following dicoumarol poisoning. Dicoumarol is a vitamin K antagonist produced by a mould found in sweet clover hay. If ingested it causes vitamin K deficiency.

B vitamins

The water-soluble vitamins are synthesized by bacteria present in the caecum. Three instances when B vitamin supplementation may be warranted include rations for young, rapidly growing horses, horses in heavy training, and debilitated horses which do not have a normal caecal microflora. The B vitamins are involved in the release of energy and formation of red blood cells. B vitamins of concern in equine nutrition are niacin, riboflavin (B_2), thiamine (B_1), pantothenic acid, biotin, folic acid, pyridoxine (B_6) and cyanocobalamin (B_{12}). If supplementation is necessary a B-vitamin premix, brewers' yeast or dressing the feed with a B-vitamin supplement is recommended. Although evidence from controlled studies is lacking, field experience would suggest that hoof horn may be improved by the daily addition of 15 mg of biotin to the ration. The vitamin needs of most classes of horses are easily met by inclusion of a vitamin premix at the rate of 1 kg per metric tonne in the grain mix portion of the ration as shown in Table 1.4. Over-supplementation is a more significant problem than vitamin deficiency and unless supplementation is designed to meet specific needs, it is unnecessary and may be harmful (Figure 1.2).

Table 1.4 Recommended vitamin premix for horses

Vitamin	Per kg premix
Vitamin A	2 200 000 I.U.
Vitamin D	220 000 I.U.
Vitamin E	88 000 I.U.
Thiamin	2.64 g
Riboflavin	1760 mg
Pantothenic acid	1760 mg
Vitamin B_{12}	11 mg

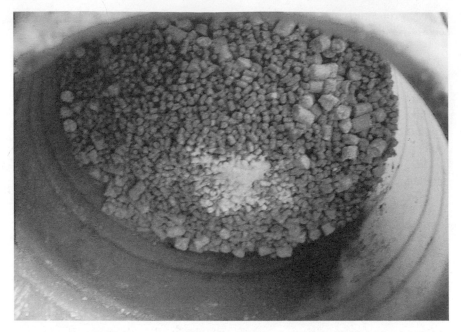

Figure 1.2 Random use of supplements to top-dress feeds is not warranted and may be harmful.

Sources of nutrients in equine diets

Protein sources for horse diets should be evaluated by the following criteria: total crude protein content, digestibility of protein, amino acid profile, availability, price and content of nutrients other than protein. Although there are numerous protein sources of plant and animal origin, only a few are of practical significance, the most important of which are discussed below.

Vegetable protein sources

Soyabean meal

The most widely used protein supplement in horse diets is soyabean meal, produced when the oil is removed from whole soyabeans during processing. Soyabean meal, sometimes referred to as soyabean oil meal, is extracted mechanically, with solvents or extruded as full-fat bean meal. The predominant type used in horse feeds is solvent extracted, which contains 44 or 48%

crude protein depending on the amount of soyabean hulls in the finished product. Raw soyabeans should not be fed to horses as they contain an anti-trypsin factor that inhibits the digestion of protein; this is destroyed by 'toasting' the meal. Soyabean meal is the most widely used protein source in livestock feeds due to its relatively high lysine content, its distribution, price and quality (protein quality is the amino acid profile of a protein). Soyabean meal has a higher lysine content than any other vegetable protein and many animal sources, including dried skim milk.

Linseed meal

Linseed meal is produced in much the same manner as soyabean meal but is derived from flax seeds. Once a favourite of horse owners as a protein source for their animals, linseed meal or flaxseed meal is of less importance in the manufacture of modern horse feeds. Linseed meal's popularity was due to its high oil content which made it an excellent coat conditioner, similar to the way maize oil is used today. When the method of oil extraction changed from using a mechanical press to a chemical solvent, the resulting product had a lower fat content, and the advantage of linseed meal was reduced. The lysine content of linseed meal is significantly lower than that of soyabean meal and so it is of less value as a protein source in horse diets. In many areas of the world it is common practice to feed whole soaked flax seed to horses as a gruel. This practice is acceptable if the flax seeds are soaked in boiling water, which inactivates the enzyme linase. Cold water soaking activates the enzyme allowing release of the highly toxic hydrocyanic acid from glycosides present in the flax.

Other vegetable protein sources

Cottonseed meal may be used as a protein source if it is low in gossypol. The toxin, gossypol, is inactivated to a large extent by heating, although this binds lysine so reducing the protein quality. Cottonseed meal containing over 60 ppm gossypol should not be used in horse rations. The lysine concentration of the total feed should be monitored if cottonseed meal is included as it is low in lysine compared to soyabean meal. If cottonseed meal is included in the diets of young horses supplementation with lysine is required. Rapeseed meal currently does not make up a very high percentage of the protein supplements used in horse diets. However, its widespread distribution indicates that it may become a more important source of supplemental protein in the future. Only rapeseed meal from varieties low in glucosinalates should be used for feeding to horses. Lupins are used extensively as a protein source in Australia and though lower in protein than soyabeans are an excellent source of supplemental protein. Other plant protein sources including sunflower meal and peanut meal are rarely used because of their lower lysine content and higher cost. If included, especially in feeds for young horses, supplementation with lysine is necessary. Peanut meal has a high content of unsaturated fatty acids, which become rancid and reduces palatability as well as causing oxidation of fat-soluble vitamins.

Animal protein sources

Animal protein sources used in horse rations are: milk products, fish meals and meat-and-bone meal, but their use in horse rations is limited due to the high cost when compared to soyabean. Protein quality is generally good and so their primary use is in rations for young horses where protein quality is critical. Dried skimmed milk is included in foal milk replacers and creep feeds. It is not suitable for inclusion in the diets of adult horses because of their inability to tolerate high lactose levels. Fish meal is a good quality protein but is too expensive to be an ingredient of equine diets. It is significantly higher in lysine than most vegetable protein and may be used to supply lysine in the diet of young horses. Although the protein quality of meat-and-bone meal is generally high it is infrequently used as a source of protein in equine diets due to the possibility of contamination with salmonellae. If this protein source is used care should be taken to ensure that it is heat treated to minimize bacterial contamination.

Feed grains for horses

Cereal grains and cereal grain by-products are used extensively in horse feeds primarily as a source of energy. Their high energy density makes them suitable for supplementing forage when a forage diet alone is not capable of meeting a horse's nutrient needs or when forage availability is limited. The major grains used in the formulation of equine diets are oats, corn (maize), milo (sorghum), barley, wheat and wheat by-products, and to a limited extent rye, spelt and triticale.

Oats

Throughout the world oats are by far the most commonly used feed ingredient for horses. Oats have a lower energy density compared to other cereals but a higher fibre and protein content. Oats may be fed whole, crimped, rolled or steam flaked although the extra cost of processing is difficult to justify. Crimping or rolling increases digestibility only a small per cent compared to whole grains. Oat groats (oats with the hulls removed) are a good feed ingredient and have greater energy density and lower fibre content compared to whole oats. Oat-mill feed (an oat by-product feed) is used in pelleted feeds but is not readily available. Oats are often sold by the bushel with heavy 'race horse oats' weighing 34 lb/bushel commanding a higher price than lighter weight oats (1 bushel = 36.37 litres).

Corn (maize)

Corn has the highest energy density but lowest crude protein of cereal grains. It is excellent as a source of energy in textured or pelleted feeds, with an average energy density of 3.4 Mcal/kg. Unlike oats, corn should be processed prior to feeding and may be fed cracked, rolled, steam flaked, micronized or ground if used in a pelleted ration. Processing breaks the kernel increasing the surface area exposed to digestive enzymes and raising the digestibility. Corn is lower in fibre than oats and should be fed by weight based on its energy density rather than by volume. An equivalent volume of corn is twice as high in energy as oats due both to greater bulk density and higher energy content per unit weight. Mouldy corn should not be fed to horses due to the risk of mouldy corn disease or leukoencephalomalacia, a disease fatal to horses caused by the mycotoxin fumonisin released by *Fusarium moniliforme*.

Barley

Barley, after corn (maize) and oats is the third most common cereal grain included in horse rations and is intermediate to oats and corn in energy value, protein and fibre content. The availability of barley is limited for use in horse feeds but its price is competitive with oats and corn. Barley needs to be crimped or steam rolled prior to feeding to maximize its digestibility.

Wheat

Most of the whole wheat produced is for human consumption and is too expensive to be included in horse rations. There are times when damaged or surplus wheat is available and is included either textured or pelleted not to exceed 30% of the grain portion of the diet. More important than wheat as a horse-feed ingredient are the by-products of the wheat milling industry, referred to under a variety of names including middlings, shorts, mill run, mill feed, and bran. Wheat-mill feed consists of the bran, broken grains, flour and other large particles associated with the making of flour. Due to its small particle size and dustiness, with the exception of bran, wheat by-product feed is generally used in pelleted rations.

Milo (sorghum) grain

In the southwest USA a significant amount of milo is used in horse feed. Milo is grown in areas where rainfall is inadequate to produce corn or other cereal grains. It is a small, hard, round grain that should be cracked, rolled or ground prior to being fed to horses and is similar to corn in its energy density.

Rye, spelt, triticale and other grains

Rye grain, spelt and triticale along with rice and millet seeds can be used as energy sources in horse grain mixes but their availability is limited. Of importance is the possible presence of ergot in rye. Ergot is an abortigenic compound that has a potent vasoconstrictive effect and may cause sloughing of the distal extremities including the tail, ears and hooves if present in sufficiently high concentrations. Ergot-infected grain should not be used as a source of feed for horses. Rye is not very palatable to horses and may reduce intake if it constitutes more than 20% of the grain mix. Rice-mill feed, a by-product, is more important as a feed ingredient than whole rice grain. Rough rice—rice with the hull still on the grain—can also be used as a feed ingredient for horses. Triticale is a hybrid of wheat and rye and has a similar feeding value but is susceptible to ergot.

By-product feeds

By-products are an important source of nutrients in the manufacture of horse feeds. As competition for cereal grains for human consumption increases the livestock feed industry is looking more carefully at by-product feeds in the formulation of rations. The term by-product has a negative connotation for some horse owners; this is a misconception as they are a superior source of nutrients. Wheat mill, oat mill and rice mill have been discussed but other by-product feeds used primarily as energy sources include sugar beet pulp, brewers' and distillers' dried grains, citrus pulp, sugar cane and sugar beet molasses and hominy feed.

Sugar beet pulp

Beet pulp is a by-product of sugar manufacture from sugar beets. It is high in calcium and digestible energy as readily fermentable fibre, mainly fruit pectin.

Beet pulp is available either shredded or pelleted, the former being most used in horse rations, especially for horses with chronic obstructive pulmonary disease (COPD). COPD horses are allergic to dust and mould spores in hay, and beet pulp is used to meet fibre requirements when hay is contraindicated. Horses in intensive training benefit from beet pulp in the diet as a method of maintaining energy balance. It may cause faeces to become loose and should not exceed 30% of the grain mix ration. Many horse owners consider that beet pulp must be soaked in water prior to feeding but it is not necessary.

Brewers' and distillers' dried grains

Brewers' dried grains are a by-product of the brewing industry and distillers' dried grains of the distilling industry. They are a good source of protein, fat, fibre and digestible energy but may be lacking in palatability especially if damaged by heat during processing. Diets with brewers' dried grains as high as 40% of the grain mix can be fed to older horses, and diets containing up to 20% distillers' grains are appropriate. For young horses 10% for both products is the maximum above which the diet must be supplemented with lysine. Brewers' dried grains consist primarily of the residues of barley, corn or maize, and rice. Occasionally wet brewers' grains are available in areas where brewing is undertaken, but it is not a good choice of feedstuffs for the horse. A disadvantage of brewers' and distillers' dried grains is the variation in the nutrient content and heat damage.

Molasses

Both wet and dehydrated molasses are frequently used in horse feeds. Wet molasses is included in textured feeds to increase palatability, reduce dustiness, bind sources of vitamins and trace minerals and as a source of energy. Molasses averages 75% dry matter so is not as wet as might be imagined. Most textured 'sweet feeds' contain 7–10% molasses, which contributes significantly to the energy value of the feed. Dehydrated molasses may be used in both textured or pelleted feeds as a flavour enhancer, but is most useful as a binding ingredient to make a good pellet. Molasses is derived from sugar beet or more frequently sugar cane. Molasses-oil blends have been used recently in colder climates to keep feed from freezing and maintain flow in automated feed delivery systems. Propionic acid, a mold inhibitor is frequently used in sweet feeds during the summer and may be added to the molasses.

Hominy

Hominy is a by-product of the maize milling industry and is similar to maize in feeding value but has a high fat content with a tendency to become rancid. If hominy is fed fresh it is an excellent source of energy.

Stored forage

Stored forage, predominantly dry cured or conventionally cured hay, is utilized extensively to meet the nutrient needs of horses. Haylage or silage may also be used if care is taken in their preservation. When selecting stored forage for horses the most important criteria are: stage of maturity at which the forage was cut, species of plant, freedom from mould and other debris, smell, colour, leafiness (Figure 1.3), freedom from insects, especially blister beetles, and dust

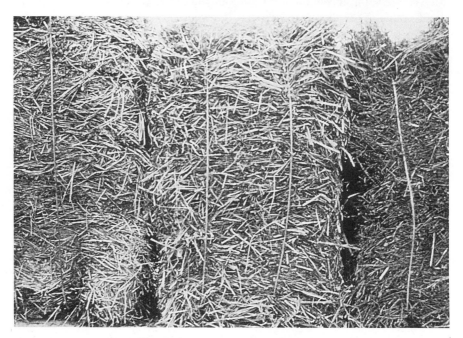

Figure 1.3 An important aspect of quality determination of stored forage is visual appraisal for colour, leafiness and maturity.

and nutrient content as determined by chemical analysis (Figure 1.4). Maturity of the plant at harvest has the most profound effect on quality and suitability for use as horse feed. As the plant matures the percentage of cell wall constituents including lignin, hemicellulose and cellulose increase and cell contents such as soluble carbohydrates decrease. The cell wall constituents are less digestible than the cell contents and as the plant matures digestibility decreases. With maturity the acid detergent fibre (ADF) and neutral detergent fibre (NDF) content of the plant increase and the crude protein falls, which

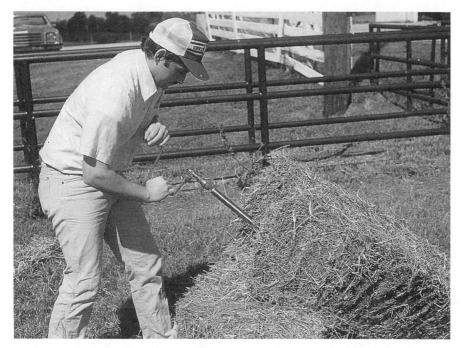

Figure 1.4 Core samples of hay should be taken and analysed for chemical composition.

has a negative impact on digestibility and voluntary intake. Maturity can be determined by analysing the ADF, NDF and crude protein concentrations in a forage sample. In the absence of a chemical analysis the maturity of forage can be assessed by looking at stem size, leaf:stem ratio and the number of flowers of legumes and seed heads of grasses. Stem size increases with maturity, there are fewer leaves and the plant flowers and produces seed heads. The nutrient contents of a variety of forages are shown in Table 1.5. It is a common misconception that horses should not be fed 'same year hay.' Hay that is put up or cured properly at appropriate moisture levels is perfectly safe for feeding and need not be stored for a prolonged period of time. The characteristic heating that occurs after baling is due to continued respiration of the plant material and is related to the moisture level at baling. Hay that 'heats up' excessively during storage is more likely to develop moulds and become unsuitable for feed.

Forages stored for use as hay, haylage or silage are either grasses or legumes or mixtures of the two. Legumes are higher in crude protein, digestibility and calcium than grasses, and mixed grass-legume forages are intermediate in nutrient value. A greater quantity of a legume hay can be harvested from a given amount of land and as a consequence good quality grass or mixed

Table 1.5 Nutrients in feeds used in horse diets[1]

Feed	Dry matter (%)	Digestible energy (Mcal/kg)	Crude protein (%)	Lysine (%)	Ether extract (%)	Fibre (%)	Ash (%)
Alfalfa							
Hay, sun-cured, early bloom	90.5	2.25	18.0	0.81	2.6	20.8	8.4
Meal, dehydrated, 17% protein	91.8	2.16	17.4	0.85	2.8	24.0	9.8
Bahiagrass							
Hay, sun-cured	90.0	1.74	8.5	–	1.8	28.1	5.7
Barley							
Grain	88.6	3.28	11.7	0.40	1.8	4.9	2.4
Beet, pulp	91.0	2.34	8.9	0.54	0.5	18.2	4.9
Bermudagrass, Coastal							
Hay, sun-cured	93.0	1.96	10.9	–	2.4	28.0	6.2
Bluegrass, Kentucky							
Hay, sun-cured	92.1	1.59	8.2	–	3.0	29.9	5.4
Brome, Smooth							
Hay, sun-cured, mid-bloom	87.6	1.87	12.6	–	1.9	28.0	9.5
Canarygrass, Reed							
Hay, sun-cured	89.3	1.78	9.1	–	2.7	30.2	7.3
Canola							
Seed meal, solvent-extracted	90.8	2.82	37.1	2.08	2.8	11.0	6.4
Clover, Ladino							
Hay, sun-cured	89.1	1.96	20.0	–	2.4	18.5	8.4
Clover, Red							
Hay, sun-cured	88.4	1.96	13.2	–	2.5	27.1	6.7
Corn, Dent, Yellow							
Grain	88.0	3.39	9.1	0.25	3.6	2.2	1.3
Distillers' grains	92.0	3.22	27.8	0.81	6.6	11.3	3.1
Cottonseed meal, solvent-extracted	91.0	2.76	41.3	1.68	1.5	12.2	6.5
Fats and oils							
Fat, animal, hydrolysed	99.2	7.96	–	–	98.4	–	–
Oil, vegetable	99.8	8.99	–	–	99.7	–	–
Fescue, Kentucky							
Hay, sun-cured	91.9	1.90	11.8	–	5.1	23.9	7.6
Linseed meal, solvent-extracted	90.2	2.76	34.6	1.16	1.4	9.1	5.9
Lespedeza, Kobe							
Hay, sun-cured	93.9	1.96	10.0	–	2.8	26.2	3.8
Milk							
Skimmed, dehydrated	94.1	3.81	33.4	2.54	1.0	0.2	7.9
Millet, Pearl							
Hay, sun-cured	87.4	1.34	7.3	–	1.8	32.2	8.9
Molasses and syrup							
Beet	77.9	2.65	6.6	–	0.2	0.0	8.9
Sugar-cane, dehydrated	99.4	3.22	9.0	–	0.8	7.1	12.0
Sugar-cane	74.3	2.60	4.3	–	0.2	0.4	9.9

Table 1.5 (*continued*)

Feed	Dry matter (%)	Digestible energy (Mcal/kg)	Crude protein (%)	Lysine (%)	Ether extract (%)	Fibre (%)	Ash (%)
Oats							
Grain	89.2	2.87	11.8	0.39	4.6	10.7	3.1
Groats	89.6	3.09	15.5	0.55	6.1	2.5	2.0
Hay, sun-cured	90.7	1.74	8.6	–	2.2	29.1	7.2
Orchardgrass							
Hay, sun-cured, early bloom	89.1	1.94	11.4	–	2.6	30.2	7.6
Pangolagrass							
Hay, sun-cured 29–42 days growth	91.0	1.63	6.7	–	1.8	29.5	7.3
Rice							
Bran with germs	90.5	2.62	13.0	0.57	13.6	11.7	10.4
Grain, ground	89.0	3.40	7.5	0.24	1.6	8.6	5.3
Mill run	91.6	0.62	6.3	0.26	5.2	28.9	15.7
Rye							
Grain	87.5	3.37	12.0	0.41	1.5	2.2	1.6
Ryegrass, Italian							
Hay, sun-cured, late vegetative	85.6	1.57	8.8	–	2.1	20.4	9.4
Sorghum, grain	90.1	3.22	11.5	0.26	2.7	2.6	1.7
Soyabean							
Seed meal, solvent-extracted, 44% protein	89.1	3.15	44.5	2.87	1.4	6.2	6.4
Seed meal without hulls, solvent-extracted	89.9	3.37	48.5	3.09	1.0	3.5	6.0
Sunflower, common							
Seed meal without hulls	92.5	2.58	45.2	1.68	2.7	11.7	7.5
Timothy							
Hay, sun-cured, early bloom	89.1	1.83	9.6	–	2.5	30.0	5.1
Wheat							
Bran	89.0	2.93	15.4	0.56	3.8	10.0	5.9
Grain, hard, red winter	88.9	3.44	13.0	0.40	1.6	2.5	1.7
Grain, soft, red winter	88.4	3.42	11.4	0.36	1.6	2.4	1.8
Mill run, less than 9.5% fibre	89.9	3.13	15.6	0.57	4.1	8.2	5.1
Whey							
Dehydrated (cattle)	93.2	3.79	13.1	0.94	0.7	0.2	8.7
Yeast, brewers'							
Dehydrated	93.1	3.09	43.4	3.23	1.0	3.2	6.7

[1] Adapted from 1989 NRC report on *Nutrient Requirements of Horses*.

grass-legume hay is difficult to obtain in some areas. Legumes, especially alfalfa (lucerne), can be irrigated and produce as many as six cuttings of high-quality hay. As land resources become more scarce the availability of high-quality grass hay will become more difficult.

Legume hays

World-wide there is more alfalfa (lucerne) hay harvested than any other type of forage. Alfalfa grows well under irrigation and tolerates lack of water better than most forage crops. Alfalfa is a good horse feed especially as stockpiled forage to horses at pasture. Stockpiled forage is grass that is allowed to grow to provide roughage during the winter months. Forage kept in this way loses some of its nutritional value but remains a viable source of nutrients even in the coldest climates. There is some controversy as to which cutting of alfalfa is best for horse hay. The manner in which the hay is made is more important than which cutting is taken. Second and subsequent cuttings of alfalfa are of greater quality, lower in crude fibre and acid detergent fibre than the first cutting. Alfalfa ranges from 13 to 21% crude protein, 1.8 to 2.4 Mcal/kg digestible energy and 1.0 to 1.6% calcium. It is best utilized as a high-quality source of nutrients rather than the sole source of roughage. The majority of haylage and silage for horses is made from alfalfa. Clover hays for horses include red, ladino and white, with red clover being the most popular to harvest. Sweet clover is not appropriate for feeding to horses due to the presence of the vitamin K antagonist dicoumarol. The primary concern when purchasing clover hay is to ensure it is free from mould. The second and subsequent cuttings of red clover hay may cause a condition known as salivating disease due to the presence of a fungus. It causes no serious health problem but can be disconcerting to those not aware of the condition. Lespedeza hay is similar in quality and nutritive value to alfalfa hay but yields and availability are significantly less.

Cool season grass hays

Timothy grows vigorously in temperate climates during the spring and fall and is a favourite of many horse owners. Timothy hay that is properly cured and put up in an early stage of maturity provides an excellent quality horse feed, is palatable and a good source of nutrients. There is a tendency to allow timothy to become too mature prior to cutting and baling, when it is a poor source of nutrients and is less palatable. Orchardgrass makes excellent quality horse hay and properly cured is higher in protein than timothy, is greener, softer in texture and leafier. Orchardgrass present in a mixed sward with alfalfa or clover is frequently found in a mixed grass-legume hay. Brome grass is similar in quality and nutrient content to other cool season grasses. Brome is found widely distributed in temperate areas of the world and makes excellent grazing as well as hay. In addition to the cool season grasses listed above other grasses including reed canarygrass, bluegrass, fescue and ryegrass are suitable as horse hays.

Warm season grasses

In terms of tonnage and distribution the predominant warm season grass for horse hay is bermudagrass and its various cultivars. The most important cultivar in the USA is coastal bermuda and under irrigation and nitrogen fertilization, excellent yields of high-quality very palatable hay can be obtained. Although not generally used as a hay, bahiagrass cut in early stages of maturity will provide a significant percentage of a horse's energy requirements. Bahia is stemmy and makes a poorer quality hay than coastal bermuda and is more frequently used as a pasture grass. Properly cured pangolagrass can also be fed to horses.

Oats, wheat and rye along with their hybrids such as triticale can be used to make forage. Most cereal grain hays should be cut when the grain is in the dough stage to maximize the nutrient content and the tonnage to be harvested. In addition to long hay, oat or wheat chaff is used extensively in Australia and New Zealand. Chaff is made by chopping oaten or wheaten hay into small pieces. Chaff adds bulk to the diet and provides a very useful fibre source. From a management point of view chaff is useful to slow down the aggressive eater and reduce overconsumption of the grain mix. It is recommended that if a chaff feeding system is used an additional source of long stem fibre or fresh pasture is provided to reduce the risk of colic.

Silage

Silage is one of the most universally used forage feeds for cattle but is of minor significance in feeding horses. Properly preserved silage may be fed to horses but the problems that are associated with spoiled silage makes it a practice that is seldom used. In order to make good silage, forage must be stored in an anaerobic manner, at a low pH to eliminate the formation of moulds.

There is considerable interest in baled hay ensiled in plastic bags. Known as horsehage it is of high quality but tends to be inordinately expensive. If fed to horses care must be taken to ensure that it is not spoiled, mouldy, or contains soil, faeces and animal remains, as the anaerobic environment may lead to the production of clostridial toxins which result in cases of botulism.

Physical form of feeds

Grain mixes may be fed in a textured, pelleted or occasionally in an extruded form. However, the primary consideration is not the physical form but ensuring that the ingredients are of a high quality. There is little difference in the feeding value whichever form it is presented in.

Textured or loose feeds

Textured feeds are far and away the most common form of horse feed. They consist of whole or processed grains with or without a protein-vitamin-mineral pellet and are presented dry or with molasses added. In the USA feeds are commonly molassed using cane molasses or a molasses-vegetable oil mixture with a preservative such as propionic acid. While molasses is not essential it does make a feed more uniform and palatable (Figure 1.5). Outside the USA

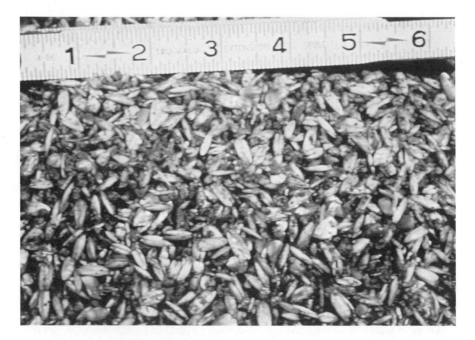

Figure 1.5 A typical textured or loose feed with molasses added to increase palatability and reduce the sorting of fine ingredients.

molasses is included less often. Compared to pelleted feed, textured feed has the advantage that the quality of ingredients can be more easily assessed, and it is easier to add supplements or medication. Textured feeds are more readily consumed by finicky eaters, there is less possibility of choke and horses are less inclined to bolt their feed.

Pelleted feeds

Pelleted feeds have greatly increased in popularity and are manufactured by grinding the ingredients and forcing them through a die to bind them together. Pellets are the form of choice if many finely ground ingredients such as wheat-mill feeds are to be used or ingredients of questionable palatability are to be included. The advantages of pelleted over textured feed are that the nutrients are more uniformly distributed, there is less wastage and dust, and feed can be stored for a longer period (Figure 1.6). The most common complaint about pellets is that some feed manufacturers include inferior ingredients. Pellets have a greater bulk density than loose feed and there is a tendency to overfeed pellets if rations are dispensed by volume rather than weight. Overall, pellets are a safe, economical and effective way to feed horses.

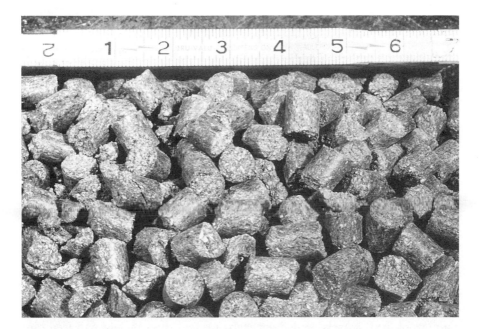

Figure 1.6 A pelleted feed that ensures more even distribution of ingredients and longer shelf life.

Extruded feeds

Extrusion of feed is in some ways very much like pelleting in that ingredients are ground prior to being forced under extreme pressure through a small die. Extruded feeds have been used for some time in the pet food industry, but only recently in the manufacture of horse feeds. They are readily consumed and are of benefit to horses prone to colic as they are consumed more slowly than textured or pelleted feeds. Extruded feeds are more expensive than other forms but it is likely that they will be used more extensively when manufacturing costs are reduced.

Hay cubes and grass nuts

Hay cubes or grass nuts of various sizes are made in the same manner as pelleted feeds and are of particular significance in some parts of the USA, where alfalfa (lucerne) cubes and pellets are popular. Hay cubes or grass nuts are of particular benefit when hay supplies are short or when storage space is limited. The nutrient composition is the same as the raw material used in their manufacture unless a vitamin-mineral premix is added. Although a good source of nutrients, cube nuts and especially pellets made from finely ground grass or alfalfa may not satisfy a horse's requirement for bulk or long-stem fibre. Horses consuming them as the sole source of fibre are more prone to develop vices such as wood chewing or cribbing.

Feed storage

The considerable emphasis on quality ingredients and proper formulation is meaningless if the feed is not stored in a manner which preserves its quality. The most important aspect of storage is keeping the feed dry. Moisture provides an ideal environment for the growth of moulds, which are the biggest single detriment to feed quality. Feed should be stored in a cool, clean, dry area that is protected from rodents, birds and insects. Watertight grain bins are convenient for storing large quantities of bulk grain or pelleted feeds but are not appropriate for storing molassed textured feeds, which have a tendency to bridge or cake together. If a bulk storage facility is used the feed should contain no more than 12% moisture to prevent mould development. For small amounts of feed, barrels, sealed garbage cans and sheet metal-lined feed bins provide an economical means of storage. It is often convenient to store feed in bags, which should be placed on pallets off the floor, but the room must be kept free of rodents and insects. In tropical or very warm, humid environments it may be necessary to air-condition the storage area to prevent feed from going mouldy. Storage areas should be cleaned regularly and fumigated if there is any indication of insects. Grain weevils not only damage grain but create conditions which favour the growth of moulds. Improper storage may result in feed becoming rancid reducing its palatability and nutritional value due to oxidation of fat-soluble vitamins. To prevent loss of quality the oldest feed should be used first. In many cases digestive problems can be traced to improper storage and handling.

The requirements for the storage of hay are the same as for grains or mixed feeds. Ventilation and air flow are important aspects, especially when hay is placed in the storage area. When stacking hay the first bales should be placed on edge with the cut ends on the ground or floor. This allows air to flow between the floor and the hay and facilitates drying. If conventionally cured and preservative-treated hay are to be stored in the same facility they should not be stacked together. Propionic and acetic acid are used to inhibit mould growth in hay that has a moisture level greater than 17%. When the two are in contact the moisture diffuses resulting in mould development. If hay is properly stored there is no reason why year-old or older hay cannot be fed without problems. Length of storage will impact most significantly on the vitamin A level, which decreases as storage time increases, but as most feeds are over-fortified with vitamin A this is not a great concern.

Further reading

Cunha T J (1980) *Horse feeding and nutrition*. Academic Press, New York.
Ensminger M E (1977) *Horses and Horsemanship* 5th edn. Interstate Publishing Company, Davisville IL.
Frape D L (1986) *Equine nutrition and feeding*. Longman, London.
Maynard L A, Loosli J K, Hintz H F, Warner R G (1979) *Animal nutrition* 7th edn. McGraw-Hill, New York.
Morrison F B (1951) *Feeds and feeding*. Morrison Publishing Company, Ithaca NY.
National Research Council (1989) *Nutrient requirements of horses* 5th edn. National Academy Press, Washington DC.
Swenson M J (1977) *Dukes' physiology of domestic animals* 9th edn. Cornell University Press, Ithaca NY.

2 FEEDING THE HORSE
STEPHEN G. JACKSON, PhD

Summary

Mares are divided into four categories for the purpose of discussing their nutrient requirements, barren and maiden mares, early pregnant non-lactating mares, late pregnant mares and lactating mares. Appropriate feeding regimes for each class of mare are discussed and example rations included.

The young horse should be fed in a manner that optimizes growth. Growth rate and change in body weight should be monitored to achieve maximum mature size while minimizing skeletal anomalies which may result from too rapid growth. Specific differences in nutrient requirements of nursing foals, weanlings and yearlings make it prudent to design feeding programmes that address the varied nutrient needs of young horses. Example grain mixes for young horses are given along with suggested feeding levels that result in desirable growth and optimization of athletic potential.

Energy is the most critical nutrient for the performance horse. The protein requirements are generally over-emphasized. If adequate feed is provided to meet the horse's energy requirement the protein requirement is met as well.

Mature idle horses and stallions can be fed good quality pasture or hay if adequate quantities are available. When grain feeding is necessary because of restricted pasture availability or reduced turn-out time, it is important to provide adequate fibre intake to maintain normal gut function. Rations that emphasize energy and mineral intake rather than protein intake should be utilized.

With a basic knowledge of nutrients plus an understanding of feedstuffs and forage derived from Chapter 1 it is possible to formulate feeding programmes for different classes of horses. The nutrient requirements differ depending on age, use and physiological state of the horse. Classes of horses to be considered include the broodmare, the foal and yearlings, the performance horse, the mature idle horse and the stallion.

Weighing to determine energy balance and body condition

In designing feeding programmes for all classes of horses it is important to be aware of body condition and weight. Knowing a horse's weight should be a routine part of a stable or farm operation and will result in improved efficiency in the farm's feeding programme, training and racing schedules. Weight can be a useful indicator of health problems and determining the correct amount of medication to be administered.

Over- and under-feeding are the most common nutritional problems of most animal species including the horse. Weight gain or loss is the single most effective measure of determining whether a horse's energy requirements are being met. Energy intake and growth rate are particularly important in the young horse. Young horses that grow rapidly are at greater risk of developmental orthopaedic disease than their slower growing contemporaries. Accurate monitoring of weight change allows the opportunity to control growth rate more effectively than casual visual observation. The stresses on the immature skeleton are lessened if a moderate growth rate is encouraged from an early stage by frequent weighing and adjustment of feeding levels.

Recent work at Texas A&M and Colorado State Universities has indicated a direct relationship between body-fat stores and reproductive efficiency in broodmares. Mares maintained in a positive energy balance were more likely to get in foal than mares allowed to lose weight. As subtle changes in weight of growing and mature horses are difficult to determine, weighing on a routine basis as illustrated in Figure 2.1 is the best way to assess how horses are responding to feeding and management programmes.

Young horses should be weighed every two weeks and broodmares and mature horses monthly. The condition of racehorses and performance horses can also be monitored more accurately and the optimum performance weight established.

Broodmares

When formulating rations for the broodmare, the maintenance requirement, the nutrition of the developing foetus, milking production, the health and

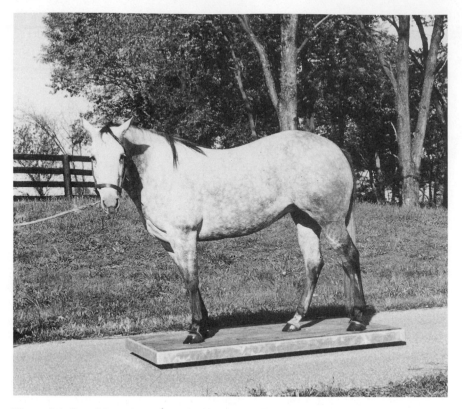

Figure 2.1 Portable scales are a valuable means of assessing growth rate in young horses and body-weight changes in mature horses.

viability of the foal and the subsequent reproductive performance of the mare must all be considered. Mares can be divided into four categories with respect to their nutritional requirements: the maiden mare; the barren mare; the pregnant mare during the last trimester of pregnancy; and the lactating mare. Each category has different nutrient requirements and the practical aspects of feeding differ in terms of the amount required and when and how it should be provided. A feeding programme which strives to keep mares in a positive energy balance will ensure optimum performance. A mare in positive energy balance gains weight, whereas a mare in negative energy balance loses weight. Each mare has an optimum body condition and productivity will be greatest when the mare is maintained in that condition year-round. To establish the optimum condition, each mare must be evaluated individually and conformation will play an important part. The optimum condition for a 16-hand, angular, thin mare will be different from that of a shorter, heavier muscled mare. The big mare will never appear to be carrying as much flesh as the shorter mare.

The mare should never be allowed to be in a negative energy balance so that it loses excessive amounts of body weight. To prevent this happening the amount of feed at different times of the mare's reproductive status will vary. During periods of nutritional demand and physiological stress in late pregnancy and lactation extra care should be taken to ensure the mare does not slip into a negative energy balance. There are several indicators in addition to regular weighing to determine if the mare is carrying adequate condition and is in energy balance. The mare should have fat covering the ribs so they are not easily seen, but readily felt by running the hands down the side of the ribs. The mare should carry weight directly behind the shoulder and above the flank giving a roundish appearance through the fore rib. Over the croup, along the hip and down the midline there should be adequate fat cover to make visualization of the vertebral column difficult. Some mares appear 'hippy' and bare over the croup and tail head, but will carry some fat over the ribs and around the shoulder and be in optimum condition. Once the 'optimum condition' has been established, it should be maintained throughout the year.

Maiden mares

Maiden mares entering the broodmare band fall into two categories. The mature race or show mare being retired after a successful campaign and the filly retired due to lack of ability or injury. Many maiden mares are extremely thin, in negative energy balance, and suffering from chronic fatigue. While on the racetrack, 2- and 3-year-old fillies have yet to reach maturity and for the young filly brought to the farm, it is important to supply the amount of nutrients as illustrated in Table 2.1 for continued growth, a moderate amount

Table 2.1 Minimum percentage of nutrients and digestible energy requirements in the total diet of mares

	Crude Protein %	Digestible Energy Mcal/day	Calcium %	Phosphorus %	Vitamin A I.U./kg
Barren mares and early pregnancy	8.0	16.5	0.27	0.19	1650
Pregnancy (last 90 days) and maiden mares	10.0	18.5	0.45	0.30	3300
Lactating mares (1st 3 months)	13.2	28.3	0.45	0.30	2480
Lactating mares (3 months to weaning)	11.0	24.3	0.40	0.25	2700

of fattening and reproduction. The maiden filly should receive as much good quality hay or pasture as she will eat plus a 14% crude protein grain mix containing 0.7% calcium and 0.6% phosphorus as shown in Table 2.2. The amount fed per day should represent 0.75–1.0% of body weight. Maiden 4-year-old fillies should receive a 12% protein grain mix. It is important that fillies off the racetrack and young maiden mares enter the breeding season gaining weight. During early pregnancy the amount of feed allowed 3- and 4-year-old mares should be greater than older mares but young mares should receive the same as older mares during late pregnancy. A grain mix appropriate for maiden mares is shown in Table 2.3 and the amount allowed according to forage quality is given in Table 2.4.

A filly on the racetrack or in training for performance events has probably received 5.5–7.0 kg of grain mix per day in addition to liberal quantities of good quality hay. This amount allows her to meet nutritional demands for work, but does not allow excess for fattening. When horses are taken out of training it is the established practice to dramatically reduce feed intake. The filly at this stage does not need a physical let down, rather she needs to become mentally relaxed. Care should be taken that the filly gets adequate forage and/or grain mix to allow her to build energy stores. Re-setting the shoes of fillies with flat plates and turning her out with a quiet gelding or older mare allows the filly to 'let down' and relax in preparation for the visit to the breeding shed.

Barren mares

Although it may have little to do with the feeding programme, it is important to ascertain why the mare is barren. The reasons may include severe dystocia during foaling, foaling too late in the season, uterine infection and old age. Some mares are barren due to nutritional mismanagement, including the heavy milking mare that was allowed to slip into negative energy balance, the young mare that foaled and failed to come into season, the thin mare exhibiting lactational anoestrus and the mare that slipped after being pronounced in-foal due to lack of proper feeding. These mares should be allowed to regain condition and Table 2.2 provides the minimum nutrient requirements of the mature barren mare. The nutrient requirements of most barren mares can be met with ad libitum intake of good quality hay or pasture alone plus a trace mineralized salt block and fresh, clean water (Figure 2.2). The emphasis should be on quality pasture or hay; if the pasture is merely an exercise lot, the nutritional requirements must be met using hay or a grain mix. The amount needed with hay of varying quality is shown in Table 2.4 and the ingredients of a grain mix appropriate for barren mares are given in Table 2.3. Barren and maiden mares generally benefit from flushing—i.e. increasing the plane of nutrition just prior to the breeding season—at about the same time they are put on an artificial lighting programme. With barren mares it is important to

Table 2.2 Nutrient concentrations[1] in grain mix for mares

	Crude Protein[2] %	Calcium %	Phosphorus %	Copper ppm	Zinc ppm
Barren mares and early pregnancy	12	0.7	0.6	30	90
Maiden mares and pregnancy (last 90 days)	14	0.7	0.6	30	90
Lactating mares (1st 3 months)	15	0.7	0.6	30	90
Lactating mares (3 months weaning)	15	0.7	0.6	30	90

[1] Concentration refers to the percentage of listed nutrients in the grain mix.
[2] Protein may be lowered if a high quality legume hay is fed.

Table 2.3 Grain mix for barren, maiden, late pregnant and lactating broodmares[1]

Ingredient	% of diet	Inclusion rate (kg/tonne[2])
Crimped oats	37.5	375
Cracked corn (maize)	20.0	200
Rolled barley	15.0	150
Molasses, cane	9.0	90
Soyabean meal (48%)	11.0	110
Salt	0.5	5
Dicalcium phosphate	1.5	15
Calcium carbonate	0.5	5
Wheat bran	4.5	45
KER 5X[3]	0.5	5

[1] For use in lactating mares with legume or mixed hay.
[2] 1 metric tonne = 1000 kg.
[3] KER 5X = trace mineral vitamin premix manufactured by Kentucky Equine Research, Versailles, Kentucky, USA 40383.

maintain condition and in the case of the thin mare to gain weight until the optimum condition is reached. Although there is no good evidence to suggest that overweight mares are prone to infertility and dystocia, barren mares that are overweight should not be allowed a grain mix.

Pregnant mares

The mare in the first two trimesters of pregnancy should be fed in a similar manner to the barren mare. When the mare enters the last 90 days of

Table 2.4 Amounts of grain mix to be fed with hay[1]

	500 kg mare		600 kg mare	
	Average hay: kg grain mix	Good hay: kg grain mix	Average hay: kg grain mix	Good hay: kg grain mix
Barren mare and early pregnancy	1.5	0	1.8	0
Pregnancy (last 90 days) and maiden mares	3.7	2.3	4.0	2.7
Lactation (1st 3 months)	6.4	5.0	6.8	5.5
Lactation (3 months weaning)	4.0	2.7	4.5	3.2

[1] Hay or pasture fed free-choice in addition to indicated amounts of grain.

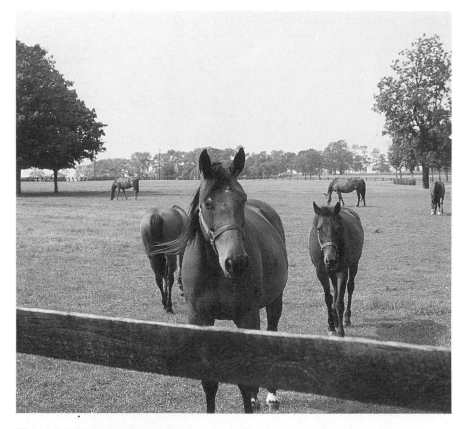

Figure 2.2 Barren mares' nutrient needs can be met by good quality pasture, trace mineralized salt and free choice water.

pregnancy, her protein, energy, calcium and phosphorus requirements increase significantly, as shown in Table 2.1. The bulk of foetal growth occurs late in pregnancy and the pregnant mare is more efficient with respect to nutrient utilization than the non-pregnant mare. The increased demand for energy during the last 3 months of pregnancy is approximately 12% above maintenance. Recent evidence suggests that if mares are fed to gain weight during pregnancy, their reproductive performance after foaling is enhanced.

It is possible for the mare to meet her nutrient requirements with good quality legume hay during late pregnancy. However, a common practice is to feed 2.5–3.5 kg of a good quality grain mix as described in Table 2.3. Table 2.5 indicates how to vary the protein percentage of the grain mix depending on

Table 2.5 Per cent of crude protein in grain mix for broodmares fed different forages

	Percent crude protein in grain mix[1]			
	Alfalfa hay	Timothy hay	Timothy hay 65: clover hay 35	Timothy hay Bluegrass pasture[2]
Barren mares (maintenance)	0	12.5	0	0–12.5
Pregnancy (last 90 days) and maiden mares	9	13.5	11	9.0–13.5
Lactation (1st 3 months)	12.5	16.0	15	15
Lactation (3 months to weaning)	12.0	14.0	13	13

[1] Forage to be provided free-choice along with grain mix.
[2] Depends upon time of year. Greater intake is indicated when cool season grasses are dormant.

the type of forage the mare is consuming. By increasing the amount fed during late pregnancy, it is possible to minimize the loss of body condition that occurs at foaling. If mares are fed a high-quality grain mix fortified with the macro and micro minerals, the chances of *in utero* foal abnormalities are also minimized.

Lactating mares

The nutrient requirements of the lactating mare are greater than those of any other type of horse, with the possible exception of the horse in hard training (Figure 2.3). The lactating mare that has just produced a foal weighing 40–

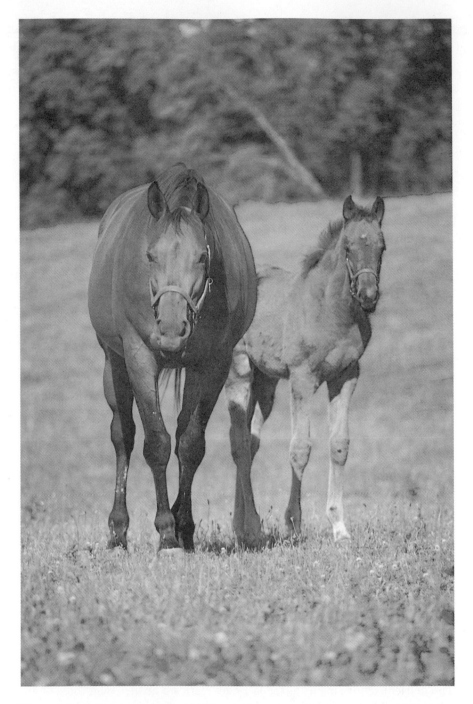

Figure 2.3 Lactating mares have higher nutrient requirements than any other class of mares.

65 kg, 27–40 kg of placenta and fluids will have lost approximately 100 kg. The lactating mare will be mated and is expected to become pregnant within a short period of time. Understanding the relationship of nutrition to these major physiological changes is very important.

During the time the mare is milking, she has an increased requirement for all nutrients, especially energy. The average mare will give 3% of her body weight per day in milk during the first 3 months of lactation and 2% during the last 3 months. A 500 kg mare will produce 15 kg of milk per day during early lactation. The composition of mare's milk is shown in Table 2.6, which indi-

Table 2.6 Composition of mare's milk (wet basis)

Constituent	Amount
Protein %	2–3
Fat %	1–3
Gross energy Kcal/kg	475
Calcium mg/100 ml	80–120
Phosphorus mg/100	45–90
Magnesium mg/100 ml	6–12
Copper mg/kg	0.15–0.4
Selenium mg/kg	0.01–0.03
Zinc mg/kg	2–4
Iron mg/kg	0.5–0.9

cates that the mare is secreting a substantial amount of nutrients in milk. These must be provided in the feed or there will be a resultant loss in weight. If undernutrition is severe during lactation, there will be a greater effect upon the condition of the mare than on milk production and she is less likely to conceive. Any adverse effect on milk production will be evident by the amount of milk produced rather than on its composition as studies have indicated there is little effect of diet on the fat and protein content of mare's milk.

The requirements of the lactating mare are shown in Table 2.1, with details of the grain mix contained in Tables 2.2–2.5. A grain mix for the lactating mare on poor quality pasture or receiving poor quality hay is illustrated in Table 2.7.

As with all types of horses, the condition of the mare will dictate the amount of feed provided on a daily basis. Maintaining the mare's weight during lactation will be rewarded in the breeding shed. It is the exception rather than the rule for a mare to become too fat during lactation if she is taking proper care of her foal. Extreme weight loss may occur in the very heavy milking mare if feed intake is insufficient, and one must be suspicious of the mare that becomes fat with a foal by her side. This mare is not giving sufficient milk which will result in poor development of the foal. One week prior to weaning and for several weeks after weaning it is necessary to reduce the feed intake of the mare to

Table 2.7 Grain mix for lactating mares receiving poor quality grass hay or grazing poor quality pasture

Ingredient	% of diet	kg/tonne
Oats	39.0	390
Cracked corn (maize)	20.0	200
Rolled barley	10.0	100
Molasses, cane	9.0	90
Soyabean meal (48%)	18.5	185
Salt	0.5	5
Dicalcium phosphate	1.75	17.5
Calcium carbonate	0.75	7.5
KER 5X[1]	0.50	5

[1] KER 5X = trace mineral vitamin premix manufactured by Kentucky Equine Research, Versailles, Kentucky, USA 40383.

curtail milk production. It is common practice to turn the mare out on pasture with little or no additional feed at this time. For the mare in good condition or the fat mare, this approach is valid depending upon the quality of available forage. However, if the mare is thin it will be necessary to improve her condition.

Foals and yearlings

Feeding the young horse is the most challenging area of horse nutrition. The horse owner is faced with uncertainty with respect to the impact that early nutrition has on future performance and soundness. There are an abundance of supplements and feeding programmes purporting to eliminate developmental problems in the young horse. Many factors determine the feeding programme for young horses including economics, availability of feed ingredients, labour and amount and quality of forage available. Nevertheless, there are some absolutes to keep in mind in order to meet the young horse's nutrient needs. First, and foremost, the young horse should be considered as a potential athlete. Second the young horse is growing rapidly and feeding errors can become greatly magnified. Third, all classes of nutrients must be considered when formulating the rations of young growing horses.

Prior to a discussion of nutrient requirements it will be of value to examine development of the young horse and how it may be assessed in both a qualitative and quantitative manner. It is dangerous to assume that maximum and optimum growth are one and the same. Recent research has indicated that very rapid growth can result in a myriad of developmental disorders. The question arises as to how fast one can stimulate growth in the young horse and not compromise proper skeletal development. Unfortunately there are no valid and easily applied methods to assess the quality of early development. The manner in which horses respond to nutritional challenge varies between individuals and is strongly influenced by heredity. High rates of growth in some breeds or types of horse such as draft horses and European warm bloods appear to cause no problems while similar rates of growth in other horses such as Thoroughbreds may be catastrophic. Therefore genetic factors and the predisposition to growth anomalies must be considered in the formula designed to determine growth rate and the level of feeding.

Table 2.8 Expected growth rates of 500 and 600 kg horses

| | Expected mature weight | | | |
| | 500 kg | | 600 kg | |
Age of horse	BW (kg)	ADG (kg)	BW (kg)	ADG (kg)
Weanling 4 months	175	0.85	200	1.0
Weanling 6 months; moderate growth	215	0.65	245	0.75
Weanling 6 months; rapid growth	215	0.85	245	0.95
Yearling 12 months; moderate growth	325	0.50	375	0.65
Yearling 12 months; rapid growth	325	0.65	375	0.80
Yearling 18 months	400	0.35	475	0.45

BW = body weight in kg.
ADG = average daily gain in kg.

Table 2.8 shows data from various studies reflecting rates of growth in the horse. Growth expressed as average daily gain is most rapid early in life and slows down as the horse reaches 18 months of age. Weight gains in excess of 1.7 kg/day are not uncommon during the first 30 days while growth rates of 0.4 kg/day are more common for yearlings. Over the years several studies have assessed the growth of young horses as a percent of their final mature size as illustrated in Figure 2.4. Rate of increase in bone length assessed as height to the withers progressively decreases as the horse gets older. In a study by Hintz in 1979 it was observed that Thoroughbred foals attained 83, 90 and 95% their mature height at 6, 12 and 18 months of age respectively. Routine monitoring of changes in body weight and wither height is an effective way to assess

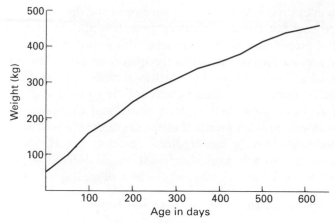

Figure 2.4 Normal growth curve for the horse (500 kg mature weight).

growth rate especially when it is compared to expected mature weight or height. Average daily gain (ADG) can be calculated using the following formula:

$$\text{ADG (kg/day)} = \frac{\text{Wt 2} - \text{Wt 1}}{\text{T 2} - \text{T 1}}$$

Where Wt 2 = current weight, Wt 1 = previous weight; T2 = age in days at second weighing and T 1 = age in days at first weighing. For example, for a foal weighing 140 kg at 60 days and 165 kg at 90 days, the ADG would be:

$$\text{ADG (kg/day)} = \frac{165 - 140}{90 - 60} = \frac{25}{30} = 0.833$$

Figure 2.4 shows a growth curve constructed from the data in Table 2.8. The rate of growth is represented by the slope of the line such that the steeper the slope the more rapid is the rate of growth. This same curve could be constructed for the response of any variable as a function of time, for example withers or hip height. The factors which determine the rate at which a particular horse grows include the genetic capacity for growth, the nutrient intake and quality of the ration, and environmental factors such as weather and disease incidence.

Particular care should be taken to meet the nutritional needs of the young horse for energy, protein and macro-minerals.

Energy requirements

Energy is provided to the young horse by milk, supplementary feeds and forage. Inadequate energy is reflected by an unthrifty appearance and below-normal rates of growth. Horses receiving inadequate energy are also less efficient in the utilization of other nutrients. The NRC's *Nutrient Requirements of Horses*, published in 1989, expresses the digestible energy (DE) requirements of the young horse as:

DE (Mcal/day) = Maintenance DE (Mcal/day) + (4.81 + 1.17x − 0.023 × 2) (ADG)

Where ADG = average daily gain (kg), and x is age in months. The digestible energy requirements for maintenance are calculated using the equation:

DE (maintenance) = 1.4 + 0.03 (body weight in kg).

The digestible energy requirement per kilogram of gain is calculated as:

DE req./kg of gain = 4.81 + 1.17x − 0.023 × 2.

DE requirement per kilogram of gain increases as the foal gets older due to an increase in maintenance requirement and a decrease in the efficiency of gain when the ration consists of more fibrous feeds and less milk. The optimum rate of gain for foals has not been established and several studies have indicated that excessive rates of gain or high energy from carbohydrate compromise skeletal development. To calculate energy requirements for growth using the above equation it is important to know the exact rate of growth so that periodic weighings must be taken. In the absence of weighing, figures contained in Table 2.9 may be used to estimate the energy requirements of young growing horses.

Table 2.9 Daily digestible energy (DE) requirements (Mcal) of young horses

Age of horse	Mature weight	
	500 kg	600 kg
Weanling 4 months	14.4	16.5
Weanling 6 months; moderate growth	15.0	17.0
Weanling 6 months; rapid growth	17.2	19.2
Yearling 12 months; moderate growth	18.9	22.7
Yearling 12 months; rapid growth	21.3	25.1
Yearling 18 months; not in training	19.8	23.9
Yearling 18 months; in training	26.5	32.0

The impact that excessive energy intake has on skeletal development and the incidence of developmental orthopaedic disease (DOD) is not fully understood. A conservative approach to the young horse's energy requirements is appropriate until the relationship of energy intake and DOD is elucidated. A method of reducing the intake of energy is to maximize the proportion of the daily diet that comes from forage and increase the frequency of feeding while decreasing the quantity of the ration. Another option is to provide energy in the form of fat; it has been shown that as much as 15% of the DE can be provided as vegetable oil with no adverse effect. Studies at Texas A&M University have successfully used tallow to replace energy from carbohydrate. This method of supplying part of the horse's energy requirement results in lower insulin peaks and a lower feed intake due to the high energy density of fat. Regardless of the approach taken to satisfy the energy needs of the young horse it is best to encourage a moderate growth rate. Horses are not sold by weight and seeking maximum daily weight gains and feeding excessive amounts of energy is unnecessary.

Protein requirements

The protein requirements of the young horse should take into account the total crude protein intake and the protein quality or amino acid profile. As mentioned in the previous chapter the provision of amino acids is especially critical during the first 12 months with the formation of muscle and bone. The concentration (%) and amount (expressed as grammes per day (g/day)) of protein required by the young horse are greater than for any other type of horse. The crude protein and lysine requirements of the young horse are shown in Table 2.10. Ultimately it would be valuable to know the requirement for all essential amino acids but this is currently not the case. The fact that the requirement for other essential amino acids is not known does not negate their importance. The most commonly used protein source in horse rations is soyabean meal because its amino acid profile is superior to other sources such as linseed meal. Until further research is undertaken the most appropriate way to consider the protein requirements of the young horse is by using an assessment of crude protein plus lysine.

The crude protein requirements of the young horse can be determined using the following nutrient/calorie relationships.

For weanlings:

Protein required (g/day) = 50 × (Mcal of DE required)

For yearlings:

Protein required (g/day) = 45 × (Mcal of DE required)

Table 2.10 Crude protein and lysine requirements (g/day) of young horses

| Age of horse | Expected mature weight | | | |
| | 500 kg | | 600 kg | |
	Protein	Lysine	Protein	Lysine
Weanling 4 months	720	30	825	35
Weanling 6 months; moderate growth	750	32	850	36
Weanling 6 months; rapid growth	860	36	960	40
Yearling 12 months; moderate growth	851	36	1023	43
Yearling 12 months; rapid growth	956	40	1127	48
Yearling 18 months; not in training	893	38	1077	45
Yearling 18 months; in training	1195	50	1429	60

[1] Adapted from 1989 NRC report, *Nutrient Requirements of Horses*.

For example if a 6-month-old weanling requires 17 Mcal of DE per day it would have a protein requirement of 50×17 g/day or 850 g crude protein/day.

The requirement for lysine can be calculated using the following equations:

For weanlings:

$$\text{Lysine required (g/day)} = 2.1 \times (\text{Mcal of DE required})$$

For yearlings:

$$\text{Lysine required (g/day)} = 1.9 \times (\text{Mcal of DE required})$$

There is concern with overfeeding protein in respect to the occurrence of developmental orthopaedic disease although there is no substantive data to support this suggestion. Overfeeding protein is costly and does not result in more rapid growth. It is more appropriate to restrict growth rate by reducing energy intake than protein intake. Protein consumed above requirement is used as an energy source, with excretion of excess nitrogen in the urine.

Protein is provided from a variety of sources; besides cereal grains and soyabeans, these include alfalfa (lucerne), distillers' grains, linseed meal and fish meal. Assuming that care is taken to meet lysine requirements this is one area where formulation of rations may be undertaken on a least cost basis.

Mineral requirements

The most important minerals in formulating diets for young horses are calcium and phosphorus. The young horse's requirement for several of the important macro-minerals, including calcium and phosphorus, are shown in Table 2.11, and levels of several important micro-minerals are given in Table 2.12. Factors

Table 2.11 Requirements (g/day) of young horses for calcium, phosphorus, magnesium and potassium

Age of horse	500 kg Mature Weight				600 kg Mature Weight			
	Ca	P	Mg	K	Ca	P	Mg	K
Weanling 4 months	34	19	3.7	11.3	40	22	4.3	13.0
Weanling 6 months; moderate growth	29	16	4.0	12.7	34	19	4.6	14.5
Weanling 6 months; rapid growth	36	20	4.3	13.3	40	22	4.9	15.1
Yearling 12 months; moderate growth	29	16	5.5	17.8	36	20	6.4	20.7
Yearling 12 months; rapid growth	34	19	5.7	18.2	41	22	6.6	21.2
Yearling 18 months; not in training	27	15	6.4	21.1	33	18	7.7	25.1
Yearling 18 months; in training	36	20	8.6	28.2	44	24	10.2	33.3

Ca = calcium; P = phosphorus; Mg = magnesium; K = potassium.

Table 2.12 Trace mineral concentrations (ppm) in the total diets (forage plus grain) of young horses (ppm)

Copper	Zinc	Selenium	Iron	Manganese
20	60	0.2	50	40

to be considered when assessing the mineral adequacy of the diet include type and amount of forage fed, amount of minerals in the grain mix, total amount of feed and age of the horse. Regardless of the type of forage the grain mix should not contain more phosphorus than calcium. It is common for phosphorus intakes to be marginal and rations may contain as much phosphorus as calcium at a ratio of 1:1. This is appropriate for use with a wide range of forages and reduces the difference in the calcium and phosphorus ratio of the total diet when a legume hay high in calcium is fed. It is important that young horses are fed diets containing sources of inorganic phosphorus such as dicalcium phosphate or monosodium phosphate since the digestibility of organic phosphorus sources is inhibited by complexes formed with phytate. Estimates of digestibility for phytin phosphorus in diets of horses is 30%.

The precise role of trace minerals remains unanswered although they have been the focus of considerable interest in recent years. Selenium, copper, zinc, molybdenum, manganese and aluminium have all shared the spotlight and been implicated as deficiencies or excesses in abortion, tying-up syndrome, OCD, physitis, wobbler syndrome and many other problems. It is probably accurate to assume that trace minerals are involved in some of these conditions but random and wholesale supplementation is not warranted. The levels of trace minerals given in Table 2.12 are in many instances greater than those recommended by the NRC but reflect current practice.

Vitamins

Far more emphasis than is warranted is placed on vitamin nutrition of the horse, due in part to the constant barrage of advertisements which suggest that vitamin supplementation for the horse and human is a necessary aspect of nutrition.

The vitamin premix shown in Table 1.4 (Chapter 1) should meet or exceed the young horse's requirements. There are instances in which supplementation above the level recommended is warranted, as when biotin at 15 mg per day is included to promote hoof growth.

Mare's milk and lactation

Colostrum produced in the first 36 hours following parturition is higher in protein, fat and many minerals than normal milk. Most important is the concentration of antibodies to a variety of pathogens that provide the foal with temporary passive immunity. Failure of passive transfer (FPT) as a result of the foal's inability to obtain sufficient colostrum during the first 24 hours is discussed in more detail in Chapter 9. It is essential that consumption of colostrum occurs within the first 24 hours of life as after this time the foal is unable to absorb the large immunoglobulin (IgG) molecules from the gastrointestinal tract. Even though absorption of colostral antibodies may occur up to 24 hours post foaling, the health status of foals that have not received colostrum within the first 6 hours of life is compromised. Following 'gut closure', when IgG can no longer be absorbed, it may be necessary to supplement with intravenous infusions of plasma to provide passive protection. Checking the foal's blood IgG level at 24 hours to establish that passive transfer has been accomplished (as discussed in Chapter 9) is an investment in the foal's future health and well-being.

During the first 2 months of life the foal's nutrient needs are entirely met by milk and there is no need for supplemental feed. If a mare is a poor milk producer the foal should be encouraged to consume dry feed. Peak lactation occurs at 5–7 weeks post parturition after which milk production begins to fall away.

Orphaned and early weaned foals

Mare owners at some stage are faced with raising an orphaned foal due to the loss of a mare, a mare not accepting a foal or a mare that has no milk. Even when mares are healthy and producing milk there may be instances when it is appropriate to wean a foal at an early age. It is not uncommon to wean foals from mares that are old or have to be transported a long distance for breeding. Early weaning, either voluntarily or involuntarily, may occur at the time of birth or at any time prior to what would be considered a normal weaning age. There are two methods for raising an orphan—the use of a foster or nurse mare, or feeding a milk replacer.

Nurse mares

In areas with a high mare concentration, there are farms which specialize in keeping nurse mares. Particularly popular as nurse mares are heavy, draft breed mares such as Belgians, Shires and Percherons due to their even temperament and ability to produce large quantities of milk. Where nurse mares are not available, a mare might be found that has lost her foal and is available as a nurse mare. Regardless of the origin of the mare, there are several criteria that must be met before a mare is brought on the farm. Nurse mares should have been on a stringent vaccination and de-worming programme and preferably come from a closed herd and are free from strangles. Mares should be healthy and in early rather than late stages of lactation and producing an adequate supply of milk.

Nurse mares should be brought to the foal as soon after weaning their natural foals as possible. The mare may be sedated prior to presenting the foal. A way to mask the smell of the foal should be devised such as rubbing the foal with a blanket that has been on the mare's natural foal or rubbing camphorated oil, Vick or other pungent material in the mare's nostrils and on the foal. When initiating the bonding process the foal should be hungry to increase its instinctive urge to suckle. The mare should be allowed to sniff the foal but adequately restrained so that she does not savage the foal. The use of a partition that allows the foal access to the mare's udder but protects the foal is recommended. In some instances the nurse mare will immediately allow the foal to nurse but some kind of physical separation should be in place for at least 24 hours. Once the mare is comfortable with the new foal and shows no aggressive behaviour, the partition can be removed but the mare should still be watched very carefully to avoid injury to the foal. After 48 hours have passed and the mare has accepted the foal, the pair may be turned out in a small paddock. Introduction of the pair into the broodmare band should be delayed until it is sure the mare has adopted the foal. Adoption can be checked by removing the foal from the nurse mare and observing the mare's behaviour. If the mare nickers and becomes anxious as a natural mother might do then adoption has been successful.

Foal milk replacer

When a nurse mare is not available, foals may be raised successfully on milk replacer. In the USA there are several products available and collected data indicate that the growth rate of milk replacer-raised foals is equivalent to that of conventionally reared foals. The formulation of the milk replacer should be as close to the composition of mare's milk as possible. Particularly important are protein, fat and total solids. Foals that are to be raised on milk replacer should be fed using a bucket rather than a nippled bottle. Foals learn very quickly to drink milk replacer out of a bucket if the product is palatable. The foal should always receive colostrum as soon as possible after birth. Successful artificial rearing of foals depends on good hygiene and husbandry practices. All equipment used should be disinfected daily and foals should be kept in a warm, dry, clean, draught-free environment. The biggest dangers in raising foals on milk replacer are the development of diarrhoea (scours) and failure of transfer of passive immunity. If foals have an adequate IgG level and are not overfed initially these problems can be minimized.

Table 2.13 Feeding of orphan foals

Age of foal	Feedings per day	Amount to be fed daily (litres)
1 day	—	Colostrum
2–7 days	8	4–8
2nd week[1]	6	6–12
3rd and 4th weeks	6	8–15
5th week	4	8–15
6th–8th weeks	4	6–12

[1] Begin feeding a small quantity of high quality foal creep ration and fresh clean water at all times. Gradually increase creep feed until foals are consuming 0.5 kg per month of age.

Table 2.13 shows a feeding schedule appropriate for use in raising foals on milk replacer. The sooner a foal can be encouraged to consume solid feed the earlier weaning from the milk replacer can be accomplished. The schedule applies to a 24% protein, 16% fat product which is made up by adding 1 cup of powdered milk replacer to 1 litre of warm water. The characteristics of a good milk replacer are ease of mixing, a formulation similar to that of mare's milk and palatability. If the foal should start to scour a veterinarian should be consulted.

When raising a foal on milk replacer the following guidelines should apply. Make sure the foal is hungry when milk replacer is introduced. If the foal does not start drinking quickly, consult the veterinarian about nasogastric intubation. Keep all equipment and facilities clean. Feed small quantities frequently rather than large quantities infrequently. Do not feed free choice. *Do not spoil the foal.* Orphan foals that are incorrectly handled develop behavioural problems that are hard to correct as the foal gets older. React to the onset of scours by reducing the amount of milk per feeding and increasing the frequency of feeding. Encourage foals to eat solid feed. To encourage socialization, turn orphan foals out with quiet older horses. Discard milk replacer not consumed within one hour of feeding. Most foals will drink their allotment in a matter of minutes.

Creep feeding

It is not recommended that creep feed be provided as free choice (Figure 2.5). When creep is offered ad libitum there is often an increased incidence of physitis, osteochondrosis, enterotoxaemia and other growth-related problems among heavier more robust foals. As a general rule the amount of creep feed should not exceed 1.5% of body weight per day, or expressed another way the foal should receive a maximum of 0.5 kg per day per month of age. Adjustments in creep intake should be based on the condition of the individual foal and the availability of forage. This is particularly true where there is an abundant supply of high-quality forage, when it may be prudent to restrict the consumption of creep feed to as little as 0.5 kg/day of a protein, mineral and vitamin supplement. The nutrient requirements for a creep feed are provided in Table 2.14 and a recommended grain mix is given in Table 2.15. Creep feed intake and the condition of the foal should be monitored carefully and adjustments to the amount of feed should be based on these two criteria.

Weaning

Prior to looking at feeding the weanling it is appropriate to discuss the weaning process. Weaning involves removing the foal from the mare and is accomplished in a number of ways. The method chosen should minimize the stress

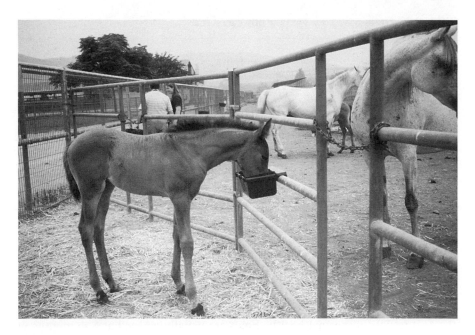

Figure 2.5 Supplemental feed available to the foal using a creep feeder.

Table 2.14 Nutrient requirements of a creep feed for unweaned foals

Nutrient	Inclusion level
Digestible energy, Mcal/kg	3.0
Crude protein, %	16.0
Calcium, %	0.9
Phosphorus, %	0.8
Copper, ppm	40.0
Zinc, ppm	100.0
Selenium, ppm	0.2
Potassium, %	0.7
Magnesium, %	0.25
Vitamin A, I.U./kg	2200.0
Vitamin D, I.U./kg	220.0
Vitamin E, I.U./kg	80.0
Thiamin, mg/kg	2.7
Riboflavin, mg/kg	1.75
Vitamin B_{12}, µg/kg	11.0

on mare and foal and be convenient for the farm, bearing in mind personnel
and facilities. If weaning is undertaken with adequate preparation there is no
need for the mare or foal to suffer adverse effects. Regardless of the method
chosen it is important that the foal is in good health and consuming adequate

Table 2.15 Grain mix creep feed for unweaned foals[1]

Ingredient	% of diet	Inclusion level (kg/tonne)
Crimped oats	37.5	375
Cracked corn (maize)	18.25	182.5
Rolled barley	10.0	100
Molasses, cane	8.0	80
Soyabean meal (48%)	22.5	225
Salt	0.5	5
Dicalcium phosphate	2.00	20.0
Calcium carbonate	0.75	7.5
KER 5X[2]	0.50	5

[1] For best results all ingredients except oats, maize, barley and molasses should be pelleted.
[2] KER 5X = trace mineral vitamin premix manufactured by Kentucky Equine Research, Versailles, Kentucky, USA 40383.

amounts of feed. If a foal is sick the weaning process should be postponed until the foal returns to normal health. Foals are usually weaned at 5–6 months of age, at which time the mare is producing insufficient milk to meet the foal's nutrient requirements. Foals can be weaned at an earlier age if the mare is not producing adequate milk. It may be necessary to wean early if the foal is causing an older mare to lose weight, thereby jeopardizing her chances of becoming or remaining pregnant. Some foals will benefit from early weaning if they are growing at a rate that might lead to skeletal problems or if they must be confined for an extended period due to an injury and the mare would be better outside. It is easier to carefully regulate nutrient intake in the weaned foal than in the foal nursing its dam.

In the opinion of the author the least traumatic method of weaning is the mare elimination technique, which requires removal of mares from a group one or two at a time, leaving the weaned foals to run with the group of unweaned foals (Figure 2.6). The oldest foals are weaned first and become accustomed to the absence of their mares while still in the company of other foals. It is important that the last mares in the herd have a good temperament and tolerate several foals around them. Using the mare elimination, or pasture weaning technique it is beneficial to place an old gelding or barren mare in the herd to serve as a babysitter when all the mares have been removed. This reduces the amount of running by the foals and lessens the likelihood of injury. The method works best when foals are eating creep feed in the pasture and so removal of the mare necessitates that creep feed is available. It is important that foals are handled prior to weaning so they can be caught and taught to lead, otherwise it becomes difficult to catch weaned foals once the mare is removed.

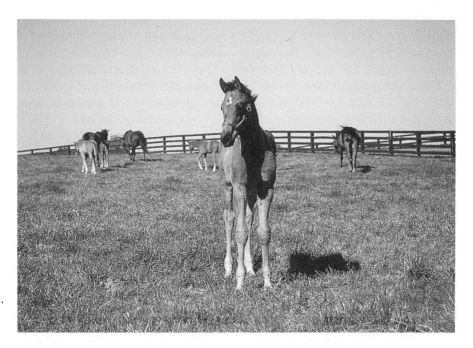

Figure 2.6 An older, weaned foal with a group of unweaned foals and their mothers.

Another method is stall weaning when foals alone or in pairs are taken from their dams and placed in box stalls. The mares should be removed to another part of the farm out of view and hearing distance so as to reduce the stress on both mare and foal. If the foal can neither hear nor see its dam it will call and fret a minimal amount of time. Care should be taken to ensure the weaning stall is safe and contains no sharp objects that could injure the foal. If the single foal method is used it has the advantage of weaning from the mare as well as from other foals. The disadvantage is that it is more stressful. A variation of the stall weaning technique is to separate the foal from the mare for short periods and return the foal to the mare. The time the foal is removed is increased gradually until the foal is removed entirely. This method is more labour intensive and increases the total time taken to wean the foal but reduces the degree of stress.

Weanlings

In the period immediately following weaning there is a period of weight loss or slowed growth followed by a growth spurt, which has been shown to result in an increased incidence of acquired limb deformities. If the foal was consuming creep feed prior to weaning there should be little interruption in growth rate. A smooth uninterrupted growth curve will reduce the likelihood of developmental disorders. The suggested nutrient requirements of a ration for weanlings are shown in Table 2.16; this may be adjusted depending on forage quality, although in practice this is rarely done. The weanling should be allowed 1–1.5% of their body weight per day of grain mix plus liberal quantities of good quality forage. An example of a grain mix for weanlings is shown in Table 2.17. The weanling expected to mature at 500 kg should be eating 2.5–4 kg of grain mix per day depending on weight and body condition. Although it is possible to exceed this amount the adverse consequences resulting from a too rapid growth rate must be considered. Weanlings should have free access to good quality forage and be allowed as much voluntary exercise as they desire. Exercise has been shown to increase bone density and cortical thickness producing a more durable athlete. Calcium levels in the diet should exceed those of phosphorus but at the same time ensuring that adequate phosphorus is present.

The following guidelines will permit weanlings to maximize their genetic potential for growth without adverse effects:

1 Minimize the post-weanling slump and feed a maximum of 1.5% of body weight per day in grain mix depending on the condition of the weanling.
2 Allow a liberal intake of good quality hay and pasture and ensure the total intake of calcium is greater than that of phosphorus.
3 Monitor the growth rate carefully, avoid growth spurts and allow plenty of exercise.

Yearlings

Assuming that the nursing foal and weanling were fed correctly, the growth rate should have slowed down by the yearling stage. Once a horse attains 12 months of age there should be fewer problems associated with bone development. It is important to remember, however, that in terms of growth priority, bone is first, muscle second and fat third. The challenge in feeding the yearling is to ensure that growth of skeletal and muscle tissue continues while avoiding excess deposition of fat. This is achieved by an adequate intake of protein and minerals but avoiding an excessive intake of energy. The yearling's nutrient requirements are shown in Diet 2 of Table 2.16 with a suggested grain mix in Table 2.17. The protein concentration in the grain mix can be adjusted according to the type of forage fed, as illustrated in Table 2.18. The amount the yearling should receive must be adjusted according to the individual's growth rate, condition and maturity. Table 2.19 shows the amounts of grain mix to be fed depending on hay quality or pasture availability. The yearling's energy needs are met by feeding 0.75–1.5% of body weight per day as grain mix plus

Table 2.16 Nutrient requirements in a grain mix for weanlings

Nutrient	Diet	
	1[1]	2[2]
Crude protein, %	16.0	14.0
Calcium, %	0.90	0.75
Phosphorus, %	0.80	0.65
Magnesium, %	0.25	0.25
Potassium, %	0.70	0.60
Copper, mg/kg	50.0	50.0
Zinc, mg/kg	90.0	90.0
Selenium, mg/kg	0.3	0.3
Vitamin A, I.U./kg	11 000.0	11 000.0
Vitamin D, I.U./kg	1100.0	1100.0
Vitamin E, I.U./kg	80.0	80.0

[1] Diet 1 to be fed to weanlings and yearlings up to 14 months of age or until 18 months of age if a poor quality grass hay is being fed.
[2] Diet 2 to be fed to yearlings and long yearlings, may also be fed to 2-year-olds in training.

Table 2.17. Grain mix for weanlings

Ingredient	% of diet[1]	Inclusion rate (kg/tonne)
Crimped oats	45.0 (39.0)	450 (390)
Cracked corn (maize)	20.0	200
Rolled barley	11.25 (10.0)	112.5 (100)
Molasses, cane	8.5 (9.0)	85 (90)
Soyabean meal (48%)	12.0 (18.5)	120 (185)
Salt	0.5	5
Dicalcium phosphate	1.75	17.5
Calcium carbonate	0.50 (0.75)	5 (7.5)
KER 5X[2]	0.50	5

[1] If yearlings are on poor quality pasture and/or receiving legume hay, figures in brackets should be substituted.
[2] KER 5X = trace mineral vitamin premix manufactured by Kentucky Equine Research, Versailles, Kentucky, USA 40383.

liberal quantities of high quality forage. As an example, a 14-month-old year-ling weighing 365 kg should receive 14% protein in the ration. The minimum amount of grain mix would be 2.75 kg (365 × 0.75), the maximum 5.5 kg (365 × 1.5). Table 2.20 provides guidelines for estimating the approximate amounts of grain mix to feed young horses.

If oats are the preferred grain portion of the ration special mixes can be

Table 2.18 Crude protein % in grain mixes when feeding grass or legume hays[1]

Age of horse	Grass hay	Legume hay
Weanling	16–18	14–16
Yearling	15–17	12–14
Long yearling	14	12

[1] Examples of grass hays include timothy, orchardgrass, coastal bermuda, brome and prairie. Examples of legume hays include alfalfa (lucerne), clover and lespedeza.

Table 2.19 Amount[1] of grain mix (kg) to be fed to yearlings relative to hay[2] quality

	Digestible energy requirement (Mcal/kg feed)	Weight of Horse at Maturity			
		500 kg		600 kg	
		Average hay	Good hay	Average hay	Good hay
Weanling	2.75	3.6	3.0	4.0	3.6
Yearling[3]	2.64	4.0	3.6	4.5	4.0
Long yearling[3]	2.42	4.5	4.0	5.0	4.0

[1] Amounts of grain fed should be adjusted according to the condition of the horse.
[2] Hay fed free choice.
[3] Figures reflect greater forage consumption by the long yearling.

Table 2.20 Grain-mix feeding schedule for young horses

	Rate of feeding[1]
Creep feed	0.75–1% of body weight
Weanling	1–1.5% of body weight
Yearling	0.5–1.5% of body weight

[1] Amounts of grain mix may be varied if good quality pasture is available or liberal amounts of good quality hay are fed.

formulated. Most contain 25–30% protein, 3% calcium and 2% phosphorus compensating for their low level in oats. One of the reasons why young horses develop bone deformities is that they are on a high intake of grain without adequate amounts of calcium. Adjusting the intake of calcium and phosphorus will eliminate the problem. The calcium and phosphorus levels are greater than the requirements listed in Table 2.16, but provide greater flexibility in the forage feeding programme and allow the special mix to be fed with a variety of hays.

Performance horses

For all the emphasis placed on selecting, breeding and feeding the performance horse, very little is currently known about the nutrient requirements of the horse engaged in strenuous work. Folklore abounds and special 'tonics' are used extensively—feeding the performance horse is far from being an exact science. When the difference in a winner of a graded stakes or group race and a placed horse is a fraction of a second, it is no longer possible to rely on outdated methods. Renewed interest and funding for research into the nutrient needs of the performance horse is beginning to show promising results. Although more is known about the science of feeding the horse, even the most capable scientist recognizes that the skill of the trainer is a vital ingredient in developing the horse to optimum fitness.

The performance horse has a basic need for water, energy, protein, minerals and vitamins, the amount provided being a function of age and type and amount of work to be undertaken. The energy utilized by the horse is a function of work intensity, training, genetics and environment. Training enhances the horse's capacity for energy metabolism, yet energy utilization and storage remain factors that limit performance. Energy storage is primarily in the form of adenosine triphosphate (ATP), creatine phosphate, muscle glycogen and stored body fat. The form of energy utilized during exercise depends upon the amount of anaerobic work undertaken. Anaerobic work is performed without utilizing oxygen, whereas aerobic work requires a supply of oxygen to the tissues. Most exercise that horses undertake is a combination of aerobic and anaerobic work. Light work of a long duration such as walking and trotting represents the highest percentage participation of aerobic metabolism. Maximal racing effort represents the highest degree of anaerobic work. The horse's anaerobic and aerobic capacities are enhanced by training as is the ability to utilize the energy involved in each type of metabolism. During anaerobic work the energy available, via glycolysis, is stored ATP, creatine phosphate and muscle glycogen. For aerobic work these same energy sources plus fat are utilized. When designing a feeding programme for supplying energy it is therefore important to identify the type of work to be undertaken.

An accurate method for estimating the dietary energy intake to ensure that stores are optimal for the attainment of work performed is not available. In the human, glycogen storage can be increased by a process referred to as glycogen packing. This is accomplished by depleting glycogen stores in the muscles by exercise in conjunction with a high-protein, high-fat/low-starch diet that is followed by feeding high levels of starch. This regime results in higher levels of glycogen storage in muscle than were present before the depletion process. For horses doing a great deal of work, sufficient energy in the form of carbohydrate should be included in the diet.

The anaerobic threshold describes the point at which the horse relies on anaerobic metabolism to supply its energy needs. This varies between horses and among breeds, but is characterized by heart rates of greater than 180 per minute and by the accumulation of lactic acid, the end-point of anaerobic glycolysis. Through continued interest in exercise physiology it should be possible to obtain a better understanding of the physiology of the exercising horse and make subtle changes in diet or training which will result in enhanced performance.

Energy

Contrary to popular belief, the greatest increase in nutrient requirements of the performance horse concerns energy. The energy required at high work intensity is more than twice that required for maintenance. Table 2.21 illus-

Table 2.21 Energy requirements of horses in various types of work

Type of work	Digestible energy (Mcal)	Digestible energy concentration (Mcal/kg)
Light[1]	21.89	2.2
Medium[2]	28.69	2.65
Strenuous[3]	34.00	2.75

[1] Includes horses used in western pleasure, hacking, equitation, pleasure riding.
[2] Includes horses used in ranch work, roping, cutting, barrel racing, jumping.
[3] Includes horses in endurance racing, polo, combined training.

trates the horse's requirement for DE for various types of work. The amount of energy and the energy density (Mcal/kg) of the diet increase dramatically as work intensity increases. The most common sources of energy are cereal grains such as corn (maize), oats, barley and milo. The addition of fat to the diet also enhances its energy value. The digestible energy value of the feed does not tell the whole story as the energy source in the diet should depend on the type of work performed. The more strenuous the work, the greater the amount of energy that should be supplied as soluble carbohydrate. Corn (maize) is by far the best source of starch because of its higher DE value and lower fibre content. Starch or other soluble carbohydrates are needed to replace muscle glycogen. Fat digestion results in energy stored as triglyceride or body fat. Fibre digestion by microorganisms in the caecum results in the formation of the volatile fatty acids, acetate, propionate and butyrate. Only propionate is utilized in the formation of glucose and the synthesis of glycogen stored in muscle or hepatic tissue. Because of the large amount of energy required for work and the small capacity of the gastrointestinal tract, the working horse cannot meet its energy needs by forage alone. The horse in training should receive 1–1.75% of its body weight per day in the form of grain mix in addition to the minimum of 1% of body weight per day as good quality forage. Energy deficiency is manifest by weight loss, loss of vigour, chronic fatigue and a disinterest in strenuous work. Weight gain in the mature horse indicates that energy in excess of requirements is being consumed.

Protein

There is no evidence to indicate that the horse in training has a protein requirement greater than that required for maintenance. The protein requirements of the horse in work are shown in Table 2.22. The protein requirements

Table 2.22 Total crude protein requirements of performance horse

Type of horse	Crude protein, (g/day)	Crude protein, (%)
2-year-old	1117	10
Mature horse[1]		
Light work	820	8
Medium work	984	8
Heavy work	1320	8

[1] Descriptions of work are the same as in Table 2.21.

for work are generally met with a cereal grain and medium quality hay diet. The protein needs of the 2-year-old horse in training are provided by a 13–14% protein grain mix plus good quality hay with a minimum crude protein of 8%. For the mature horse the protein requirement is met by feeding a 12–13% protein grain mix plus good quality hay with at least 8% crude protein. By increasing the amount of feed the horse consumes to meet its energy needs, the protein intake is also increased. Nitrogen lost from sweat or through muscle catabolism must be replaced. Protein provided in excess of what is required is deaminated, the nitrogen excreted in urine and the carbon skeleton of the amino acids utilized for energy. Protein is provided by most dietary constituents. However, corn (maize) and oats—the primary energy sources—are not good sources of protein. Consequently, it is common practice to use soyabean meal to provide an adequate source of protein.

Vitamins

In order to assess the vitamin adequacy of the diet, it is important to know not only the overall requirement, but the contribution from natural sources, the ability of the horse to synthesize vitamins and an understanding of specific physiological states that increase the horse's requirement for one or more vitamins. Although it is generally perceived that the horse in heavy work has an increased demand for vitamins, the practice of supplementation with vitamin 'tonics' is not warranted and indeed may be dangerous due to possible toxicity.

Vitamin E from natural sources is adequate to meet the needs of most classes of horses. However, the performance horse may benefit from higher levels and the NRC's *Nutrient Requirements of Horses*, published in 1989, recommends that the performance horse in hard training receives a minimum of 80 I.U. of vitamin E in the total diet. Wheatgerm oil, properly cured hay and cereal grains are good sources of vitamin E. Daily levels of 1000 I.U. are adequate to meet the horse's needs but evidence of increased performance has been observed following supplementation with vitamin E. A feed fortified with B-vitamins using a premix as shown in Table 1.4 (Chapter 1) or a B-vitamin supplement is warranted for horses in hard training because of the involvement of this vitamin group in energy metabolism.

Minerals

The primary minerals of concern when considering the performance horse are calcium, phosphorus, sodium and chloride. The role of calcium and phosphorus in the formation and maintenance of bone, nerve conductivity, muscle contraction and energy metabolism make them especially important to the performance horse. Regardless of the calcium and phosphorus content of hay or forage, a grain mix should *never* be formulated containing more phosphorus than calcium. Forages are a good source of calcium and cereal grains a good source of phosphorus. If a good quality alfalfa (lucerne) or other legume hay is being fed, a 1:1 calcium:phosphorus ratio should be included in the grain mix. Sodium and chloride are of utmost importance to the performance horse due to their role in maintaining osmotic and acid–base balance. During strenuous exercise, horses may lose as much as 90 g of salt (sodium chloride) through sweat. These losses must be replaced by the inclusion of salt as 0.5–0.75% of the diet and/or providing trace mineralized salt as a free choice. As long as an adequate supply of fresh clean water is available, there should be no problems with salt toxicity. Potassium losses in sweat may be high and there is evidence that potassium loss increases with exercise. The loss of electrolytes via sweat causes a decrease in water intake resulting in dehydration. For horses consuming a reasonable amount of forage, the potassium intake should be adequate as most forages contain in excess of 1.5% potassium. Excessive potassium loss through sweat and urine may result in post-exercise fatigue and diaphragmatic flutter or 'thumps'. In addition to the minerals mentioned above, trace minerals are necessary and are provided by access to a trace mineralized salt block. The primary concern in feeding the performance horse is that as exercise increases there is a need to increase the amount of energy. Nutrient concentrations that should be provided in the grain mix portion of performance horse diets are shown in Table 2.23. As a general rule, 1–1.75% of body weight per

Table 2.23 Nutrient concentration of grain mix for performance horse diets

Nutrient	Type of horse			
	2-years-old	Light work	Medium work	Heavy work
Energy (Mcal/kg)	3.0	2.8	3.0	3.3
Protein (%)	14	13	13	13
Calcium (%)	0.7	0.6	0.6	0.6
Phosphorus (%)	0.6	0.5	0.5	0.5
Potassium (%)	0.7	0.7	0.7	0.7
Sodium (%)	0.45	0.45	0.45	0.45
Chlorine (%)	0.35	0.35	0.35	0.35
Magnesium (%)	0.25	0.25	0.25	0.25
Iron (ppm)	60	60	60	60
Zinc (ppm)	40	40	40	40
Copper (ppm)	20	20	20	20
Selenium (ppm)	0.2	0.2	0.2	0.2
Vitamin A (I.U./kg)	2380	2380	2380	2380
Vitamin D (I.U./kg)	230	230	230	230
Vitamin E (I.U./kg)	100	100	100	100
Riboflavin (ppm)	4.8	4	4	4
Thiamin (ppm)	6	6	6	6
Pantothenic acid (ppm)	20	20	20	20

day should be fed as grain mix plus liberal amounts of good quality hay. The horse has an absolute requirement for long-stem forage. Not only does roughage promote efficient function of the gastrointestinal tract, it also decreases the likelihood of horses developing stable vices due to boredom. Fifty per cent of the performance horse's needs can be met with good quality hay and/or pasture at light and moderate workloads. It follows that the remaining 50% should be provided as grain mix. Although many trainers worry about developing a 'hay belly' on their horses, if good quality, highly digestible hays cut in early stages of maturity are fed, this should be of little concern. When horses are at high work intensity, meeting 50% of their energy needs with hay may not be practical due to limitations in the capacity of the intestinal tract. The horse is unable to consume adequate forage to meet its DE requirements and so 70% of DE requirements must be met by the grain mix portion of the diet. An example of a grain mix appropriate for performance horses is shown in Table 2.24.

Table 2.24 Grain mix for performance horses

Ingredient	% of Diet	Inclusion rate (kg/tonne)
Crimped oats	38.0	380
Cracked corn (maize)	20.0	200
Shredded beet pulp	15.75	157.5
Molasses, cane	10.0	100
Soyabean meal (48%)	8.5	85
Salt	0.5	5
Dicalcium phosphate	1.5	15
Calcium carbonate	0.75	7.5
Soyabean oil	4.5	45
KER 5X[1]	0.50	5

[1] KER 5X = trace mineral vitamin premix manufactured by Kentucky Equine Research, Versailles, Kentucky, USA 40383.

Mature idle horses

The nutrient requirements of the mature idle horse are shown in Table 2.25. Horses in this category do well on good quality hay or pasture alone provided that forage availability is not limited. Voluntary dry matter intake of fresh forage in the mature horse has been estimated to exceed 3.5% of body weight per day. Assuming a 500 kg horse ate this amount of a forage containing 1.9 Mcal/kg DE and 6% crude protein then his intake of DE and crude protein per day would be 34 Mcal and 1050 g respectively. This intake far exceeds requirements and emphasizes that horses can obtain a significant part of their nutrient requirements from forage. If on the other hand forage is limited,

Table 2.25 Nutrient requirements of the mature horse and stallion at maintenance (500 kg mature weight) as a concentration of the total diet (90% dry matter basis) and Total Required Per Day

Nutrient	Concentration in diet	Amount per day
Digestible energy	1.8 Mcal/kg	16.4 Mcal
Crude protein	7.2%	656 g/day
Calcium	0.21%	20 g/day
Phosphorus	0.15%	14 g/day
Magnesium	0.08%	7.5 g/day
Potassium	0.27%	25 g/day
Sodium	0.10%	10 g/day
Sulphur	0.15%	14 g/day
Iron	40 ppm	370 mg/day
Manganese	40 ppm	370 mg/day
Copper	10 ppm	92.6 mg/day
Zinc	40 ppm	370 mg/day
Vitamin A	2 000 I.U./kg	18 000 I.U./day
Vitamin D	300 I.U./kg	2 800 I.U./day
Vitamin E	50 I.U./kg	500 I.U./day

either by space restrictions or environmental factors, a grain mix such as shown in Table 2.26 can be fed in addition to good quality hay to maintain body condition. The general tendency is to overfeed rather than to provide too little feed. In most cases when horses on a maintenance diet are turned out to pasture the only supplementation they need is a free choice of water and trace-mineralized or plain salt.

Stallions

Specific information on the nutrient requirements of the breeding stallion is lacking. Most published reports have assessed the effects of vitamin and mineral supplementation on semen quality and are inconclusive. It is therefore necessary to utilize a combination of experience and data collected from other types of horses to arrive at a best estimate of the nutrient requirements of the breeding stallion. There is no reason to believe that the stallion's nutrient needs differ from those of the mature horse at maintenance as shown in Table 2.25, at least during the non-breeding season. The NRC's most recent *Nutrient Requirements of Horses*, published in 1989, recommended that the stallion's requirements increase 25% during the breeding season. Even though the basic

Table 2.26 Grain mix for mature idle horses and stallions

Ingredient	% of diet	Inclusion rate (kg/tonne)
Crimped oats	45.0	450
Cracked corn (maize)	19.0	190
Rolled barley	20.0	200
Molasses, cane	8.0	80
Soyabean meal (48%)	5.0	50
Salt	0.5	5
Dicalcium phosphate	1.0	10
Calcium carbonate	0.75	7.5
KER 5X[1]	0.50	5

[1] KER 5X = trace mineral vitamin premix manufactured by Kentucky Equine Research, Versailles, Kentucky, USA 40383.

recommendations for feeding the stallion are similar to those of the mature idle horse, there are several factors that may necessitate adjustment to keep the stallion in proper condition. Feeding rates for stallions will vary due to activity, age, temperament, dental condition, forage availability, time turned out to pasture and environmental conditions. The nutrient of greatest concern is energy; the requirements for protein, vitamins and minerals are unlikely to vary. The stallion should be fed to maintain a specific body condition year-round. Stallions that are allowed to become overweight are at greater risk of laminitis, colic and heart disease. It is critical that stallions receive adequate exercise if they are to have a long career at stud. One major stud farm in central Kentucky uses a strict regimen of riding and exercise in an attempt to prolong the useful life of their stallions.

Table 2.26 illustrates a grain mix that can be fed to stallions in both the breeding and non-breeding season. For most light horse breeds the average stallion can maintain suitable condition on 4–6 kg of grain mix and 8–10 kg of good quality hay. This amounts to about 1% of body weight per day of grain mix and 1.3–1.6% of body weight per day of hay. Actual feed needs will vary depending on pasture availability and the factors relating to individuality mentioned above.

It is of paramount importance to remember that horses are individuals and vary greatly in their requirements for feed. Some horses will tend to become overweight when fed according to 'the book' while others will lose weight. It is imperative to constantly monitor the horse's condition and feed accordingly. Regardless of what the 'average' horse is thought to require, the person responsible for feeding the horse must be the final judge in making sure the horse receives adequate feed to meet its needs. Expressed in another way, the 'eye of the master fattens the ox'.

Further reading

Cunha T J (1991) *Horse feeding and nutrition*, 2nd edn. Academic Press. New York.

Evans J W (1989) *Horses*. W H Freeman, New York.

Evans J W, Borton A, Hintz H F, Van Vleck L D (1990) *The horse*. W H Freeman, New York.

Glade M J (1983) Nutrition and performance of racing Thoroughbred horses. *Equine Veterinary Journal* **15**: 31–6.

Henneke D R, Potter, G D, Krieder J L (1984) Body condition during pregnancy and lactation and reproductive efficiency of mares. *Theriogenology* **21**: 897–909.

Hintz H F, Hintz R L, Van Vleck L D (1979) Growth rate of Thoroughbreds, effect of age of dam, year and month of birth, and sex of foal. *Journal of Animal Science* **48**: 480–7.

Lewis L D (1982) *Feeding and care of the horse*. Lea & Febiger, Philadelphia, PA.

Pagan J D, Hintz H F (1986) Equine energetics I. Relationship between body weight and energy requirements in horses. *Journal of Animal Science* **63**: 815–21.

Pagan J D, Hintz H F (1986) Equine energetics II. Energy expenditure of horses during submaximal exercise. *Journal of Animal Science* **63**: 822–30.

Ralston S L (1988) Nutritional management of horses competing in 160 km races. *Cornell Veterinarian* **78**: 53–61.

Raub R H, Jackson S G, Baker J P (1989) The effect of exercise on bone growth and development in weanling horses. *Journal of Animal Science* **67**: 2508–14.

3 COMMON NUTRITIONAL DISORDERS
STEPHEN G. JACKSON, PhD

Summary

It is not uncommon to ascribe many of the disease states in horses to a nutritional aetiology. Although there are problems that are a result of nutrient deficiencies, excesses or toxic factors, one must guard against blaming nutrition when other factors may be in operation. Currently more problems are associated with nutritional excess rather than as a result of inadequate nutrition. Developmental orthopaedic disease (DOD) has a multifactorial aetiology due to genetics, nutritional excesses, deficits and imbalances, and faults of conformation. Major nutrients to evaluate in the face of a DOD problem are energy intake, and mineral status of the diet. A discussion of DOD including physitis, osteochondrosis, wobbler syndrome and acquired flexural deformities must begin with an evaluation of the ration being fed and how the feeding programme is being administered.

Toxic factors in forages are responsible for several of the more commonly seen nutritional disorders of the horse. Fescue toxicosis affects the pregnant broodmare, making fescue an inappropriate forage for this class of horse. Sudangrass and sudangrass hybrid forages cause cystitis in horses and should not be grazed. Blister beetle-infested alfalfa (lucerne) is lethal to horses. Ingestion of only traces of the toxin cantharidin is fatal to the horse. Mouldy corn disease is caused by contamination of corn (maize), barley or milo with *Fusarium moniliforme*.

Ingredients intended for other classes of livestock such as ionophores and urea can be toxic to the horse depending on the amount consumed. Deficient or inappropriate balances of several nutrients can cause nutritional secondary hyperparathyroidism, goitre, white muscle disease and exertional rhabdomyolysis.

Inadequate fibre intake is one of the predominant causes of colic in horses and may also encourage wood chewing.

Many of the disorders dealt with by horse owners and veterinarians may be of nutritional origin. Beyond the simple nutrient deficiencies there are a number of disease states or syndromes that have at least a nutritional component to their aetiology. It is not the intention to consider each nutrient and the deficiency symptoms associated with them, but rather, in concise terms discuss common problems seen in the horse that may have a nutritional cause or component. As a word of caution, many health problems in horses are erroneously ascribed to mistakes in the feeding programme. It is the responsibility of the horse owner or manager to ensure the horse is properly fed, the veterinarian to accurately diagnose, treat and prevent disease conditions, and the nutritionist to formulate feeds that will minimize the occurrence of the conditions described below.

Developmental orthopaedic disease (DOD)

Developmental orthopaedic disease, sometimes referred to as metabolic bone disease, consists not of a single but of several related disorders affecting the young horse during the critical developmental stage. Included are: epiphysitis (physitis), osteochondrosis, osteochondrosis dissecans, wobbler syndrome and acquired flexural deformity. All these conditions are multifactorial in cause and are for the most part related. There is a strong genetic component which must not be ignored. Whether the genetic component is a specific gene or several genes which as a result of selection pressure have resulted in an increase in the incidence of the problem is not well understood. It is recognized that faster growing, earlier maturing, larger horses exhibit a greater tendency toward DOD than their slower growing smaller counterparts. The selection for early and rapid growth along with speed seems to have increased the prevalence of DOD creating a greater need to understand the condition. In other species the problem has been diminished by careful genetic selection but this approach is not so feasible in the horse partly because of the slow generation rate and small number of offspring. The solution rests in a better understanding of the possible causes, a recognition of the genetic component and establishment of management and feeding programmes that minimize the expression of these conditions.

Epiphysitis

The term 'epiphysitis' is in itself a misnomer. The condition should more appropriately be referred to as physitis or metaphysitis. 'Epiphysitis' is an inflammation of the physis or growth plate which constitutes a centre of cartilaginous growth in the long bones of all mammalian species. Growth plates, as illustrated in Figure 3.1, are found both at the proximal and distal ends of all of the long bones and are the means by which longitudinal growth occurs. The growth plate is dynamic and new cartilage is being formed as old cartilage cells are converted to bone. 'Epiphysitis' occurs when the cartilage growth plates become inflamed or when normal maturation of cartilage to form bone is disrupted. Although any growth plate can be affected those most commonly observed are those at the distal ends of the metacarpal bones, metatarsal bones, radius and tibia. The lesion appears as a bony enlargement and is more frequently seen on the medial rather than lateral side, as shown in Figure 3.2. Figure 3.3 shows a radiograph of the normal physes most commonly affected. 'Epiphysitis' may be accompanied by palpable heat in the affected areas and lameness, although many young horses show clinical physitis without exhibiting lameness. The list of causes includes, but is not limited to, angular limb deformity, very rapid growth, injury, nutritional deficiencies, nutritional excess, nutritional imbalance, trauma and genetic predisposition.

It is important to appreciate changes in joint architecture and distinguish between normal changes and physitis, which is potentially threatening to development. Treatment of physitis varies depending on the severity and cause if diagnosed. In most instances it is advisable to reduce energy intake so the rate of growth is slowed. A common error is to slow growth by not only reducing the intake of energy but also other nutrients critical to normal bone development. It is more prudent to meet the horse's requirement for protein, minerals and vitamins than to stop feeding altogether. One of the ways in which this can be undertaken is by utilizing a protein, vitamin and mineral supplement fed at approximately 1 kg per day. The feeding rate will depend upon the type of supplement and how it is formulated. In addition good

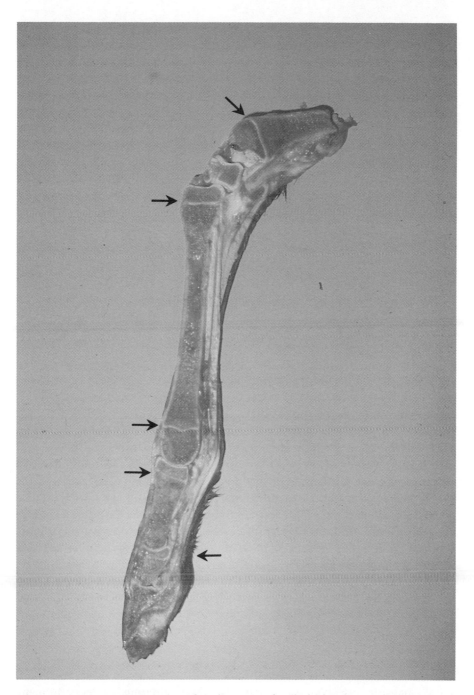

Figure 3.1 Longitudinal section of the immature forelimb showing cartilaginous epiphyseal plates as indicated by arrows.

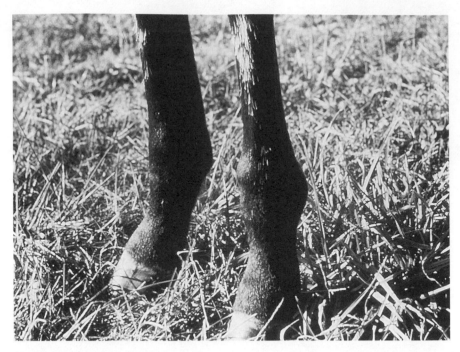

Figure 3.2 Physitis recognizable as enlargements on the inside of the fetlocks (seen on the medial side of distal third metacarpal bone).

quality hay should be offered ad libitum. Once feed intake has been reduced, an assessment of the diet should be undertaken. Nutrients of critical concern in rations for young horses include: protein, calcium, phosphorus, copper and zinc and the reader is referred to the section on feeding the young horse in Chapter 2 for appropriate levels of these nutrients. If after evaluation of the ration there is no evidence of a nutritional problem then other causes should be considered. Even if the ration appears to be balanced it is advisable to reduce the feeding rate until the problem is resolved. On many occasions it appears that mild 'epiphysitis' goes away in 60 days if it is treated and 2 months if it is not. In the final analysis it is not particularly alarming to observe inflammation prior to closure of a specific physis. The major concern is that it may be the visual indicator of a more serious metabolic problem.

Osteochondrosis (OC)

One of the more serious aspects of the DOD complex is osteochondrosis. Unlike physitis, osteochondrosis may result in debilitating lameness, in many instances reducing or eliminating any chance of an athletic career. Osteochondrosis is a disorder involving the maturation of joint cartilage. Aberrant carti-

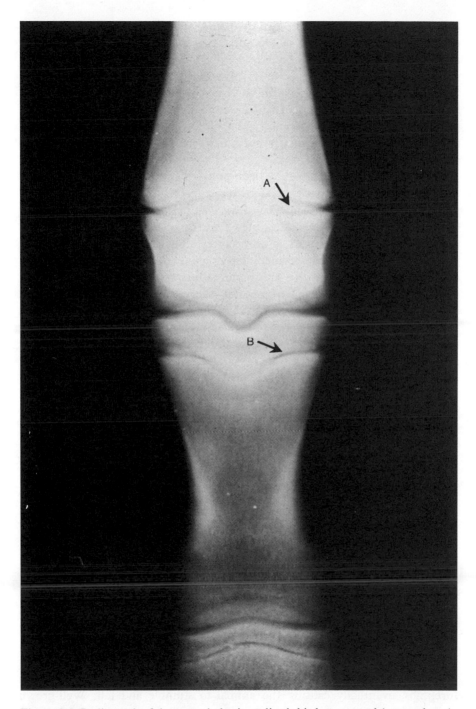

Figure 3.3 Radiograph of the normal physis at distal third metacarpal (cannon bone) (A) and proximal phalanx (long pastern bone) (B) as indicated by arrows.

lage formation results in the separation of cartilage from the subchondral bone resulting in the formation of subchondral cysts and cartilaginous flaps. When these lesions are observed, usually by taking X-rays, the condition is referred to as osteochondrosis dissecans (OCD). It is most frequently seen in the ankle, hock and stifle joints, as shown in an X-ray in Figure 3.4. The lesions may involve the articular or non-articular surfaces, with the former posing the greatest immediate risk of lameness. Articular lesions which become detached from the subchondral bone may be surgically removed with variable degrees of success.

A number of causes of OC have been proposed, yet the specific aetiology of the disease is far from understood. Interest in OC has been generated by a perceived increase in the incidence of the condition and a recent report from Ohio State University which suggested that the occurrence of OC may be a result of mineral deficiencies or imbalances. It is difficult to determine if indeed the incidence of the problem has increased or if the condition is being diagnosed more frequently due to superior radiographic techniques and equipment. With respect to the micro-mineral theory, careful balancing of rations containing liberal concentrations of copper and zinc have resulted in only a slight alteration in the occurrence of OC, emphasizing the multifactorial cause of the problem. Other factors currently under consideration include hypercalcitoninism as a result of high calcium intake in mares and hyperthyroxaemia due to excessive carbohydrate intake. It is likely that genetic, nutritional and endocrine components contribute to the aetiology and to obtain a decrease in incidence all must be considered.

Until the cause of OC is better elucidated it is appropriate to take a conservative approach to the nutritional management of affected populations of horses. Rations should be designed that meet but do not significantly exceed the horse's requirements for all nutrients, with specific emphasis on copper, zinc, manganese, calcium and phosphorus. Once formulated the ration should be fed in a manner that results in moderate growth rates and maximizes the forage rather than the grain part of the diet.

Wobbler syndrome

One of the earliest accounts of the wobbler syndrome was written in 1939 by members of the Department of Veterinary Science at the University of Kentucky. They described 47 cases which had occurred in central Kentucky between 1937 and 1939. Cases occurred particularly among Thoroughbreds and Saddlebreds, breeds which have long necks. Foals around weaning developed a lack of coordination in the hindlimbs, which progressed to include the forelimbs, eventually causing the animal to stumble and fall. Well-grown

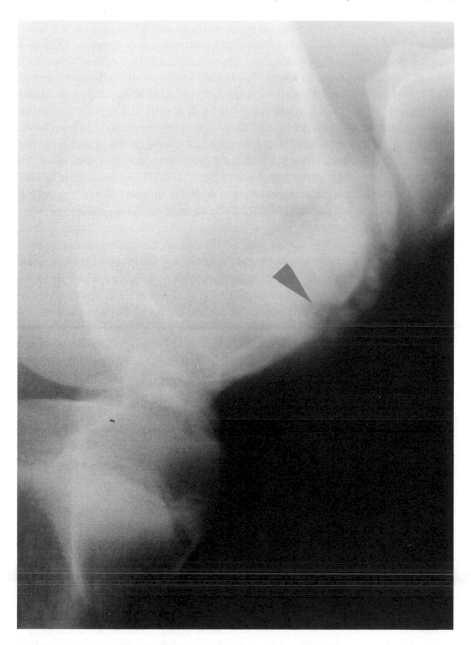

Figure 3.4 OCD lesion of stifle joint as indicated by arrow.

weanling and yearling colts seemed particularly prone, with three colts affected to every one filly. As a result of necropsy studies, it was suggested the condition was related to abnormalities of the vertebrae of the neck, which caused damage to the spinal cord. These observations were confirmed some 20 years later by Dr James Rooney, also from the University of Kentucky, who identified more precisely the sites and nature of the lesions in the cervical vertebrae. Rooney suggested the overgrowth of the articular processes on which vertebrae move upon each other causes distortion and narrowing of the spinal canal and results in pressure and damage to the cord. The most frequent sites of lesions are between cervical vertebrae C3 and C7, although the presence of lesions does not always result in clinical signs of wobbler disease. When the neck is flexed, the lesions may cause pressure to be exerted on the spinal cord.

Clinical signs associated with wobblers may be related to other causes, including trauma, parasitic infection of the spinal cord, and infection with equine rhinopneumonitis virus. In terms of prognosis it is therefore important to differentiate and establish an accurate diagnosis. Currently a true wobbler—the condition of which has recently been given the name cervical vertebral malformation (CVM)—is confirmed by taking X-rays of the neck region. To do this, the horse must receive a general anaesthetic so that a technique known as myelography can be performed. This involves the injection into the spinal canal of a contrast fluid so that the space between the cord and the surrounding bony mass of the vertebra can be readily visualized. Narrowing of this space due to lesions of CVM can then be located. The procedure is not without its hazards and should only be undertaken by those who are experienced with the technique and its interpretation. Two types of lesions have been identified. The first typically affects horses from 4 to 12 months of age and occurs most frequently between vertebrae C3 and C4, and C4 and C5. It causes pinching of the cord only when the neck is flexed. The second affects horses between 12 and 36 months of age and occurs between vertebrae C5 and C6, and C6 and C7. Compression of the spinal cord is not relieved or exacerbated by flexion or extension in this region. Injury to the cord results from pressure which interferes with blood flow, causing damage to the cells comprising the cord. It is this injury which results in signs of incoordination, the severity of which is related to the extent and site of damage.

In the young horse destined to become a wobbler, osteochondrosis intervenes allowing cartilage within the vertebra to develop in the absence of bone formation. The blood supply becomes inadequate leading to death of the surrounding tissue and the subsequent development of chronic joint lesions between the cervical vertebrae. What triggers these pathological changes at this critical growing period is still a matter of considerable debate. The initial suggestion that wobbler syndrome was an inherited condition linked to certain families has not been proven although genetic influence has not been eliminated. By breeding two wobbler parents it has not been possible to increase the incidence of wobblers in their offspring. It was noted, however, that the incidence of other bone deformities was increased.

It is interesting to compare the development of similar bone lesions, including spinal deformities in other species, particularly in poultry and pigs, both of which have been subjected to intensive genetic selection and high planes of nutrition to improve growth rate and feed conversion. It is apparent that within these populations, genetic selection has contributed to an overall increase in skeletal problems. A similar situation may well have evolved in the Thoroughbred with the current commercial incentive to produce a well-grown but nevertheless skeletally immature yearling in time for the summer and autumn (fall) sales. Foals and yearlings receive a diet high in protein and energy, which has a critical demand for the correct balance of vitamins and minerals. This feeding level occurs at a time when the skeleton is still not capable of bearing increased muscle mass, nor is it able to respond to the strains and pressures imposed upon it. As a consequence, lesions of osteochondrosis may develop, causing CVM. The prognosis for a wobbler has always been poor because of the progressive nature of the condition. However, within the last ten years a number of wobblers have been treated surgically. Two techniques have been developed. The first involves inserting a plug of bone between the ventral aspect of the affected vertebrae in an attempt to fuse and thereby fix the vertebrae and thus prevent them from pinching the spinal cord. The second involves removal of bone from the dorsal aspect of the affected vertebrae to relieve pressure on the cord. Both approaches require heroic surgery, and even though it has been reported that clinical improvement does occur in a proportion of cases, there is still considerable concern as to whether such animals should be allowed to participate in athletic competition. An alternative but less dramatic approach is to try to eliminate factors which might promote the wobbler condition, primarily by reducing the level of nutrition in the young horse.

Research workers at the New Bolton Centre, Pennsylvania, have developed criteria for the early recognition of 'potential' wobblers using radiographic techniques devised by Mayhew of the Animal Health Trust, Newmarket. Treatment of the 'suspect' horses includes complete stall rest and a level of nutrition only slightly in excess of maintenance requirements. Horses on this programme with which the author has had contact appear neurologically normal after completion of the treatment regime and by late in their two-year-old year have achieved growth similar to that of their contemporaries.

Acquired flexural deformities

Acquired flexural deformities, also referred to as acquired contracted flexor tendons, appear frequently as a sequel to DOD, as illustrated in Figure 3.5.

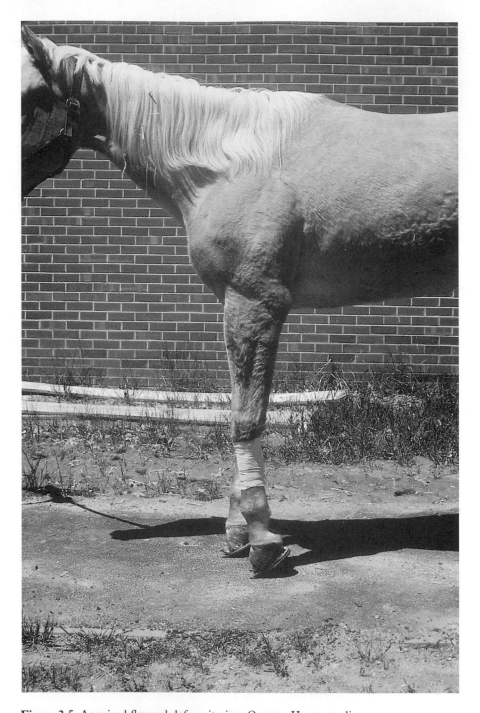

Figure 3.5 Acquired flexural deformity in a Quarter Horse yearling.

Rapidly growing horses that are erect in their pasterns are at most risk. The exact cause and an effective treatment remain elusive. Reducing growth rate, bandaging, surgery and tetracycline therapy have all been tried with varying degrees of success. The incidence of acquired contractures is high among horses that have been on a restricted diet and are then fed more liberally, a trend observed among horses in the USA and UK.

Fescue toxicity

Fescue toxicity is a condition affecting pregnant mares grazing endophyte-infected tall fescue pastures. Fescue (*Festuca arundinacea*), as shown in Figure 3.6, is a cool season grass found in Midwestern, Southern and Atlantic Coast

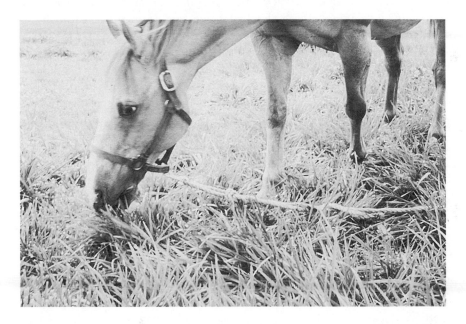

Figure 3.6 Tall fescue pastures are inappropriate for pregnant mares during the last third of gestation.

regions of the USA that has desirable agronomic properties such as drought resistance, resistance to over-grazing and insect damage and yields greater than most pasture species. The toxin, as yet unidentified, is produced by the endophytic fungus, *Acremonium coenophialum*. Unlike many fungal infections of forage, *A. coenophialum* is symptomless because the mycelia are located within the cell of the plant and do not affect the appearance of the tall fescue. The fungus is identified by taking basal stems of tall fescue and examining under the microscope using special stains to demonstrate the presence of mycelia. It is of considerable significance that the fungus is seed transmitted and does not spread on pasture from plant to plant. This is borne out by the observation that plots of endophyte-free fescue have remained so for many years despite being separated from infected fescue by only a fence.

Studies at the Universities of Auburn, Clemson, Kentucky and Missouri in the last 10 years have provided evidence of the deleterious effects of endophyte-infected tall fescue on pregnant mares. Signs of fescue toxicosis in mares are restricted to the reproductive system and include abortion during the latter stages of pregnancy and prolonged gestation, sometimes up to 13 or 14 months. At parturition, dystocia, premature separation of the chorion with neonatal asphyxia and retained placenta can occur. Large foals may require assisted delivery and the chance of injury to the mare's reproductive tract is greatly enhanced. An abnormally thick, tough placenta—the 'red bag' syndrome—may be present with the foal being unable to break through the membranes and consequently dying of suffocation if unattended. One of the more frequently reported problems is lack of udder development resulting in very little colostrum let down when the foal is born. Unless they are supplemented with colostrum these foals are more susceptible to septicaemia caused by bacterial infection. The damage that occurs to the mare's reproductive tract can delay or prevent the ability of the mare to conceive again.

Various ergot alkaloids produced by the fungus have been incriminated as the toxic agent responsible for causing signs among cattle and horses consuming infected fescue. The specific toxic compound has yet to be identified making the demonstration of a cause and effect relationship difficult. However, the mechanism by which this as yet unidentified toxin exerts its effect has to some extent been elucidated. The toxin appears to suppress the release of prolactin—a hormone produced by the pituitary gland in the brain. Normally, levels of prolactin in the mare's blood rise markedly during the last week of pregnancy and help promote milk secretion. Prolactin is not involved in the onset of parturition so the toxin or toxins are exerting a much broader effect on the mare's physiological reproductive mechanisms than is currently recognized.

If pastures containing tall fescue are found to be heavily infected with the endophyte fungus especially during the spring months, pregnant mares should be moved off the pasture. Each pasture should be tested individually; most animal diagnostic laboratories in the USA have facilities for determining endophyte levels. County agricultural agents or agronomy advisers should be consulted with regard to the sampling methods and where samples are to be submitted. If a high proportion of samples are found to be positive, two options are available: to minimize the effect or eliminate infected fescue and re-establish the pasture. The best option is determined by the extent of the problem and how well the solution fits the management of the farm. The effect of the endophyte can be minimized by keeping plants young and leafy by grazing and/or topping (clipping). Hay made from endophyte-infected tall fescue is potentially toxic and should not be fed or used as bedding. The addition of other forages in the diet, especially legumes, will provide a dilution effect. Sowing white clover at a seed rate of 1–2 kg per acre (2.5–5.0 kg/ha) is a good companion crop for fescue.

The alternative is to kill the infected fescue and replant with low or endophyte-free seed. In some US states fescue seed labels indicate the percentage level of endophyte infection. If the label does not specify a percentage it should be assumed that the seed is infected. When selecting a new variety of fescue it is important to know whether it is productive in the area in which it is to be planted.

As a general rule late summer or early autumn (fall) is the preferred time for sowing grass seed. Spring-sown forages are more susceptible to weeds interfering with the early stage of growth compared with autumn sowing. It is important to graze, top or apply herbicides to prevent seed production in pastures that are to be replanted as the endophyte fungus remains viable in seed for a year or more.

There are several methods of replacing endophyte-infected fescue, including rotation with other crops, preparing a new seedbed or herbicide treatment. Whichever method is selected it is important that grass waterways and fence rows are maintained to avoid soil erosion. Rotation with other crops such as corn (maize) or alfalfa (lucerne) is the method of choice but is not always practical. Weed control and tillage necessary to produce the rotated crop will usually kill the infected fescue. Herbicides that persist in the soil and might subsequently harm the fescue or other forages to be sown should be avoided. Destruction of the infected fescue by tillage alone is the second choice but does not always ensure a complete kill. If neither rotation nor tillage is feasible, chemical treatment followed by direct drilling (no-tillage planting) is a third alternative. To achieve maximum effect with herbicide treatment, it is essential that the label instructions are followed. The herbicide should be used at the period of optimum environmental and plant conditions to give greatest effectiveness. Herbicides of choice are Roundup (Monsanto) or Gramoxone Extra (ICI); these should be applied when fescue growth is small but actively growing, preferably in the late summer or early autumn (fall). Horses must be removed from the pasture prior to application and not return for at least 60 days and until the new forage has become established. When reseeding, the inclusion of annual summer or winter grasses should be considered as they will smother any old fescue which may have escaped chemical treatment or tillage. A combination of autumn-applied herbicide plus direct-drilled summer annual grasses is often the most effective means of eliminating most of the old tall fescue. It is important to ensure that the old fescue is sufficiently suppressed before proceeding with reseeding. Cattle or horses grazing these newly established pastures should not be fed hay harvested from infected fescue pastures. Infected seed that has passed through the digestive tract of animals can remain viable in their manure and survive to reinfect the pasture.

In the past it has been recommended that pregnant mares should be removed from endophyte infected pasture from 90 to 30 days before foaling. This wide range is a reflection of the inadequacy of our knowledge regarding the true effects of 'fescue toxicosis' on pregnant mares. If alternative pasture is not available feeding of mares in a dry lot with endophyte-free hay will be necessary.

Pharmacological studies have been undertaken in an attempt to reverse the inhibition of prolactin among mares exposed to endophyte-infected fescue. Several pharmacological agents that stimulate prolactin release, including phenothiazine tranquillizers such as acepromazine, have been tested but on a somewhat empirical basis. A considerable amount of further study is required before any of these agents can be recommended with confidence.

The logical approach is that farms with pastures containing a high percentage of fescue should have them tested. If they are found to be heavily infected with the endophyte fungus a systematic long-term programme of elimination and reseeding should be undertaken. In the short-term, pregnant mares should not be allowed to graze endophyte-infected tall fescue during the last third of pregnancy.

Nutritional secondary hyperparathyroidism (NSH)

Nutritional secondary hyperparathyroidism, also known as miller's disease, bran disease or big head disease, is caused by excessive mobilization of calcium from bone under the influence of parathyroid hormone. The maintenance of blood calcium homeostasis is critical to the function of the muscular and nervous systems and is under close regulation of the hormones parathormone and calcitonin. When blood calcium levels fall below normal, calcium is mobilized from the bone under the influence of parathormone to re-establish normal blood levels. If this occurs over an extended period of time the bones become depleted of calcium and lose their structural integrity. The facial bones, depleted of calcium become fibrotic and enlarged, hence the name big head disease.

The condition occurs due to a dietary calcium deficiency, excess levels of phosphorus, an inverted calcium:phosphorus ratio in the total diet and high levels of oxalates in forages, which interfere with digestion and absorption of calcium. In bygone days, millers fed their horses wheat bran, a by-product of the milling process. Bran is very high in phosphorus and low in calcium and many millers' horses developed NSH. In modern times the problem occurs when high levels of grain are fed without calcium supplementation, when there is an inadequate intake of good quality forage or when horses are grazing pastures high in oxalate, including tropical grasses such as para and guinea, kikuyu grass and many cultivars of alfalfa (lucerne). Due to the homeostatic mechanism controlling blood calcium, analysis of blood for calcium is not of value as a diagnostic tool. The most accurate method of diagnosis is evaluating the ration. The calcium intake should be determined and compared with the requirement of the specific class of horse in question. Additionally the phosphorus content of the diet should be determined to make sure it is not greater than the level of calcium. Unless an inverted calcium:phosphorus ratio is being fed and providing calcium levels are adequate NSH should then be limited to areas with high levels of oxalates. Horses respond to supplemental calcium in the form of calcium carbonate and NSH should not be of concern on the well-managed farm feeding a properly formulated ration.

Blister beetles

Blister beetle poisoning is confined to horses eating hay produced in the southwestern USA, where beetles are found in large concentrations. The toxin responsible, cantharidin, is relatively stable over extended periods of storage. It takes only a few blister beetles, once ingested by the horse, to cause a fatality. Beetles are baled with hay and eaten resulting in severe illness or death. The problem has become more pronounced since the replacement of the sickle bar mower with mower conditioners; the latter crush the beetles rather than allowing them to crawl from the windrow as was the case with the older mowing machines. Cantharidin is an extreme irritant to the digestive tract causing necrosis of the gut mucosa, including the lining of the oesophagus, as well as irritation to the urinary tract. Affected horses show severe colic and discomfort, an elevated respiratory and heart rate, diarrhoea and dehydration. Death usually occurs within 48–72 hours after ingestion of the beetles. The way to control the problem is not to feed hay produced in areas where blister beetles are present.

Colic

It is beyond the scope or intent of this chapter to cover colic in its entirety and the reader is advised to consult the texts listed at the end of the chapter. However, some mention of colic with respect to nutrition-related causes is warranted. Since the advent of modern anthelmintics the most important cause of colic in horses is nutritional mismanagement. Nutritionally induced colic can be grouped into two categories—improper forage:grain ratios or inadequate amounts of forage and the use of contaminated feedstuffs, with the former by far the most important.

As was mentioned in earlier chapters, the horse evolved as a wandering herbivore, a continuous grazer, and it has an absolute requirement for long stem hay or pasture. Failure to realize this simple fact probably results in more colics than any other single cause. When hay or pasture is limited the situation is made worse by the fact that many horses have a high level of grain in their diet. On high-grain diets the rate of passage of ingesta is increased allowing more readily fermentable carbohydrate to reach the hind gut. Fermentation of this material results in a lowering of caecal and colonic pH following the production of lactic acid. This decrease in gut pH causes an alteration of the microflora of the hind gut, resulting in the release of bacterial toxins and the onset of colic. There is frequently an increase in gas production in the hind gut that may also lead to signs of colic. The most effective way to reduce the incidence of colic is to feed liberal quantities of good quality forage, limit grain intake to that which is necessary to maintain body condition and feed the grain portion of the daily ration in small quantities and as frequently as is practical. Hay should be available to mares even in the spring or other times when pasture growth is lush. In many instances there is simply not enough 'gut-fill' in young lush growth. This, combined with the increased rate of passage associated with a low dry-matter feed, leads to the presence of more soluble forage constituents in the hind gut resulting in a build-up of gas and abdominal discomfort. There are very few instances when overfeeding dry hay can lead to a problem, but there are numerous problems that can result if hay is limited.

Feeding mouldy hay or grain to horses is not nearly as important as a cause of colic as the underfeeding of forage. However, the gastrointestinal tract of the horse is very sensitive to a variety of toxins produced by moulds. Mouldy hay and/or grain should not be fed to horses as the risk of colic is considerably increased. It is currently a fairly common practice in various parts of the world to feed large round bales of hay and/or silage to horses. Whilst only rarely do problems arise there is an increased risk of intestinal upset. Horses generally will not ingest mouldy feedstuffs if given a choice, but mouldy hay or spoiled silage can be fatal if the horse consumes them. Feedstuffs fed to horses should be free of mould and other foreign debris including soil, faeces and animal remains and should be properly cured and stored in a manner that will prevent contamination.

Mouldy corn poisoning (equine leukoencephalomalacia; mycotoxic encephalomalacia)

Sudden unexplained deaths among horses are always a source of considerable concern requiring prompt and authoritative action to identify the cause and eliminate it as quickly as possible. Such is the situation with mouldy corn poisoning or equine leukoencephalomalacia, a condition which has been recognized for many years under several different names, including blind staggers, foraging disease and corn stalk disease. Cases were first reported in the USA during the middle of the last century and subsequent reports indicated that many thousands of horses died during major outbreaks in Maryland at the turn of the century and in the mid-Western states during the 1930s. The disease is not restricted to the USA and cases have been reported in other countries including South Africa, South America, and several Mediterranean countries. In virtually all the reports the disease is associated with the feeding of mouldy corn (maize), corn screenings or chaff to horses. Confirmation of the cause of death in horses which have consumed mouldy corn is provided by postmortem examination of the brain, in which lesions characteristic of the disease and unique to the horse are observed. More recently mouldy corn poisoning has been referred to in the veterinary literature as mycotoxic encephalomalacia, indicating its cause—a fungal toxin—and encephalomalacia describing the lesion in the brain.

The toxin, recently identified as fumonisin B (FB), is produced by a whitish-pink mould, *Fusarium moniliforme*, which is normally found in soil but under appropriate environmental conditions of moisture and high humidity grows on vegetable matter, including corn (maize). When mouldy corn is consumed the toxin is released within the digestive tract, absorbed into the body and reaches the central nervous system exerting a lethal effect on cells of the brain. Horses which have died from mouldy corn poisoning develop lesions, which may be observed by the naked eye and vary from pea-sized to ones engulfing an entire lobe of the brain. The changes cause swelling, liquefaction and cavitation due to damage the toxin exerts on blood vessels supplying the brain.

Clinical signs develop from 10 to 90 days after the ingestion of mouldy corn, their onset depending on the amount of toxin released. The disease is invariably seasonal, occurring from late autumn (fall) to early spring and coinciding with the consumption of contaminated feed. Corn which has been damaged by drought, insects or disease and harvested under conditions of high moisture and humidity is particularly prone to become contaminated with moulds. Initial signs in horses include loss of appetite and colic, which are followed within 48 hours by damage to the central nervous system causing drooping of the lower lip, blindness in one or both eyes resulting in the horse bumping into obstacles, muscle tremors and an unsteady gait. The horse rapidly becomes recumbent and death quickly ensues.

Other diseases with which it may be confused include rabies, the paralytic form of equine rhinopneumonitis and Eastern, Western or Venezuelan equine encephalomyelitis. The time of year, a history of recent consumption of corn, other cases occurring on the premises and examination of the feed to determine its quality are all important in determining a diagnosis, which will be confirmed on postmortem examination. Once a case is confirmed or even if a case is suspected it is imperative that the contaminated feed is promptly discarded.

Corn (maize) may be checked on the farm or at the grain elevator by the 'blacklight' test which causes samples to fluoresce if moulds are present. However a negative blacklight test does not preclude presence of *Fusarium*. *Fusarium* may also be grown in the laboratory from samples of mouldy corn. However, neither of these procedures provide absolute evidence of mouldy corn poisoning. Now that the toxin has been identified various analytical laboratory tests are available to measure the amount of FB_1 in feed samples. Corn of good quality that is not damaged or has been stored with a moisture content lower than 15% is unlikely to be mouldy. Reputable manufacturers of horse feeds take particular care to monitor their supplies to ensure mouldy corn is not included in the ration. The risk of problems occurring remains with horse owners who choose to feed their animals poor quality corn or corn products which have been home or locally produced and improperly stored.

Cystitis

The consumption of certain sudangrasses and sudan-sorghum hybrids may cause cystitis, an inflammation of the urinary tract. Cystitis is characterized by an increase in urination or a dribbling of urine, incoordination and continuous oestrus behaviour in mares. The problem is most severe when horses are allowed to graze pastures that have been subjected to drought, freezing temperatures and excessive trampling. Cystitis is caused when a glycoside in the plant is converted to prussic acid in the intestine. Besides cystitis, prussic acid poisoning causes muscle tremors, nervousness, respiratory distress and ultimately respiratory failure and death. Signs of prussic acid poisoning are also seen when wilted wild cherry leaves are ingested. To prevent the problem horses should not graze sudan or sudan-sorghum pastures such as sudex. Hays made from these pastures are not toxic to the horse, but they are stemmy and of poor quality when compared to more traditional hays fed to horses. If sudangrass or sudan-sorghum pastures are grazed every attempt should be made to discontinue grazing during a drought or immediately following freezing temperatures.

Enteroliths (intestinal calculi or stones)

Enteroliths stones or calculi, may form in the intestine in the presence of a foreign object such as a nail, stone or ball of hair. These objects serve as foci for the formation of the enterolith, which is composed of salts—usually magnesium ammonium phosphate. The enterolith may cause signs ranging from weight loss and mild abdominal discomfort to an obstruction requiring surgical intervention. The size of the stone can range from a pea to a bowling ball. Smaller stones may be passed by the horse and cause no signs, but larger ones tend to cause an obstruction at the pelvic flexure of the large intestine or at the interface of the large and small colons. Affected horses may have one enterolith or a number of variable size. The exact reason for their development is uncertain and no specific dietary cause has been identified. It appears to be of the greatest magnitude in areas where access to fresh forage is limited.

Wood chewing

Horses that chew wood should be distinguished from the classical cribber in that they actually eat wood from fences, barns and other wooden structures rather than grabbing hold and sucking in air. Wood chewing, as illustrated in Figure 3.7, may result from boredom, or from a nutritional inadequacy. Experience suggests that frequent and vigorous exercise of stalled horses will minimize wood chewing if it is boredom induced. Isolation of wood-chewing horses from the rest of the herd in a paddock lined with an electric fence will reduce the behaviour in the offending horse and prevent other horses from picking up the habit. The majority of horses that eat fences, trees and other

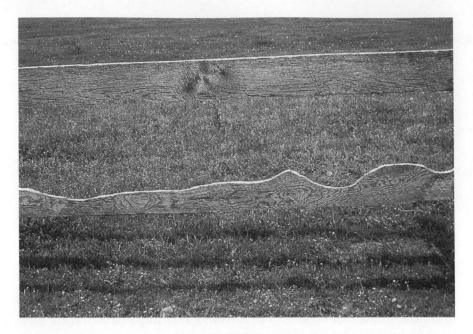

Figure 3.7 Damage to a plank fence caused by wood chewing.

wooden objects do so for other reasons besides boredom and nutritional inadequacy. As previously discussed, horses have an absolute requirement for long stem hay or fibre and if deprived the frequency of wood chewing increases. Stalled horses that are allowed a minimal hay intake are most inclined to begin chewing wood. There is a direct relationship between wood chewing and the amount of fibre in the diet. Horses fed a grain mix ration low in fibre have been shown to eat significantly more wood than horses allowed hay. Horses grazing high quality pasture may also chew wood. These horses have access to plenty of fibre, are not in a stall and get plenty of exercise, so why do they chew wood and, more intriguingly, why does this behaviour seem to be season related? Horses are most apt to exhibit wood chewing during the time of the year when forage growth is rapid and lush grass is available. When this occurs the dry matter content of the forage is low, the crude fibre content low and the rate of passage is high. The fibre content of the forage is inadequate to meet the horse's requirement and in an attempt to increase the amount of fibre in the diet the horse eats fences, tree bark and other wooden objects. One way to reduce the frequency of wood chewing is to provide hay to horses during the period when rapid growth of low dry-matter forage is taking place. It is surprising how much hay horses will continue to eat when there is an abundance of lush pasture growth available. In addition to reducing wood chewing it has been the author's observation that colic associated with horses grazing lush pastures is reduced when hay is offered free-choice during extreme pasture growth phases.

Urea toxicity

Urea and biuret are non-protein nitrogen sources commonly used in the diets of ruminants. They provide nitrogen to the ruminal microflora for the synthesis of microbial protein which is used to meet a significant portion of the ruminant's protein requirement. The horse's gastrointestinal tract makes the use of urea questionable in terms of contributing to their nitrogen requirements. Horses receiving a marginal protein intake benefit from urea, especially mature horses on a forage diet but urea is also toxic to the horse. Contrary to popular belief horses show a greater tolerance to urea than ruminant animals. Urea is broken down in the stomach and small intestine of the horse, absorbed and excreted via the kidneys prior to the time it arrives in the caecum. However, when a ration containing 25% of urea was fed to ponies a number died. Signs attributed to urea toxicity in the horse include incoordination, wandering and head-pressing (horses will stand pressing their heads against solid objects). Urea should not be fed to young horses.

Ionophores

Ionophores are antibiotic-like compounds included in ruminant diets to alter rumen fermentation. They cause a shift in the volatile fatty acid (VFA) ratio that favours the production of propionate and reduces the molar percentage of acetic acid, the net result of which is greater feed efficiency. The two most common ionophores are monensin sodium and lasalocid, both of which are extremely toxic to the horse and should never be included in equine rations. There have been instances in the USA and Europe where ionophores have mistakenly been included in horse feeds and have resulted in the death of horses. Levels of monensin as low as 2–3 mg/kg body weight have resulted in mortality. Affected horses show signs of colic, sweating, incoordination and die within 12–36 hours. Postmortem examination indicates severe damage to heart muscle; among horses that recover, cardiac damage is frequently so severe that a return to athletic performance is questionable. Monensin and other ionophores are frequently included in cattle and poultry feeds as a coccidiostat. The toxicity of ionophores to horses makes feeding cattle or poultry feed to horses extremely risky. Many feed mills that make a significant amount of horse feed will not manufacture ionophore-containing feeds due to the possibility of contamination.

Heaves (chronic obstructive pulmonary disease: COPD)

Heaves has long been associated with a horse that is not sound in the wind. It is an allergic response similar to asthma in humans. Affected horses develop a nasal discharge, cough and a heave line at the base of the ribs associated with muscular hypertrophy caused by the effort of expelling air. The lungs lose their elasticity, which results in a raised respiratory rate, and athletic ability is impaired especially in events where maximal effort is required. Horses with COPD should be kept outside on pasture rather than in a barn. Keeping the horse's environment as free from dust and mould spores as possible is the most effective way to treat the disease. COPD horses should be bedded on paper, clean wood shavings or even a rubber mat in preference to bedding on straw or hay. Hay should be soaked in water prior to feeding. These practices minimize the amount of dust, mould spores and other airborne particulate matter. The use of fibre sources other than hay can minimize the extent of COPD. Cubed grass, shredded beet pulp, and mashes made with oaten or wheaten chaff are alternatives to hay. The barn should never be cleaned while a COPD horse is inside. Sweeping, moving hay into and out of the loft, and other activity in the barn increases the amount of airborne particulate matter, which results in an allergic response by affected horses. Improving ventilation increases the flow of fresh air in the barn and helps dissipate ammonia in the stall. Ammonia is a severe respiratory irritant and causes serious problems to a COPD affected horse. COPD horses benefit from the use of expectorants to reduce coughing and bronchodilators to reduce the respiratory rate.

Goitre and iodine deficiency

Goitre, an enlargement of the thyroid gland, may occur in response to deficient (hypo-iodine goitre) or toxic (hyper-iodine goitre) levels of iodine in the diet.

Iodine is a component of the hormone thyroxine, produced by the thyroid gland. When iodine levels in the diet are inadequate the thyroid gland becomes enlarged, which is indicative of thyroid dysfunction. Thyroxine is responsible for regulation of metabolic rate and hypothyroid horses exhibit slowed skeletal growth, rough hair coat, delayed shedding of hair and muscular weakness. Foals born to iodine deficient mares are frequently dysmature, lacking hair and may exhibit an enlarged thyroid. Supplementation with iodized salt may be necessary although most modern diets contain adequate levels of iodine.

If goitre is diagnosed in the presence of adequate levels of iodine in the diet, then iodine toxicity must be suspected. Goitre has been reported in foals born to mares consuming high levels of a supplement containing kelp, a seaweed high in iodine. Levels of iodine intake as low as 50 mg/day by pregnant mares have resulted in goitrous foals. Random supplementation of mares with iodine is not a good practice and iodine provided in supplements should be critically evaluated in the overall diet. The symptoms of hyper-iodine goitre are similar to those seen in hypo-iodine goitre and so evaluation of the diet is an important diagnostic tool in determining the cause of the problem. The 1989 NRC *Nutrient Requirements of Horses* suggests the iodine requirement of the young growing horse is 0.1 mg/kg of the ration while 5 mg/kg is thought to be the potentially toxic level. Goitre may also be caused by substances in the diet that result in antithyroid activity. Feedstuffs known to exhibit antithyroid activity include uncooked soyabeans, cabbage, kale and mustard. The enzyme responsible for antithyroid effect is inactivated by heating and cooking and properly prepared soyabean meal is safe to feed. The goitrogenic effect of these feeds is not inhibited by supplemental iodine, suggesting that with the exception of properly heated soyabean meal they should be avoided in equine diets.

Selenium deficiency and white muscle disease

Selenium is a trace mineral essential in the diets of horses of all ages. In areas of the world where levels in the soil and forages are inadequate, supplementation is necessary to prevent the appearance of selenium deficiency. Although the current NRC *Nutrient Requirements of Horses* suggests the selenium level of the diet be 0.1 ppm, most well-formulated equine diets contain a level of 0.2–0.4 ppm. The most common method of selenium supplementation is by adding sodium selenite to the grain mix. Selenium deficiency is characterized by white muscle disease in foals. The skeletal muscle is pale to white and the cardiac muscle is also affected. Foals exhibiting white muscle disease are frequently weak at birth, suffer from respiratory distress and have difficulty nursing. Due to the loss of muscle function respiration is impaired and foals often die of respiratory failure. The serum selenium level and plasma glutathione peroxidase (a selenium-dependent enzyme) concentration in mares have been used as a predictive screening test to avert white muscle disease in foals produced by mares grazing selenium-deficient pastures. The normal range of serum selenium in mares is 0.06–0.15 ppm (mg/100 ml), although mares at the lower end of the expected range have been known to produce foals with white muscle disease. Plasma glutathione peroxidase concentrations of less than 20 units are indicative of marginal selenium status and horses with this low value should be treated by either the addition of dietary selenium or by injection of selenium. It is worth noting that selenium-vitamin E injections have resulted in anaphylactic shock on occasion and should be administered with care.

'Tying up' syndrome

Despite being recognized for over 100 years the cause of 'tying up' syndrome remains unresolved. It was first identified among draught horses that became stiff and reluctant to move after working on a Monday following a day of rest on Sunday, hence the description 'Monday morning disease'. It is a disease of muscle tissue which has been given many names over the years, the common as well as the various scientific descriptions are listed in Table 3.1. They all refer

Table 3.1 Synonyms for 'tying up' syndrome

Azoturia

Equine rhabdomyolysis

Exertional myopathy

Monday morning disease

Myositis

Paralytic myoglobinuria

Set fast

to the same condition, which varies considerably in the degree of clinical severity. All ages and both sexes, including geldings, are affected but a higher prevalence has been observed among young fillies in training; it is not restricted to thoroughbreds. In recent years the incidence appears to have increased among event horses, racehorses, endurance and show horses.

Exercise is the predisposing factor and following the first episode the condition may recur in the same animal; the timing of recurrence cannot be predicted. The signs may be as mild as a slight change in gait, stiffness and a shortened stride to a more severe reluctance or inability to move caused by cramping of the muscles. In a very few instances an affected horse will become recumbent and die. The muscles of the hindlimbs are primarily affected although the forelimbs may also be involved. In severe cases muscles become hard, swollen and painful. Urine assumes a dark-brown colour as a result of the excretion of myoglobin and its breakdown products resulting from damage to muscle fibres. Affected horses are often anxious, sweat, have an elevated heart and respiratory rate and a raised temperature.

'Tying up' is diagnosed on the basis of history and clinical signs supported by the results of laboratory tests on blood samples taken at various stages through the course of the disease. In cases of 'tying up' the serum levels of two muscle enzymes, creatine kinase (CK) and aspartate aminotransferase (AST), are consistently elevated. When muscle tissue is damaged, there is leakage of cellular constituents including muscle enzymes into the surrounding tissues and subsequently into the circulation. Creatine kinase is the most sensitive and specific indicator of muscle pathology in the horse. After an episode of 'tying up' serum CK levels ranging from 1000 to several hundred thousand units per litre peak within 4–12 hours and return to normal within a few days. The second enzyme, AST, is less specific of muscle damage but following an episode serum levels peak at 24 hours and decline over 7–14 days. High levels of CK and AST are consistent with muscle damage during the early phase of 'tying up'. During the recovery phase the level of CK falls below that of AST and these changes can be monitored to check the return to normal levels. The interpretation of laboratory results is, however, never straightforward and considerable caution must be exercised, as there is not a great deal of consistency between the severity of clinical signs and the degree of elevation of serum enzymes. The enzyme levels following exercise in both fit and unfit horses increase slightly reflecting a normal physiological response which is not related to muscle damage. Other conditions with which 'tying up' may be confused are overexertion, heat stress, colic, laminitis, tetanus and poisoning.

In terms of identifying the cause there appear to be more theories than facts, none of which provide a complete answer to the problem. The traditional explanation proposed 50 years ago was that exercising horses receiving a grain diet high in energy were more inclined to 'tie up'. In recent years this theory has become less acceptable for the reason that following exercise the reserves of glycogen—the energy store of muscle tissue—take several days to replenish making glycogen overloading distinctly unlikely. The accumulation of lactic acid in muscle tissue following exercise was also thought to contribute to the syndrome. However, it has been observed that following strenuous exercise blood and muscle lactate levels reach extremely high levels with no signs whatsoever of horses 'tying up'. It is generally accepted, however, that horses fed diets containing large amounts of grain and given one or more days of rest whilst on full rations are more prone to the condition when they return to training. Alterations in the blood supply to the muscles may be an important factor. Microscopic studies of muscle tissue indicate that the fast-twitch muscle fibres as distinct from the slow-twitch fibres undergo most damage when a horse 'ties up'. Fast-twitch fibres have a poorer blood supply compared to slow-twitch fibres and a reduced oxygen supply to these fibres during exercise could result in muscle damage.

In the human a deficiency of specific muscle enzymes causes signs similar to 'tying up' in the horse. Human cases are unable to maintain any intensity of activity, which is very different from the intermittent nature of the equine condition. The lack of an enzyme to metabolize fat in the body resulting in muscle stiffness and pigmented urine is also recognized in the human but no similar enzyme deficiency has been observed in the horse. Vitamin E and/or selenium have been implicated in a variety of muscle disorders in several species. Whilst some horses which develop the condition appear to benefit from vitamin-mineral supplementation of the feed there is little scientific evidence in support. It has been suggested that the stress of training may suppress the ability of the thyroid gland to respond with an increased output of thyroxine (T_4). Again the evidence is inconclusive and must be evaluated further. That 'tying up' occurs more frequently among young fillies as compared to colts and geldings has been reported extensively suggesting a possible involvement of steroid hormones. A study among a small group of 15 two- and three-year-old Thoroughbred fillies in training at Newmarket found no correlation between an elevation of serum muscle enzymes, clinical signs of 'tying up' and stage of the oestrous cycle. However, field observations linking the condition to young fillies in training have been reported from Europe, USA, Australia and Japan and merit further investigation.

Electrolyte imbalances do occur in horses following strenuous exercise especially those exposed to heat stress. Whether electrolyte disturbances affect muscle metabolism and cause signs consistent with 'tying up' has yet to be determined although fluid therapy is used extensively to treat horses suffering from the condition. Muscle stiffness has been reported among humans and horses following outbreaks of acute respiratory infection caused by influenza-virus and *streptococci* bacteria. It is conceivable that antibodies and antigens derived from these pathogens form immune complexes within body tissues giving rise to muscle damage. Following equine rhinopneumonitis infection, horses in training occasionally experience the 'poor performance' or 'loss of performance' syndrome, signs of which include muscle stiffness and slight incoordination especially of the hindlimbs. Recently an outbreak of equine rhinopneumonitis infection was reported among young Thoroughbred horses in training in England which was associated with high serum muscle enzyme levels. These two observations may be unrelated but are worthy of study. The suggestion of a hereditary link cannot be discounted. The author remembers trainers in England frequently asserting that dams of affected fillies also experienced 'tying up' when they were put into training.

Treatment is aimed at limiting further muscle damage, restoring fluid and electrolyte balance and reducing pain. Affected horses should be given complete rest and walked only the absolute minimum distance necessary to load into a trailer or returned to a stall. Veterinary assistance should be sought immediately; electrolyte fluid therapy given intravenously and orally is of considerable benefit. Horses may recommence exercise based on their clinical improvement and the monitoring of serum enzyme levels until they return to normal.

To prevent the condition a change in the pattern of exercise may be of particular value. In a recent study of a group of horses in training in England enzyme levels were noted to be highest after exercise following a day of complete rest reminiscent of the 'Monday morning disease' syndrome. The traditional pattern of exercising a Thoroughbred horse for only a very limited period of time, less than 60 minutes every 24 hours, with no exercise whatsoever on one day may not be appropriate, especially for horses that are prone to 'tie up'. Whether such horses would benefit from longer, less strenuous periods of exercise with no rest days, including a longer 'warm up' period, is worthy of consideration. Various drugs have been tried but their success tends to be based on anecdotal information. They include dantrolene sodium, which controls the release of calcium from muscle fibres, tranquillizers to relax the horse, dimethylglycine to increase oxygen utilization, thyroxine to improve exercise tolerance and thiamin to increase the rate of lactic acid breakdown.

The syndrome of 'tying up' still defies a rational explanation. Horses that suffer from the condition appear to possess an underlying abnormality that requires one or more trigger factors to initiate clinical signs. These various factors may not be the same for each horse explaining why different therapies and preventive measures work for some horses and not others. Until the nature of 'tying up' is better understood its treatment and prevention will remain empirical.

Further reading

Adams L G, Dollahite J W, Romani W M, Bullard T L, Bridges C H (1969) Cystitis and ataxia associated with sorghum ingestion by horses. *Journal of the American Veterinary Medical Association* **155**: 518–24.

Beasley V R, Wolf G R, Fischer D C, Ray A C, Edwards W C (1983) Cantharidin toxicosis in horses. *Journal of the American Veterinary Medical Association* **182**: 283.

Byars T D, Moore J N, White N (eds) (1982) *Proceedings of the Equine Research Symposium held at the College of Veterinary Medicine, September 28–30, 1982.* University of Georgia, Athens, Georgia.

Dill S G, Rebhun W C (1985) White muscle disease in foals. *Compendium of Continuing Education for the Practicing Veterinarian* **7**: 627–32, 634–6.

Donawick W J, Mayhew I G, Galligan D J, Osborne J, Green S, Stanley E (1989) Early diagnosis of cervical vertebral malformation in young Thoroughbred horses and successful treatment with restricted paced diet and confinement. In Royer M G (ed) *Proceedings of the 35th Annual Convention of the American Association of Equine Practitioners.* Boston, pp 525–28.

Driscoll J, Hintz H F, Schryver H F (1978) Goitre in foals caused by excessive iodine. *Journal of the American Veterinary Medical Association* **173**: 858–9.

Floyd K, Hintz H F, Wheat J D, Schryver H F (1987) Enteroliths in horses. *Cornell Veterinarian* **77**: 172–86.

Gerring E L, Morris D D, Moore J N, White N A (eds) (1989) Equine colic: proceedings of the Third Equine Colic Symposium held at the University of Georgia, November 1–3, 1988. *Equine Veterinary Journal* Supplement 7, June.

Glade M J, Luba N K (1987) Serum triiodothyronine and thyroxine concentrations in weanling horses fed carbohydrate by direct gastric infusion. *American Journal of Veterinary Research* **48**(4): 578–82.

Hintz, H F (1990) *Clinical nutrition.* The Veterinary Clinics of North America, Equine Practice. W B Saunders, Philadelphia.

Hintz H F, Lowe J E, Clifford A J, Visek W J (1970) Ammonia intoxication resulting from urea ingestion by ponies. *Journal of the American Veterinary Medical Association* **157**: 963–6.

Knight D A, Gabel A A, Reed S M, Embertson R M, Tyznik W J, Bramlage L R (1985) Correlation of dietary mineral to incidence and severity of metabolic bone disease in Ohio and Kentucky. In Milne J (ed) *Proceedings of the 31st Annual Convention of the American Association of Equine Practitioners.* Toronto, pp 445–61.

Matsuaka T (1976) Evaluation of monensin toxicity in the horse. *Journal of the American Veterinary Medical Association* **169**: 1098–100.

Robinson N E (1992) *Current therapy in equine medicine 3.* W B Saunders, Philadelphia.

Swartzmann J A, Hintz H F, Schryver H F (1978) Inhibition of calcium absorption in ponies fed diets containing oxalic acid. *American Journal of Veterinary Research* **3**: 1621–3.

CHAPTER

PASTURE MANAGEMENT
CHARLES T. DOUGHERTY, BSc, MS, PhD

Summary
Equine digestion and its relationship to pasture management
Eliminative behaviour of horses and its effects on pastures
Agronomy of horse pastures
Grazing systems
Further reading

Summary

This chapter relates pasture management to the evolution and function of the gastrointestinal tract, ingestive mechanics, grazing behaviour and the nutritional needs of horses.

Native and improved grasslands provide a high proportion of the energy, protein and other nutrients required by horses. Pasturage alone may not be able to meet the energy needs of draught horses, horses in training, growing horses, mares in pregnancy and lactation and horses stressed by low ambient temperatures. Pastures that cannot meet the nutrient needs of horses, especially energy and protein, are often supplemented with hays of pasture grasses and legumes, and with grains of cereal grasses.

This chapter relates practices employed in the management of horses on pasture to their grazing and eliminative behaviour (dunging and urination). Grazing behaviour is related to the ingestive mechanics and the ability of the equine gastrointestinal tract to extract nutrients from herbage. Discussion of the agronomy of pastures is limited to areas that are specific to the equine and are of direct concern to farm managers and horse owners.

Equine digestion and its relationship to pasture management

The common evolution of grasslands and animals that digest fibre

The intimate association between the progenitors of grassland plant species and equine species began about 60 million years ago. Evolution of grasslands in areas too dry to support forests was paralleled by the evolution of ungulate mammals capable of utilizing the cell wall materials of herbaceous grassland species as their primary energy source. Grasslands and grassland species co-evolved under the grazing of herbivores. Microorganisms of the gut evolved with animal fibre-digesters and played a crucial role in the life of grassland mammals.

During the Pleistocene Age, the Equidae (horses) and Camelidae (camels) departed from the North American grasslands. The continent was sub-sequently re-colonized by sheep and bison travelling across the land bridge from Eurasia. Bunchgrass species that had evolved with horses and camels were largely displaced by rhizomatous, sod-forming species, such as bluestems (*Andropogon* species), switchgrass (*Panicum virgatum*), grama grass (*Bouteloua curtipendula* and *B. gracilis*), and buffalo grass (*Buchloe dactyloides*) that sur-vived grazing by bison, antelope and sheep.

The simple gastrointestinal tracts of the early horses and ruminants were not able to directly extract energy from plant cell walls, largely composed of cellulose, hemicellulose and lignin. In spite of millions of years of evolution, mammals have not been able to develop enzymes in the gastrointestinal tract that hydrolyse the beta-1-4 linkage of the glucose subunits of cellulose, thereby freeing glucose for energy metabolism. The successful evolutionary approaches to the utilization of herbage have essentially the same end result; the extraction of energy from a plentiful, largely uncontested, but low-grade resource of plant material through the co-evolution of microorganisms of the intestine.

The strategy of the highly evolved and effective digestion processes of equids and ruminants was based on the ability of degradative enzymes secreted by microfauna and microflora to hydrolyse plant cell wall materials into simple carbohydrates. Cellulose, for example, is degraded to its glucose subunits by cellulase produced by microorganisms within the digestive tract. Fibre-digest-ing processes were concentrated in the forestomach of ruminants and in the hind gut of equids. The anaerobic environment of the gastrointestinal tract of equids and ruminants and the composition of digesta ensures similarities of intestinal microorganisms, pathways of fermentation and composition of end products. Anaerobic microorganisms that inhabit the digestive tracts of these animals are essentially unable to survive in the outside world.

The different methods of handling fibre digestion by equids and ruminants are striking but differences in the end results are small considering their evolutionary pathways diverged so long ago. In contrast, marsupials became the dominant herbivores of grasslands in the isolated Australasian continent in the absence of ruminants and equids, and their gastrointestinal tracts have considerable anatomical diversity. It is interesting to ponder on why other mechanisms of fibre utilization did not develop, or survive, during the evol-ution of the mammalian fibre digesters of Eurasia and North America.

Foraging theory predicts that successful evolutionary pathways of grassland mammals would be those that maximize the amount of energy harvested for the minimum expenditure of energy. Based on the number and populations of modern domestic livestock species one could conclude that mammals with fore-gut fibre digestion had a slight evolutionary advantage over those with hind-gut fibre digestion. Others have argued that the evolutionary strategy of equids was highly successful because the high fibre/low protein grassland niche they exploited was essentially uncontested. Given that both digestive systems are still in existence it is possible to conclude that both evolutionary solutions to cell wall utilization of herbage were successful.

Mechanics of grazing

A knowledge of grazing behaviour is essential for an understanding of the management of grazing horses. Such knowledge is particularly useful in the adaptation of the vast amount of information on the grazing management of ruminant livestock to the grazing management of horses. Grazing is a complex behaviour that involves interactions of the physiological processes of animals with the physical and chemical properties of herbage and the environment. The interface between the horse and the pasture is particularly important in our comprehension of grazing behaviour. Regrettably little is known about this interface in horses compared to sheep and cattle.

Limitations of the digestive system of horses which favoured ingestion of smaller particles and the low nutrient density of their grassland habitat may have been significant evolutionary forces that diminished the herbage-gathering capacity of the horse's tongue as compared to cattle. The flexibility of the horse's tongue is limited by the presence of the dorsal lingual cartilage embedded in its median plane. The limited function of the tongue in forage-gathering by horses may partially account for the smaller bite size of horses compared to cattle of similar body weight. The mobile prehensile lips of horses play a larger role in harvesting of herbage than cattle and may compensate for limitations of the tongue. The upper lip is particularly important in selection of herbage for biting, in the sorting of severed herbage for ingestion or rejection, and pushing ingesta to the back of the buccal cavity for chewing.

Dentition is believed to have been an important factor in the evolution of fibre digesters. Horses are superbly equipped to graze short pastures because they possess complete sets of teeth on both upper and lower jaws. In contrast, cattle have lost their superior incisors and canines and consequently, their ability to bite. Horses have a greater primary chewing capacity than cattle as evolutionary processes have resulted in the molarization of vestigial wolf teeth, the first premolars. The diet of horses is associated with high rates of teeth wear as a result of abrasions caused by the high fibre content of the diet, and the ingestion of soil and opaline deposits in the epidermal cells of grasses. Evolutionary processes apparently coped with the problem of excessive teeth wear by increasing the area of the occlusal surfaces and the durability of the enamel of these grinding surfaces. Concurrently, the root-to-crown length of teeth increased, forming the characteristic hypsodont teeth.

Factors affecting herbage intake

Horses lack the ability to ruminate, and virtually all of the particle size reduction of ingested herbage occurs during biting and chewing. Recent research suggests that chewing is promoted by diets that increase beta-endorphin production in the brain of horses. These neurochemicals are thought to make chewing a pleasurable activity and may lead to well-known stereotypic behaviour such as crib-biting and wood-chewing. Once the boli are swallowed herbage particles pass through the remainder of the digestive tract without significant reduction in size. Compared with cattle of similar body weight grazing the same swards, horses take smaller bites of herbage at slower rates of biting. It may be assumed that horses masticate herbage more than cattle, which contributes to their slow rate of biting, slow rate of herbage intake and longer grazing times per day.

Another grazing strategy employed by horses is to preferentially graze short turf and to maintain swards in a preferred state by spot or patch grazing. Obviously the shorter the sward the smaller the initial particle size of the ingested herbage reducing the need for mastication. One might assume, by invoking foraging theory, that horses would expend less energy grazing the closely cropped patches called lawns, than they would expend grazing the longer material on the ungrazed swards or roughs.

When the head of a horse is positioned in a grazing attitude, its eyes are located such that vision may be an important component in diet selection. Taste may also be an important factor in diet selection. Chewing of herbage releases cell contents and exposes them to taste sensors of the mouth and unpalatable herbage may be expelled before swallowing. Horses are seldom poisoned by toxic plants under free-ranging conditions and this is probably because of diet learning and the ability of horses to react to the phytochemical defences of plants. Horses have a limited ability to vomit, which may be the reason why taste is important in diet selection. This, however, does not always prevent horses from ingesting toxic plants.

The equine gastrointestinal tract distal to the mouth and pharynx has a considerable impact on grazing behaviour. The diameter of the horse's oesophagus is small compared to that of cattle and limits the dimensions of swallowed boli. This restricts the rate of herbage intake especially when pasture is freely available. The wall of the equine oesophagus increases in thickness and the proportion of striated to smooth muscle also increases towards the stomach, which may be related to the low incidence of vomition and inability to ruminate.

Factors affecting passage of herbage through the digestive system

Digesta entering the hind gut of the horse has already been subjected to gastric digestion and absorption. It is composed primarily of cell wall material, has low concentrations of the readily available nutrients and is considerably drier than the digesta in the reticulo-rumen of ruminants. As a consequence, the microflora and microfauna of the hind gut of horses may be substrate-limited, and digesta along with associated microorganisms is excreted with little reduction in particle size and further degradation of cell walls. The microflora and microfauna of the caecum and colon of horses are similar to microorganisms present in the reticulo-rumen of cattle and carry out similar functions. Glucose and other simple sugars released by enzymes secreted by intestinal microorganisms are available to support their maintenance, growth and replication. Acetic, propionic and butyric acids are produced from glucose and other simple sugars by anaerobic fermentation of the intestinal bacteria. These volatile fatty acids are the principal form of energy derived from herbage cell walls and are available for energy metabolism. The equine digestive tract is more efficient in the extraction and absorption of nutrients within plant cells than ruminants, but less efficient in degradation and absorption of nutrients contained in plant cell walls. Herbage cell contents, especially the cell contents of leafy tissues, are mainly soluble substances, easily hydrolysed by gastric enzymes in the stomach.

Microorganisms are not present in the digestive tract of newborn animals. Initially intestinal enzymes handle digestion and absorption of milk but the tract soon develops the capacity to digest plant cell walls. The development of fibre-digesting capacity requires the inoculation of the tract with microorganisms. Foals are coprophagous and eat dung, usually within ten days, to inoculate their hindgut with the microfauna and microflora required to digest plant cell walls. Cows, in contrast, inoculate their calves with microorganisms during the licking part of the bonding mechanism.

Rates of herbage intake and passage of digesta

The daily herbage dry matter intake requirement of horses is in the order of 2–3% of body weight, which is about the same as cattle. Horses must graze longer each day than cattle to meet their energy needs because they have slower rates of intake. When not supplemented horses graze up to 18 hours a day if herbage is scarce. They do not exhibit such a distinct diurnal grazing pattern as cattle, probably related to their slow rate of herbage intake and the time needed to meet the nutritional demands from grazing.

There are no restrictions on rate of passage of digesta through the tract of horses comparable to the reticulo-omasal orifice that prevents large particles from exiting the reticulo-rumen of cattle. However, it has been observed that about 50% of herbage particles in the boli taken from esophageal fistulae of horses have been masticated to such an extent that they passed through a 1.5 mm sieve.

The rate of passage accelerates as the quality of ingesta declines, whereas in cattle the converse applies. In a study in which mares and cows were fed similar grass hays, the retention time in the intestinal tract was 8.47 hours for mares and 20.40 hours for cows. The differences in retention time are relatively small when one considers that the gastrointestinal tract and its contents account for about 15% of the body weight of the horse and about 40% of the body weight of the cow.

Mechanisms that regulate herbage intake of horses are not well defined although they are likely to be the same as for other mammals—hunger and satiety. The recently identified role of endorphins in making chewing a pleasurable experience may also tend to increase herbage intake by delaying the onset of satiety. The act of chewing is considered to be the physiological stimulus that controls the emptying of the equine stomach, and could partially alleviate the restriction of stomach volume on herbage intake. The existence of these mechanisms places great importance on mastication to reduce particle size and release the cell contents for gastric digestion. It may be assumed that fill of the gastrointestinal tract does not limit the intake of horses as it does in ruminants. The rate of passage of digesta through the hind gut of horses is evidently not restricted unless blocked. Horses probably graze until key metabolites derived from digestion induce satiety, which stops chewing and emptying of the stomach. Such a simple, elegant mechanism accelerates passage of lower quality herbage and tends to stabilize the quality of digesta entering the caecum and colon.

Horses therefore have the ability to eat large amounts of herbage each day, albeit at a slow rate but with high rates of passage of digesta. They have a limited capacity, compared with cattle, to increase the volume of their tract when the quality of ingested material is poor. The most significant difference between ruminants and the equine in herbage digestion, however, is in the utilization of protein. Horses are more efficient users of herbage protein than ruminants. About 75% of herbage protein is located in leaves and about half of this leaf protein is present as a ribulose bisphosphate carboxylase, the primary enzyme of photosynthesis. This soluble chloroplast enzyme and the rest of the plant proteins are found in the cytoplasm and are components of the readily digested cell contents. In horses, gastric digestion hydrolyses herbage protein to amino acids, which are primarily absorbed in the small intestine.

Thus the dietary amino acids of the equine are those amino acids that are derived directly from the protein, peptides and free amino acids of herbage. Microbial protein discharged from the caecum is essentially unavailable to the host because there are no mechanisms for its hydrolysis and absorption. Protein-deficient horses may eat dung in order to obtain this microbial protein. Digestion of fibre by microorganisms in the hind gut of horses may be nitrogen-limited when the diet is of low quality. The herbage of subtropical and tropical grasses is usually quite low in crude protein and these forages may need to be supplemented with protein to improve fibre digestion and nutritional quality. There is a widespread belief amongst horse owners that the renal system of horses cannot handle the excretion of large excesses of urea generated by the intake of protein-rich herbage of legumes, such as alfalfa (lucerne) and white clover (*Trifolium repens*). It is certainly true that lush swards of these legumes have very high concentrations of protein but there is little evidence to support the view that excesses of dietary protein result in renal failure.

Eliminative behaviour of horses and its effects on pastures

Grazing behaviour of horses is much more affected by eliminative behaviour than other domestic livestock. At high stocking densities horses develop voiding areas in which they do not graze and grazing patches where they do not void. Faeces are concentrated in large dung piles in these areas by mares and stallions in a characteristic marking behaviour. This marking behaviour may be a carry-over of territorial behaviour of their progenitors and not directly related to territorial claims of modern horses. The order that dung is placed in the dung pile is an indication of the place individuals occupy in the social structure of the herd. The boss stallion is the last to defecate on the dung pile.

Herbage in voiding areas is not grazed by horses and over time it may accumulate and deteriorate. The pattern of grazing results in areas of closely grazed pastures, intermingled with areas of rank, ungrazed sward. Spot grazing and patch grazing are terms used to describe the grazing pattern of horses. These spatial patterns of grazing generally do not develop at low stocking densities, in large fields and on range. It is also likely that the patch grazing behaviour reflects limitations of the gastrointestinal tract in accordance with foraging theory. The herbage produced on lawns is young, leafy and of high quality when compared with the roughs. Short grass tillers (the physiological unit of pasture grasses) in lawns are readily prehended by horses and easily severed because their pseudostems are rigid and embedded in the sod. The particle size of herbage harvested from cropped areas by grazing horses is small and requires little chewing before swallowing, thereby reducing the energy needed for mastication. In contrast to herbage in roughs, the herbage of lawns has little or no stem, low proportions of cell wall and high concentrations of protein and metabolizable energy.

Agronomy of horse pastures

Species adaptability to soil and climate

Grass species in major horse-raising areas are those adapted to the region and available as improved grasslands for all classes of livestock. There is a wealth of information on the general agronomy of these dominant species, and consequently the reader is advised to consult regional sources. Gillian McCarthy's book *Pasture Management for Horses and Ponies* is the only recent text in English dedicated to the subject. This and Marytavey Archer's review published in 1980, are good references for temperate grasslands in the European context. For the southern hemisphere, a paper by Goold and colleagues published in 1988 describes grazing practices on a New Zealand horse farm that also applies to temperate grasslands. In the USA and Canada the wide range of climate from tropical to arctic moderated by marine and continental influence, dictates that regional sources of information should be consulted. Publications by Templeton and Baker (1986), Evans (1985) and Dalrymple and Griffith (1988) provide useful references on pasture management for horses in various parts of North America. Information on pasture management for subtropical and tropical areas is sparse and the best source is Elphinstone (1981), who discusses pasture management recommendations for subtropical Queensland in Australia.

Selection of grass species

The herbage grasses preferred by horse farmers are high quality, stoloniferous, sod-forming perennials, such as ryegrass (*Lolium* species), Kentucky bluegrass (*Poa pratensis*) and bermudagrass (*Cynodon dactylon*). White clover, the herbage legume favoured by horses, is also a short-growing, stoloniferous perennial. Grasses grown as monospecific pastures, as binary mixtures with white clover or as the base species of complex mixtures are used widely and can be established and maintained as short, leafy, permanent sods.

Probably the most oft-quoted work concerning both horses and pastures is that of Archer published in 1973 concerning the herbage species preferred by

British ponies and Thoroughbreds. The time spent grazing individual strips of 30 different species and species mixtures was used to rank grazing preference. Preference varied between horses and years, but it was evident that horses generally preferred multispecific to monospecific swards. There was little difference among varieties of perennial ryegrass (*Lolium perenne*), timothy (*Phleum pratense*), tall fescue (*Festuca arundinacea*) and cocksfoot. Browntop (*Agrostis tenuis*), red fescue (*Festuca rubra*) and meadow foxtail (*Alopecurus pratensis*) were the least palatable to horses. White clover was grazed and red clover (*Trifolium pratense*) was rejected. Common pasture weeds, including dandelion (*Taraxacum officinale*), plantain (*Plantago lanceolata*) and yarrow (*Achillea millefolium*), were found to be palatable.

A similar study was undertaken by Hunt and his colleagues on New Zealand farms in 1987 investigating 16 herbage species. They identified prairie grass (*Bromus willdenii*) as a favourite of New Zealand horses and found that Thoroughbreds preferred Italian and hybrid ryegrass (*Lolium multiflorum*) varieties over perennial ryegrasses. The Italian and hybrid ryegrasses are of better quality and contain higher levels of soluble carbohydrates. Sweetness could be the basis of choice because horses prefer sweet to salty, sour, bitter herbage. Prairie grass is very palatable, high in quality, winter-active and high yielding; however, it is not suitable for horse pastures because it lacks stolons and rhizomes and will not persist under continuous, close grazing. In the New Zealand study horses preferred white to red clover, low-oestrogen red clover to normal red clover and Nui perennial ryegrass to Nui ryegrass infected with the endophyte (*Acremonium lolii*), the cause of ryegrass staggers.

Unfortunately, information on preferential grazing is of little use when it comes to the selection of herbage species and species mixtures for horse pastures. Diet selection is essentially a learned response by foals mimicking the grazing behaviour of their dams. It follows that herbage species chosen for ingestion by horses are familiar ones.

Herbage species for temperate pastures

The agronomic worth of herbage species does not relate to the preferences expressed by the horse. The characteristics that make herbage species desirable from a management perspective may not be related to preferences of the horse.

Kentucky bluegrass, the predominant and favoured grass of Thoroughbred farms in the state of Kentucky, was among the least favoured in the study by Archer. This cool-season grass does not produce high yields of dry matter nor does it thrive in the hot, dry, late summer and autumn seasons of Kentucky. However, Kentucky bluegrass forms an easily managed association with white clover and its stolons allow it to withstand close and continuous grazing, summer droughts and winter damage. Its stolons form a resilient surface thatch that reduces the chance of hoof and leg injuries but it has a limited wear tolerance and does not survive in high traffic areas. Kentucky bluegrass grows particularly well on soils derived from marine limestone. High concentrations of phosphorus and calcium in soil and herbage favour the growth and development of young horses and Kentucky bluegrass is particularly high in phosphorus and calcium.

Ryegrasses appear to be well suited to permanent horse pastures in temperate regions and as winter grazing in bermudagrass pastures in the southeastern USA. Ryegrasses were preferred by horses in the studies quoted previously and are high yielding, of good quality and remain viable in response to close and continuous grazing, treading and poaching by the formation of underground stolons. They are also compatible with clovers and are among the most wear-resistant grasses, tolerating both high stocking rates and traffic.

A 1987 survey by Hunt revealed that the vast majority of New Zealand Thoroughbred farms were based on ryegrass-white clover pastures. About a quarter of the farms reported problems with ryegrass staggers caused by the neurotoxin lolitrem B present in ryegrass infected with the endophyte (*Acremonium lolii*). Among horses this disease causes muscle tremors which may progress to varying degrees of incoordination. Recovery occurs within 7 days once horses are removed from the pasture. Endophyte-free varieties of ryegrass are available in New Zealand but such pastures are susceptible to damage by Argentine stem weevil (*Listronotus bonariensis*) and stands of these varieties do not persist.

Ryegrass infected with *Claviceps purpurea*, may result in ergot poisoning of horses. In Brazil, mares consuming sclerotia produced on seedheads of the ryegrass *Lolium multiflorum* exhibited an extended period of gestation, poor to absent udder development, dystocia, uterine rupture and delivered dead or weak foals. Ergopeptine alkaloids may be the putative toxin and routine mowing should eliminate seedheads and reduce the occurrence of this condition amongst horses grazing contaminated pastures.

Tall fescue is ranked very high in preference studies but its lack of appreciable stolon or rhizome production accounts for its inability to recover from severe drought or spread into areas scarred by hooves. Its inability to sustain close grazing by horses may account for its lack of persistence in closely grazed patches. Tall fescue tillers succumb to close clipping when cut below the pseudostem, a management condition that is very likely to exist in the closely cropped lawns of horse pastures. It is suited to horse pastures in areas where its tolerance of high temperatures and moisture and lack of significant competition provide a unique ecological niche. Tall fescue is the dominant cool-season grass of permanent pastures of Virginia, Kentucky, Missouri and Tennessee. Unfortunately most tall fescue pastures in the USA are infected with the endophyte *Acremonium coenophialum*, associated with fescue toxicosis.

Endophyte-infected tall fescue alkaloids, the exact identities of which are not known at present, cause problems in mares including prolonged gestation, abortion and agalactia. Varieties of endophyte-free tall fescue are available but not widely used on horse farms. Cocksfoot, timothy and bromegrass (*Bromus inermis*) are often used as components of mixtures of temperate grassland pastures with ryegrass and Kentucky bluegrass.

Legumes have a place in horse pastures and, ideally, should produce as much as 25–40% of the herbage mass. Clover herbage can provide a substantial proportion of the energy, protein and vitamins required by horses. White clover is the legume of choice for temperate horse pastures because it is low-growing, stoloniferous and tolerates close grazing. Red clover, while acceptable and widely used on Kentucky horse farms, is less tolerant of close grazing and on occasions may contain toxic substances harmful to horses. As a short-lived perennial, red clover must be reseeded every 2 or 3 years to maintain a significant contribution in the pasture.

Red clover, subterranean clover (*Trifolium subterranean*), and lucerne (especially with severe leaf disease) contain phyto-oestrogens that interfere with reproductive performance. Low levels of plant oestrogens, however, may promote growth of young livestock. Red clover infected with black spot disease (*Rhizoctonia leguminicola*) contains slaframine, an alkaloid that causes excessive salivation and lacrimation in horses. Red clover and alsike clover (*Trifolium hybridum*) have been related to sporadic outbreaks of photosensitization in the USA.

Compared with grasses, herbage of legumes contains higher concentrations of calcium, phosphate and other essential minerals and vitamins needed by horses. When pastures are managed to maintain clovers by liming of soils to pH 6.2 or above, and fertilized according to soil test, symbiotic nitrogen fixation provides all the nitrogen needed for the growth of the pasture and the protein requirements of grazing horses. Clover survival is aided if the pastures are maintained between 5 and 10 cm (2–4 in) by grazing and mowing. When the clover component of pastures is less than satisfactory, it may be reintroduced with a minimum tillage seeding or broadcast into the pasture during the spring or autumn at a low cost and with reasonable success. To encourage clover establishment the sward should be maintained at a height of 10 cm by mowing and horses should be removed for 30–40 days to prevent grazing of new clover seedlings.

Herbage species for subtropical and tropical pastures

Selection of the most appropriate pasture species in subtropical and tropical climates is difficult because of the scarcity of information. However, a variety of herbage species provide satisfactory nutrition for horses throughout the year. Warm-season grasses are lower in quality than their temperate counterparts and are difficult to maintain as quality horse pastures because of weed competition, a high demand for nitrogen and the inability to maintain legumes. Low-growing, stoloniferous grasses, such as kikuyu (*Pennisetum clandestinum*), blue couch grass (*Digitaria didactyla*), bermudagrass, pangola (*Digitaria decumbens*) and the taller Rhodes grass (*Chloris gayana*) are recommended as horse pastures in Australia providing pastures are maintained in short, leafy condition by grazing or clipping. In the southeastern USA improved bermudagrass cultivars are the summer grasses of choice for horse pastures when managed as short, leafy swards.

Matching herbage legumes and grasses for horse pastures in subtropical and tropical climates is difficult because adapted legumes are generally inferior to temperate legumes and are very susceptible to competition from aggressive warm-season grasses. Herbage legumes recommended for horse pastures in Australia include lotononis (*Lotononis bainesii*), greenleaf desmodium (*Desmodium intortum*), silverleaf desmodium (*Desmodium uncinatum*), tinaroo glycine (*Glycine wightii*), siratro (*Macroptilum atropurpureum*), clovers (*Trifolium* species) and lucerne (alfalfa). In subtropical Australia and in the southeastern USA ryegrass, small grains or winter annual and perennial clovers may be sod-seeded into warm-season grass swards in the autumn to provide excellent winter pastures.

Nutritional secondary hyperparathyroidism can result in horses grazing subtropical grasses. This results from calcium deficiency because herbage calcium is present as insoluble oxalates and is not absorbed by the gastrointestinal tract of horses. Tropical grasses in pastures in Queensland, notably *Setaria anceps* cv Kazungula, kikuyu and green panic (*Panicum maximum* var trichoglume Eyles) have been associated with nutritional secondary hyperparathyroidism. Warm-season grass species, such as sorghum (*Sorghum bicolor*), sudangrass and sorghum-sudangrass hybrids that accumulate prussic acid are not recommended as pasturage for horses in the USA because they are associated with inflammation of the urinary tract.

Pastures for horses in areas with continental climates, such as north Texas and Oklahoma, depend on a combination of warm and cool-season species including annuals and perennials. For information on suitable pasture species for these and similar areas readers should refer to the article by Dalrymple and Griffith published in 1988 (see Further Reading).

Establishing new pastures

The best pastures for horses are obtained by traditional methods that have been used for centuries. These include: destroying the existing vegetation (by one or a combination of cultivation, fire, grazing or herbicides), alleviating nutritional deficiencies (by fertilization and liming), and correcting physical deficiencies of the soil (by drainage and levelling the surface). Preparation of a fine, firm seedbed provides uniform distribution and intimate contact between seed and soil for rapid water uptake and germination. High quality, preferably certified, seed should be sown at the appropriate depth, no deeper than 13 mm (½ in), and consolidated immediately with a suitable roller. Amounts of seed per hectare vary widely with species and region, and local advice should be sought.

Timing of pasture establishment is critical and poor planning has condemned many horse pastures to permanent inferiority and excessive expense. Planning of new pastures should begin several years before seeding. To prepare fields for new pastures on a minimum-cost basis requires that the pasture be preceded by one or more years of cash crops to clear the land of troublesome perennial weeds. Drainage and landshaping should also precede seeding if development of permanent pastures is the primary objective for after pastures are established there are few opportunities for improvement. Limestone should be added to soils in preparation for legume-based pastures well before seeding as it can take 6 months or more before soil acidity reaches a level to guarantee successful clover establishment, nodulation and nitrogen fixation.

Pastures of cool-season species in temperate areas should be established in the autumn to reduce competition from summer annuals and minimize the impact of heat and moisture stress. Pastures of warm-season species should be established in late spring or early summer when conditions are most favourable for growth. This also applies to bermudagrass that must be propagated vegetatively.

Pasture maintenance and restoration

Fertilization

Horse pastures require routine maintenance to ensure satisfactory productivity and quality. The management is similar for pastures used by all livestock and can be adapted to fit the requirements of the horse farm. Pasture maintenance is dependent on weather and soils and regional sources of information should be sought. Herbage productivity and pasture composition can be maintained with regular applications of fertilizer and lime according to soil tests. Soil tests, however, are of little value in determining the optimum level of nitrogen fertilization. Nitrogen is the most common nutrient deficiency of horse pastures as it is transient in the soil and must be supplied on a continuous basis by fertilization or from nitrogen fixation by pasture legumes. Maintenance of the grass base and the restoration of pastures stressed by drought or overgrazing may be achieved at a relatively low cost by a programme of nitrogen fertilization. Applications of up to 110 kg nitrogen per hectare per year, split and timed to coincide with critical periods of plant growth are recommended. For cool-season grasses nitrogen should be applied during periods of active tiller, stolon and rhizome production, which occur during the early spring and late summer.

Pastures with a good balance between grasses and clovers should not require nitrogen fertilizer but will need phosphorus and potassium. Small amounts of nitrogen may be applied to grass clover pastures if the herbage is needed quickly. Competition from grasses can be minimized if the pastures are maintained at 10 cm or less. Minor plant nutrients, such as molybdenum and sulphur, may be applied according to local recommendations to correct soil deficiencies. Trace elements, including cobalt, copper and selenium, that are required by horses but not adequately supplied by herbage may be applied to the soil although it is preferable to supply them as mineral supplements in feed.

Renovation

On occasion it may be necessary to introduce legumes and grasses into horse pastures. Red clover, a short-lived perennial, must be reintroduced into pastures every 2–3 years in order to maintain a good clover base. In Kentucky, red and white clover may be broadcast into horse pastures during late winter with a good chance of success, providing grass competition in early spring is checked by topping (clipping), grazing or herbicides, and horses are temporarily removed until the clover is established. Direct drilling of pasture legumes into horse pastures with minimum tillage or ploughing techniques, such as slot seeding, increases the chance of establishing a good clover stand. Nitrogen fertilizer need not be applied to pastures with a good clover base and should not be applied to pastures in which clovers are re-establishing because of the resulting competition from resident grasses. Nutrient deficiencies, principally phosphorus and potassium, and acidity should be adjusted by fertilizer and limestone applications before seeding.

Over-seeding of permanent pastures with grasses is often less successful than over-seeding clovers. Ryegrasses are quickly and easily established but many others, such as Kentucky bluegrass and tall fescue, are slow to establish and are less likely to result in acceptable swards even under good management. Broadcasting of grass seed into established pastures is largely an ineffective and wasteful exercise.

Reseeding

When horse pastures have deteriorated to such an extent that they cannot be renovated, the pasture should be re-established with desirable species after passing through a series of cash crops to reduce populations of perennial weeds and deplete the weed seed reservoir in the soil. Minimum tillage methods can be used to reduce the cost of reseeding and to accelerate the process. These practices are valuable when soil moisture is limited and terrain and weather are conducive to excessive soil erosion. Herbicides such as glyphosate (Roundup: Monsanto) and paraquat (Gramoxone: ICI) can be applied to actively growing pastures after grazing and/or topping (clipping) to reduce the herbage mass. Pasture seeds are best introduced into the soil with no-tillage or minimum tillage, i.e. direct drilling.

Minimum tillage practices are less effective in pasture establishment than conventional methods. Destruction of the old pasture by herbicides is usually only partially successful and many perennial weeds reappear. Soil-borne insect pests are also likely to be more troublesome because their habitat may be relatively undisturbed. Decaying plant material on the soil surface supports plant pathogens resulting in the death of grass and legume seedlings. Minimum tillage and no-tillage methods offer little opportunity of working consolidated and trampled areas and poor seedling establishment will result. No-tillage practices eliminate the opportunity to incorporate limestone and level undulations in the soil surface caused, for instance, by fencelines, furrows, trees, hedges, pathways and areas poached by hoofs. Many farm owners are reluctant to destroy old pastures in the erroneous belief that they are native pastures and it will take years to establish a satisfactory sod. However, because tillers seldom live longer than 18 months and have an average lifespan of 2 months or less, pastures become permanent by vegetative propagation or natural reseeding. Excellent pastures for horses can be established in most locations within a year using good management practices.

Weed control

Mowing is the main form of weed control practised on horse farms. Often weed control and dung management involves a combined operation using mowers and harrows. Weed control with herbicides is feasible but its effectiveness is limited in small paddocks and where patch grazing induces spatial variation in populations and species of weeds. Many of the herbicides labelled for use in pastures have restrictions that prevent or limit grazing for 60 days after application. Herbicides should be selected on the basis of the weed problem but their use is largely dependent on availability and label instructions that vary with locality.

Many Kentucky horse pastures have been invaded by nimblewill (*Muhenlenbergia schreberii*), a native, stoloniferous, warm-season grass that is rejected by horses and other livestock. Its growth and spread are favoured by clipping at

12–17 cm (5–7 in) and it cannot be controlled by selective herbicides. The only feasible way to control this weed is to place pastures in a tillage or minimum tillage crop rotation, such as maize, using appropriate herbicides until the nimblewill is destroyed.

Management of herbage by mowing

Patchy grazing is reduced when the stocking rate is increased and virtually eliminated when pastures are grazed in rotation. On most horse farms these options are not feasible and mowing as frequently as once per week during periods of active pasture growth is necessary to maintain satisfactory swards. Mowing of pastures to a height of 5–10 cm (2–4 in) favours the growth and survival of desirable pasture species, such as white clover, and controls the growth of many broadleaf weeds. The formation of ergot in the flowering stems of cool-season grasses, such as ryegrass, cocksfoot and tall fescue, is minimized by regular mowing. Routine mowing not only maintains a higher quality sward but reduces the content of biologically active substances, such as phyto-oestrogens, mycotoxins and alkaloids, which are present at higher concentrations in older, senescent and dead herbage.

Management of dung

Herbage in voiding areas is not grazed by horses and over time it accumulates and deteriorates in quality. If patch grazing is allowed to continue over several years, plant nutrients such as nitrogen, potassium and phosphorus, are transferred from the grazed to the ungrazed areas in the dung and urine, creating variations in soil fertility, sward composition, yield and quality. Methods of improving patch grazed pastures include routine chain harrowing in conjunction with mowing, co-grazing with cattle, the application of fertilizers to minimize grazing-induced field gradients in potassium and phosphorus, placing the field into a crop rotation, making hay for a number of years or a combination of these various options. Removal of manure by hand or machine sweeping also reduces parasite larvae and increases the effective grazing area.

Soil compaction

Soils under grazed pastures are subject to compaction from animal traffic. Soil compaction by hoofs of grazing animals is affected by soil type and water content, density and height of the sod and the density and type of livestock. Horse pastures are particularly susceptible to soil compaction because horses spend most of their day standing whereas cattle often lie down resting and ruminating. In a Texas study, horses spent up to 18 hours each day in grazing activities, time mostly spent on the pasture lawns. At other times horses socialize in groups along fencelines, around waterers and feeders and in shade. In these high traffic areas, only wear-resistant and/or unpalatable herbage and weeds survive. It is virtually impossible to establish permanent pastures of desirable species in these high-traffic areas. Feeders can be moved to different locations but waterers usually cannot be moved. The only feasible alternative is to reseed with a fast-establishing wear-tolerant grass, such as perennial ryegrass. It is necessary to keep horses off these seeded areas until the grass becomes established. Soils in these heavily treaded areas are characterized by high bulk density and poor aeration, infiltration and root growth. Herbage yields are low and when dry the surface is a poor shock-absorber. Compacted pastures can be slitted or aerified to alleviate compaction.

Grazing systems

Continuous and rotational grazing

The extended time spent by horses in grazing reduces the effectiveness of intensive grazing practices. The horse will adapt to grazing systems as simple as tethering or as complex as integration with other livestock enterprises. Continuous or set-stocking systems are generally favoured on Kentucky horse farms because mares and foals are maintained in small groups on large expanses of grassland at stocking rates of 1 mare per 1.2–1.6 ha (3–4 acres). This is far below the carrying capacity of the fertile soils of the Bluegrass region. Because pastures provide less than one half of the energy needs of mares, the stocking rate is not as critical as it is on other commercial livestock farms. Horses are usually housed overnight, especially during inclement weather. Individual stallions are assigned their own paddocks for grazing and exercise. Yearlings are separated into colts and fillies and housed overnight to prevent injury, especially from fighting. Because many mares are housed as temporary boarders, a variety of factors are important in determining grazing pattern. These include the area and shape of fields, design and material of fences and other features of landscaping. By resting horse pastures it is possible to promote pasture growth, maintain quality and availability of herbage. Resting will also prevent or limit the development of lawns and roughs and promote the establishment of clovers and grasses following seeding. Moving horses to fresh pastures every 4–5 days also interrupts the life cycle of intestinal parasites. Studies that have compared continuous and rotational grazing indicate that rotational grazing is superior because of greater herbage availability and the elimination of spot grazing. In the description of pasture management on New Zealand horse farms, Goold and his colleagues noted that successful pasture management entailed close matching of pasture production and animal needs. Shortfalls in pasture growth were met by utilizing preserved pastures, feeding hay and supplements, and destocking. Surplus herbage was controlled by restocking, hay conservation and mowing. Utilization of herbage averaged 50% on a yearly basis and if pasture growth was slow in the winter approached 80% when grazing was managed by electric fencing.

In comparing continuous and rotational grazing systems for horses the advantages of rotational grazing systems are seen in the higher stocking rates. Almost without exception agronomists favour controlled rotational grazing of horses whereas equine specialists favour continuous grazing. However, the success of any grazing system depends on the integration of both stockmanship and agronomic skills.

Stocking rates

Stocking rates of horse pastures are difficult to establish because they depend on factors as diverse as the yield and seasonal distribution of forage dry matter, the desired level of herbage intake and the proportion of the horse's requirement provided by supplements. Other factors include the degree of utilization of available herbage, weather, pasture growth rates and the quality of management.

Little information is available on optimizing stocking rates of horses, which may be a reflection of the historical practice of stocking farms at low densities. The stocking rate on Kentucky farms quoted above is very low considering the ample use of supplements and pasture productivity. Research on stocking rates is complex and expensive and new information on this subject with respect to horses is not likely to be forthcoming. High stocking densities, as encountered in intensive rotational grazing systems, may result in increased aggressiveness. This behavioural problem, which is common to all livestock, may be worse in young horses.

Grazing with other livestock

Horse pastures may be improved by grazing horses with beef cattle. Although the diets of free-ranging cattle and horse are similar, cattle are the most compatible of the domesticated livestock as co-grazers. When cattle and horses occupy the same pasture, cattle graze the longer herbage of the roughs while horses graze the short material of the lawns. Cattle void in roughs where they graze; unlike horses they do not establish special voiding areas. If the ratio of cattle to horses is carefully adjusted roughs can be eliminated and the pasture maintained in a favourable state for horses. Although cattle and horses are compatible co-grazers, horses are dominant. In some situations it may be better to follow horses with cattle in rotation grazing systems. Co-grazing is practised on some of the largest horse farms in Kentucky so as to maintain pastures in a satisfactory condition and minimize costs of pasture maintenance. Some farms maintain their own beef herds, whilst others lease grazing.

Sheep are poor choices as grazers with horses because they prefer the short, high-quality herbage of lawns and are competitive rather than complementary grazers. When sheep co-graze with horses they increase the disparity between swards of the lawns and roughs.

Fencing

Fences are an integral part of any livestock pasture because they are needed to control and separate animals and manage pasture growth and quality. Modern fencing technology has made tremendous advances since the introduction of barbed wire in the late 1800s. New materials and designs provide safe and secure fencing for all classes of livestock. Horse farms have some unique fencing situations because of the social and behavioural requirements of horses associated with grazing and watering. Tradition, human values and concepts of horses' needs and value are factors that influence decisions about fencing on horse farms.

The area and shape of pasture fields best suited for horses is not well defined. Horses have a need for extensive exercise in contrast to other domesticated livestock and lack of exercise has been associated with growth-related musculoskeletal disorders of young horses. The horse in its natural habitat has a vast home range and may travel up to 16 km (10 miles) each day. No other domesticated animal suffers such a great reduction in its area of natural habitat as a horse confined in a stall.

There is no minimum field size for horses when nutritional requirements are provided by supplementary feed, but there may be a minimum field size for exercise especially in young growing stock. The optimum field size for nutrition by grazing is obviously related to the level of herbage productivity and the number of horses in the group. It is important to define pasture size to ensure that the lying-down area, which may be denuded of vegetation, does not account for more than 10% of the paddock area. Larger fields may be subdivided by temporary fencing. Adjustment of the number and size of grazing groups to accommodate grazing management of fields of a fixed area may have social consequences for established groups of horses.

With respect to capital cost and maintenance of fences, fields should be square or as close to square as possible. Grazing behaviour and pasture

117

utilization is adversely affected by rectangular fields when the ratio of the longest side to the short side exceeds 8:1. When fields are long and narrow horses spend more time exploring fencelines and visiting neighbouring herds causing these areas to be adversely affected by the increased traffic.

A traditional wooden fence on a Kentucky horse farm as illustrated in Figure 4.1 costs about $US8000 per km ($13 000 per mile) although other

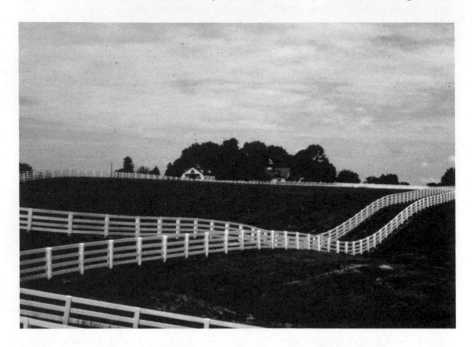

Figure 4.1 Traditional wooden fence on a Kentucky horse farm.

fencing options are now available (Figure 4.2). Although these fences are aesthetically pleasing, their attractiveness means little to horses. Plank fences are expensive to maintain, have a relatively short life and are easily damaged by chewing, rubbing and kicking. Ingested wood particles cause colic and impaction and horses may develop an addiction for creosote which is used as a preservative. Low maintenance, high tensile wires supported on driven treated wood posts are considerably cheaper to install and maintain compared to plank fences. They have an effective life at least twice that of plank fences. The topmost wire may be threaded through plastic pipe, or replaced with wooden board or wire embedded in plastic tape to improve visibility. Technology has vastly improved the utility of electric fences and they have many applications in modern horse operations. Horses learn the essential attributes of electricity very quickly but should be initially exposed to electric fences under controlled conditions. Training may be as simple as placing an electrified wire or tape across a paddock separating horses and a hay feeder for about 24 hours. Modern electric fences that are designed for horse-farm application are safe and secure. Electronic fence energizers that deliver low-energy pulses (5 J) of up to 5000 volts for a very short time (330 millionths of a second) at 1 pulse per second are recommended as they are robust and reliable and do not harm livestock.

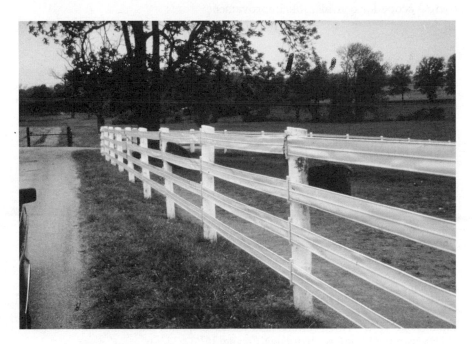

Figure 4.2 PVC plastic as a substitute for wooden railings.

Broad white tape made from polypropylene co-woven with a number of stainless steel wires as conductors, is particularly effective for temporary electric fencing on horse farms because it is highly visible. Temporary fences are especially useful in restricting horse movement on heavily treaded areas around waterers and feeders. They may be used to keep horses off reseeded or renovated areas until plants are established, to reduce the exposure of horses to herbicides and pesticides applied to pastures, trees and shrubs and separate different social groups of horses. Electric fences can also be used to secure old fences and prevent horses eating fencing materials, toxic plants, drinking dirty water and entering unsafe areas.

It is obvious from the information presented in this chapter that the association between horses and grasslands is complex and longstanding. The literature on this association is rather scant compared with the information for cattle and sheep. Many of the agronomic management recommendations described in the literature and practices on horse farms are derived from stockmanship and experience rather than scientific research. A sizeable proportion of the information applied to horse pasture management has been derived from pasture research on sheep and cattle. Based on the published literature, the quality of information on plant/horse interrelationships leaves a lot to be desired and there is scope for considerable improvement.

Further reading

Alfalfa A-2 (1991) Horse owner clinic. *Proceedings of the 21st National Alfalfa Symposium* **16**, *February, 1991, Rochester, Minnesota*. Certified Alfalfa Seed Council, P.O. Box 1017, Davis, California, 95617–1017.

Archer M (1973) The species preference of grazing horses. *Journal of the British Grassland Society* 28: 123–8.

Archer M (1980) Grassland management for horses. *The Veterinary Record* **108**: 171–4.

Carson K, Wood-Gush D G M (1983) Equine behaviour: II. A review of the literature on feeding, eliminative and resting behaviour. *Applied Animal Ethology* 10: 179–90.

Crowell-Davis S L, Houpt K A, Carnevale J (1985) Feeding and drinking behavior of mares and foals with free access to pasture and water. *Journal of Animal Science* **60**: 883–9.

Dalrymple R L, Griffith C A (1988) *Horse forage and horse forage management*. Noble Foundation Report HF-88. Noble Foundation, P.O. Box 2180, Ardmore, Oklahoma, 73402.

Elphinstone G D (1981) Pastures and fodder crops for horses in southern coastal Queensland. *Queensland Agricultural Journal* **107**(3): 122–6.

Evans J L (1985) Forages for horses. In Heath M E, Barnes R F, Metcalfe D S (eds) *Forages: the science of grassland agriculture*. Iowa State University Press, Ames, Iowa, pp 597–604.

Goold G J, Baars J A, Rollo M D (1988) Management of thoroughbred pastures in the Waikato. *Proceedings of the New Zealand Grasslands Association* **49**: 33–6.

Hintz H F (1983) *Horse nutrition*. Arco, New York.

Janis C (1976) The evolutionary strategy of the Equidae and the origins of rumen and cecal digestion. *Evolution* 30: 757–74.

McCarthy G (1987) *Pasture management for horses and ponies*. Howell Book House, New York, NY.

Templeton W C, Baker J P (1986) Utilization of forages by horses. In Smith D, Bula R J, Walgenbach R P (eds) *Forage management*, 5th edn. Kendall Hunt, Dubuque, Iowa, pp 287–95.

5 HOUSING AND VENTILATION
JOHN F. LEECH, MA

Summary
Remodelling old barns and farm buildings
Site selection
Essentials of barn design
Further reading
Appendix 5.1: Building checklist

Summary

Housing requirements for horses have evolved for the comfort and benefit of their human handlers and have not taken into consideration the welfare of the horse. Many horse barns have poor or non-existent ventilation and, especially in colder climates, horses are required to spend many hours each day in a moisture-filled, dust-laden environment.

The design of horse accommodation is a combination of art and science. In this chapter, practical recommendations are provided regarding building layout, design, safety and comfort of both horse and the people to whom their care is entrusted. Suggestions as to the minimum air exchange per hour, size and orientation of building, stall size and flooring are provided.

Many horse owners have little practical agricultural background and fail to appreciate the needs of horses. Whilst most farm owners and builders realize the necessity for ventilation for all classes of livestock its importance to the horse is not always recognized. When discussing buildings and ventilation requirements for horses, it is necessary to consider how the horse differs from other livestock. Horses are animals whose primary defence is flight, but in so doing they have the propensity to injure themselves. Thus facilities to house them should be safe and accident-proof. Horses are generally non-aggressive but when excited, frightened or in pain may strike, bite, kick, and break out of their stall or stable. Under natural conditions, horses do not spend long periods in an enclosed area, such as a stall or stable. If confined to a small space many horses will become bored and develop vices such as wood chewing, pawing holes in the floor, weaving or cribbing which are copied by other horses in the stable. Horses have lived outdoors with natural windbreaks as their only protection for centuries. Therefore, the simplest housing is the best and healthiest for the horse. A large field or paddock along with a simple shelter will provide adequate housing.

The design of horse accommodation is currently influenced by two factors. The first is that owners consider their horses are pets and need to be pampered, and secondly horse barns tend to be built for the comfort of owners and workers rather than the comfort of the horse. The majority of barns are ill-ventilated, placing the horse in a poor environment which contributes to a variety of respiratory problems. This chapter will initially consider building codes and regulations and progress through the total building layout and ventilation design.

In planning a horse facility there are several basic questions that need to be asked. What is the purpose of the facility and is there a need? What number and breed of horses are to be housed? Most farms end up needing more stalls and barn space than was originally planned. Is there sufficient room for future expansion? What are the budget constraints? Equine facilities generally cost more than was planned and changes are expensive.

The information provided in this chapter applies to horses of 14 hands or higher as it is not considered economically feasible to build facilities for the purpose of raising ponies.

Remodelling old barns and farm buildings

When examining old barns or other farm buildings as possible horse accommodation certain details need to be considered. How is the barn located, is it subject to flooding and is there a good traffic pattern? If the answers to these questions are unsatisfactory it might be appropriate to consider an alternative site. If the structure of the building is in good condition, it may be possible to move it to an alternative site. The foundation of an old barn should be straight and sound as the cost of putting in a new foundation may be more expensive than building a barn from scratch. The rafters, floor joists, structural support, walls and roof should be examined—adding to or repairing any of these is costly and makes remodelling impractical. In old barns ventilation is usually a problem; this can be determined by observing whether the paint is peeling on the outside. If it is difficult to keep a barn painted, it means that poor ventilation has allowed moisture to build up inside the barn. It is important to check whether there are openings for ventilation and if so whether they are open or blocked. If they are absent, then they need to be installed. Does the barn have a large number of dust webs or cobwebs—their presence also indicates a lack of proper ventilation. Most old barns require mechanical ventilation, which is achieved by placing inlet or exhaust fans or both in a barn so as to keep fresh air moving through the building. Tobacco barns, which are only used for drying tobacco during the latter part of the year, make excellent barns for horses and are used extensively in central Kentucky (Figure 5.1). There is plenty of inlet area at the sides and the height of the barns permits an upward movement of air allowing it to be drawn out at the ridge. This contrasts with the individual stalls or boxes to house horses present in most training establishments in Europe, as illustrated in Figure 5.2.

Site selection

It is important to check the local zoning requirements or planning laws before buying a farm or designing a new building. In the USA some local authorities place a figure on the number of acres that must be available before a livestock building can be erected. Others have regulations concerning the distance a building must be situated from boundary lines, dwellings and neighbours. If these regulations cannot be met it is necessary to obtain a variance from the zoning board before construction can commence. In other countries planning permission may be necessary from the local authority. At this early stage it is appropriate to make a detailed plan layout to ensure there is sufficient space available for all the buildings, roads, paddocks, working rings and training tracks. Details on the plan should indicate where water, sewer and electrical lines enter the building.

Essentials of barn design

Initially it is important to consider the size of the barn and the number of stalls desired as subsequent additions can prove very costly. Valuable information is obtained by examining barns designed by others to observe the good features and recognize the mistakes. Keeping horses is a very labour-intensive operation and a proper layout is one of the best means of conserving labour. If architects are employed they should be familiar with the design of livestock buildings. Many horse barns contain expensive mistakes as a consequence of

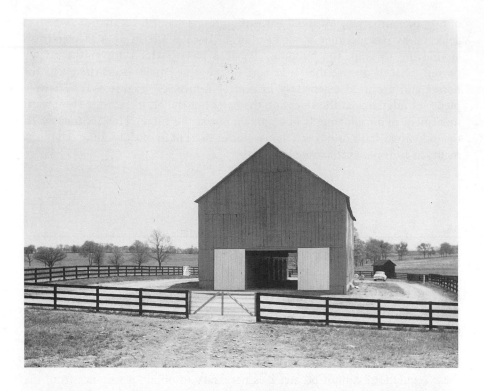

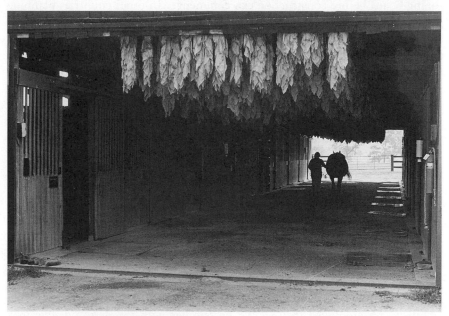

Figure 5.1 (a) (b) Converted tobacco barns to house horses in central Kentucky.

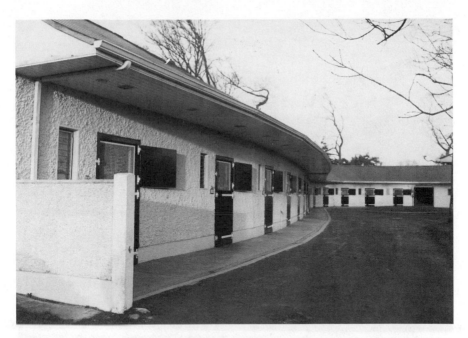

Figure 5.2 Traditional European training stable.

being designed by individuals with little or no experience of farm-building construction.

The breed of horse and activity to be undertaken must be taken into consideration when planning and laying out a new barn. The height of each stall or stable should be a minimum of 240 cm (8 ft), alley ways 275 cm (9 ft) and indoor exercise areas 425–490 cm (14–16 ft). A 300 × 300 cm (10 × 10 ft) stall should be the absolute minimum size; 300 × 365 cm (10 × 12 ft) or 365 × 365 cm is the preferred size. For stallions and foaling stalls a 365 × 425 cm or 365 × 490 cm stall is preferable. The larger size stalls are easier to keep clean, provide more room for horses to move around and alleviate some of the more common stall vices. Two stalls in the barn should share a common removable wall so as to provide a 600 × 365 (20 × 12 ft) foaling stall, or a purpose built padded stall (Figure 5.3) may be built. It is wasteful to build stalls smaller than 300 × 300 cm as they are harder to keep clean and limit the resale value.

Orientation of the building is one of the most important aspects to be considered in order to utilize the natural air flow to keep the barn ventilated in hot weather. Windows properly placed in the south side of a barn will help raise the temperature inside the building during the summer and winter using solar radiation. Ventilation will be most effective if the barn is built in an area of unrestricted air flow with air being able to move over the top of the building, drawing out warm moist air from the inside as illustrated in Figure 5.4.

In livestock housing the principal climatic elements that affect the animal's

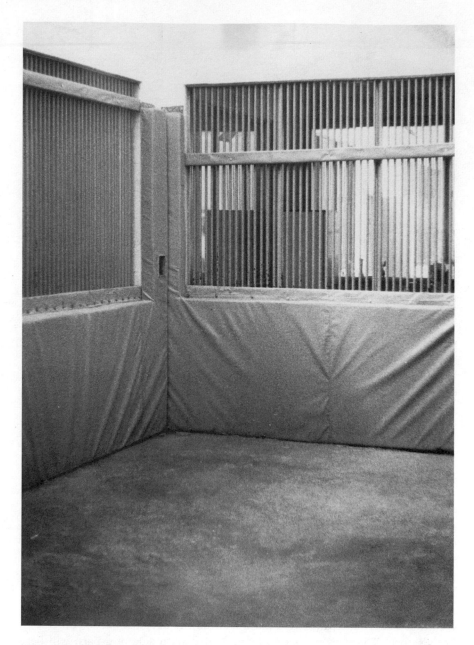

Figure 5.3 Padded foaling stall.

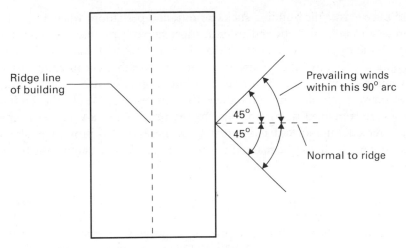

Figure 5.4 Structure orientation to prevailing wind.

well-being are ambient temperature, moisture (relative humidity), ventilation rate (air changes per hour) and air movement. A horse will do well in nearly any temperature if the humidity can be held to a comfortable level and there is enough air movement through the building to keep the air clean and free of condensation and ammonia, the latter resulting from the breakdown of faecal and urinary urea. Conditions detrimental to a horse's health, particularly affecting the respiratory system, occur when the barn is cold and the relative humidity above 70%. Very few horse barns are insulated and any attempt to reduce ventilation in order to maintain the temperature causes an increase in the level of humidity.

Feed rooms, hay storage and facilities for farm personnel should be situated in a central position to facilitate easy access and observation of animals. They should be rodent proof and have satisfactory pest control. Consideration should also be given during the planning stage to minimizing the risk of fire. Space should be available around the barn for roads, pens or paddocks, and exercise rings.

Ventilation

The most important detail in a new or remodelled barn is to ensure an abundance of natural ventilation. Most horse barns are under-ventilated rather than over-ventilated. There is a difference between a well-ventilated barn and a draughty barn. A properly ventilated barn will not have draughts, but will have an adequate air exchange to maintain horses in a healthy environment. The simplest ventilation techniques rely on the appropriate use of natural phenomena—the stack effect when warm or stale air rises; aspiration, when wind force across the building sucks air out; and perflation, when air is blown from side to side or from end to end. Most horse barns use the stack effect through the provision of an open ridge (Figure 5.5a) with inlets at the side of the building (Figure 5.5b). During hot summer weather encouraging cross-air movement by open doors at the sides of buildings (Figure 5.6) will considerably improve ventilation and reduce the temperature inside the building. Horses are contained within the stall by the provision of a wire mesh screen. When remodelling an old barn, it may be necessary to provide intake and exhaust fans which can be manually controlled or are on an automatic thermostat or humidistat control. A new barn should have a 15–30 cm (6–12 in) ridge vent with a minimum of 25–30 cm overhang at the side and a vented soffit running the full length of the building. A vented soffit is a covering with 60 mm (¼ in) holes under the overhang which allows fresh air to enter the barn. A rule of thumb guide is to provide an outlet ventilation area of 900 cm^2 (1 sq ft) and an inlet area of 2700 cm^2 (3 sq ft) per horse or stall. The recommended air movement is 0.85–2.8 m^3 (30–100 cu ft) per minute to provide a ventilation rate ranging from 6 to 30 litres per minute per kilogram body weight (0.3–0.5 cu ft/minute/lb body weight). This should be achieved with a minimum of eight air changes per hour to ensure that dust and spores are kept at a low level.

A ventilation problem occurs when hay is stored above the stall. Unless provisions are made to allow air movement above the stall area, effective ventilation becomes reduced or non-existent. An air passage of at least 30 cm must be left between the wall and bales of hay stored above each stall to allow hot, moist air to escape from the area below. The dust from hay and straw contains numerous spores of fungi and actinomycetes that are small enough to penetrate the lower respiratory tract. In horses which suffer chronic obstructive pulmonary disease (COPD), commonly referred to as 'heaves', the inhalation of spores from organisms such as *Aspergillus* and *Micropolyspora* may stimulate signs of respiratory distress similar to those associated with asthma in humans. It is suspected that these allergens in dusty environments are also a factor in reduced exercise tolerance and prolong the course of outbreaks of acute respiratory disease attributable to viruses such as influenza and equine rhinopneumonitis.

In most barn designs providing an opening under the eaves along with an outlet through a ridge opening is adequate. Where this is not possible a mechanical ventilation system may be needed, for which expert advice should be obtained.

Insulation

The most common place to use insulation in a horse barn is the roof area. Care must be taken to add a vapour barrier, which is placed on the inside and must

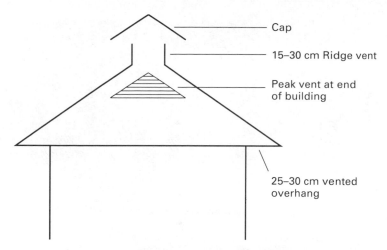

Cap

15–30 cm Ridge vent

Peak vent at end
of building

25–30 cm vented
overhang

The ridge vent should have a cap to keep out rain or snow.

The 25–30 cm vented overhang will be covered with vented
soffit or 60 mm hardware cloth to keep out birds.

(a)   The peak vent will have a screen to keep out birds.

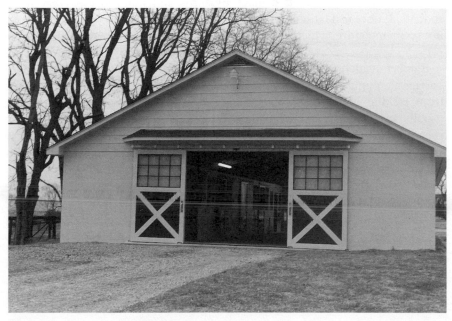

(b)

Figure 5.5 (a) (b) Barn ventilation specification.

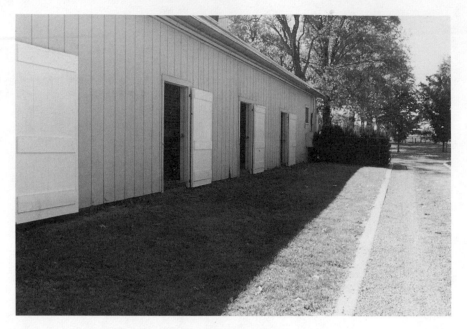

Figure 5.6 Side doors to improve ventilation during summer.

be strong enough to resist damage by birds and not provide a haven for rodents. If fibre insulation is placed in the roof care should be taken that it does not retain moisture, which would cause a metal roof to rust or a wooden roof to rot.

Blanket insulation may be installed with a kraft or aluminium paper vapour barrier although these are not usually strong enough to keep birds or rodents from making holes. Glass-wool insulation with a plastic vapour barrier is usually strong enough to keep birds from pecking holes. Rigid wood fibre sheathing may be used but over time it will absorb moisture and bow away from the underside of the roof allowing moisture to collect between the sheeting and roofing material. Birds and rodents will also make holes in this material. Expanded polystyrene with or without an aluminium foil surface may be used but without some type of rigid cover this material will become damaged by birds and rodents. A well-ventilated building will not need insulation, but if it is necessary attention needs to be given to the type of material as many insurance companies require it to be made fire resistant.

Selection of building materials

Most building materials are satisfactory as long as they are strong enough to stand up to abuse by horses. Steel and aluminium are commonly used but without insulation barns constructed with these materials are hot in summer and cold in winter. Most commercial steel buildings are designed as machinery sheds or grain stores and are not ventilated. To be satisfactory aluminium and steel buildings generally require insulation of at least the roof area.

Barns constructed with cement block and masonry are cold, have limited flexibility and need to be well ventilated. They are more costly to build because they need good footings to support the building. If cement block (Figure 5.7)

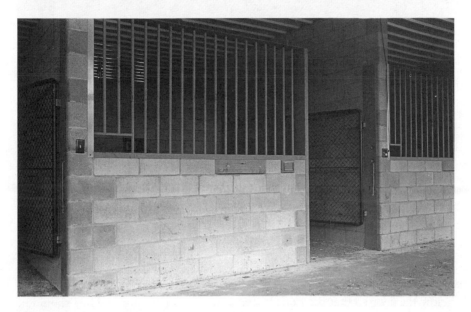

Figure 5.7 Cement block stall partition.

or poured walls are used footings are necessary for stall partitions, which should be built into the front and back walls. It is more costly to install feeders, waterers and hay racks in cement walls. Cement block partitions and walls are easy to paint and keep clean and if they are correctly built there is little maintenance involved. They will withstand abuse from horses and if the bottom 120 cm (4 ft) of the stall wall is lined with wood it will protect horse's limbs when they kick the wall. Wood is the best all-round material for horse buildings, as illustrated in Figures 5.8a, b and c, although it needs to be treated if it is to come into contact with soil or manure. If softwood is used, it needs to be protected from excessive chewing by horses. Wood is strong, attractive and is a good insulator. It is easier to install ventilation systems in wooden buildings as compared to other materials. One of the most reasonably priced materials for horse barns is 4 × 8 ft (120 × 240 cm) plywood sheets of T-111 barn siding which gives the building a rustic look.

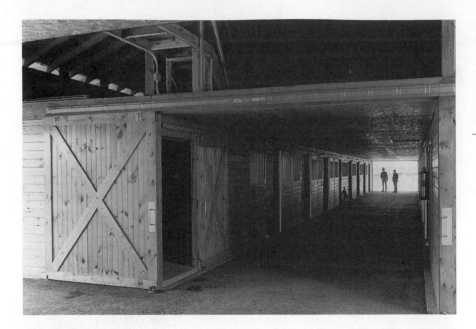

Figure 5.8 (a) Wood barn.

Construction

Interior stalls need to be of smooth, rugged material free from any projections on which a horse may get injured. Partitions need to be flush with or slightly below the floor so that the horse's legs cannot become caught. They should be solid up to 2.5 m (8 ft) from the floor with at least 30 cm (1 ft) of space between the top of the partition and ceiling to allow air movement along the full length of the barn. Some partitions may be of solid wood to a height of 1.5 m (5 ft) with a bar or screen bringing the height to 2.5 m (7–8 ft). This arrangement may cause problems if horses do not get along with their neighbours and is not suitable should a mare be next to a stallion, or two stallions next to each other. Openings in which a horse can catch its foot or leg should be avoided. If bars are used on the top of a stall, the spacing should be 9–10 cm (3½–4 in) apart. If a mesh front is used on a stall or stall door the holes should be 5 × 5 cm (2 × 2 in) or smaller.

Wooden planks for stall partitions can have a spacing of 2.5–4 cm (1–1½ in) between for additional ventilation, but this provides edges for horses to crib and chew on. The planks on the bottom 120 cm (4 ft) of the stall should be solid for additional strength. Each stall should have a window located so the bottom of the window is 180 cm (6 ft) above the stall floor. The window should be at least 90 × 120 cm (3 × 4 ft) and act as a source of ventilation. Windows should be protected by bars or wire mesh. Rough cut 2 × 6 in (5 × 15 cm) oak

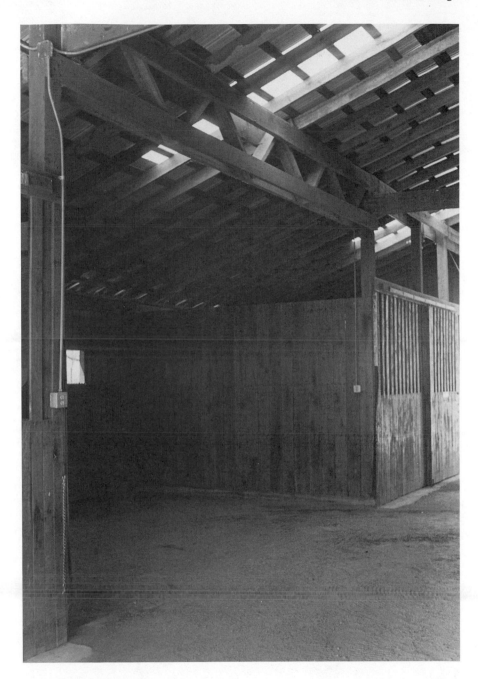

Figure 5.8 (b) Wood barn.

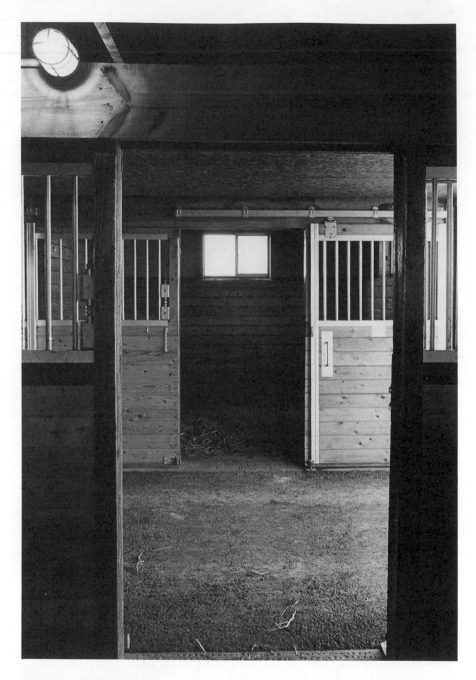

Figure 5.8 (c) Wood barn.

plank is the strongest of wooden materials, and horses are less likely to chew or destroy it. One-inch rough-cut oak is equal to the strength of two-inch finished timber of yellow or white pine. If finished oak is used, it will be more costly than treated yellow pine. Rough-cut oak is easiest to install when it is green as nails are easier to drive before it dries. If dry oak is used a nailing gun or drill to make the holes will be necessary. When green oak is used it will shrink and twist as it dries. For this reason it is preferable to use a dried finished material on the front of stalls and rough-cut oak for partitions and the back. Treated timber should be used for the bottom boards of stalls to prevent rotting where partitions come into contact with the floor or manure. Tongue-and-groove treated yellow pine is also used for stall partitions. A problem with tongue-and-groove yellow pine is that the timber tends to have more knots, and horses can kick or push off the grooves or tongue between the boards. Yellow pine is not as hard as oak, but it is stronger than white pine which splits and splinters easily. All edges should be protected to prevent horses chewing them. Any softwood timber or posts need to have the exposed surfaces covered with some type of metal to protect them from being chewed by horses. Formed aluminium, sheet metal or angle iron can be used for protecting softwood timber.

Wood preservatives

There are three types of wood preservatives: inorganic arsenicals, which include chromated copper arsenate (CCA), ammoniacal copper arsenate (ACA), and ammoniacal copper zinc arsenate (ACZA); pentachlorophenol and creosote. Neither pentachlorophenal nor cresote are recommended for use in or around livestock buildings because of their toxic effect. In the USA, chromated copper arsenate (CCA) type III is one of the most common preservatives used for treatment of soft timber. The arsenate in CCA is toxic but is tightly bound to the wood and when dried is of minimal risk to people and animals.

The effectiveness of the preservative depends on wood species, chemical type, application method, penetration and retention. In selecting treated timber check for the 'preservative retention' which is usually expressed in preservative chemical per cubic foot (PCF) of wood. The higher the PCF the better the treatment.

Stall floors

Stall floors need to be made of a durable material that is not slippery but is absorbent, easy to clean, and resistant to pawing. Floors should require the minimum of expense and time to maintain in a satisfactory condition. Some of the more commonly used materials include a clay and sand mix, clay, limestone dust, wood, cement, asphalt, and rubber floor mats. Clay and sand mix is generally the least costly and most easily obtained. A mixture of ⅔ clay and ⅓ sand will allow drainage and is easily replaced. It should be well mixed, levelled and packed before horses are allowed in the stall. Many horse owners believe clay is the floor of choice although good clay is hard to obtain and does not drain well, producing wet spots where horses urinate. This makes stalls hard to keep dry and free of odours, and the floor is difficult to replace.

If limestone dust is installed over a good base and is watered and packed down before horses use the stall it makes a good hard surface that drains well and keeps the stall odour free. If limestone dust is properly applied, the floor will be nearly as hard as cement without the disadvantages that come with cement floors. The key to a good limestone dust floor is to have it wet and well packed before horses are allowed in the stall. The thickness of the limestone needs to be 10–12 cm (4–5 in) over a base material of 15–20 cm (6–8 in) of sand, gravel or mix of sand and gravel on top of parent soil (Figure 5.9).

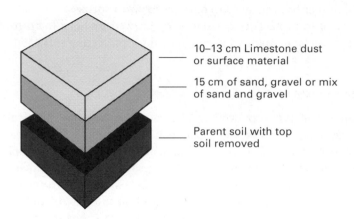

10–13 cm Limestone dust or surface material

15 cm of sand, gravel or mix of sand and gravel

Parent soil with top soil removed

Figure 5.9 Stall floor composition.

Wooden floors have been used for many years, the most suitable being a rough-cut hardwood with a thickness of at least 5 cm (2 in) that must be treated to retard decay. Wooden floors are slippery when wet and prone to attract rodents as they allow urine to accumulate and feed to fall through the cracks. Floors made of cement are easy to clean and sanitize, but bedding is needed to soak up urine, which does not drain away. Cement floors are cold and being slippery require a considerable amount of bedding. The use of cement floors is associated with an increased incidence of leg injuries. If stalls are well bedded and horses are kept outdoors for at least 4 hours per day, such injuries can be minimized however. Regular asphalt is also used for stall flooring but many of the problems associated with cement also occur with asphalt. If a finishing coat is put on the surface, it becomes slippery and cold and requires more bedding although less than for cement. If the surface is not sealed, some drainage will occur reducing the amount of bedding required.

A major consideration before installing rubber mats is to make sure the stall floor is level and packed well. The mat should be a single piece per stall or as few pieces as possible and fit close to the walls. It must be at least 1.5–1.9 cm (⅝–¾ in) thick and made of a durable rubber that will withstand pawing. The addition of bedding may be necessary as solid mats do not allow urine to drain down through the floor of the stall. Rubber floor mats can add $US500 to the cost of the stall.

One of the newer types of flooring material is interlocking rubber paving bricks recently installed in the Keeneland Pre-race Parade Ring (Figure 5.10).

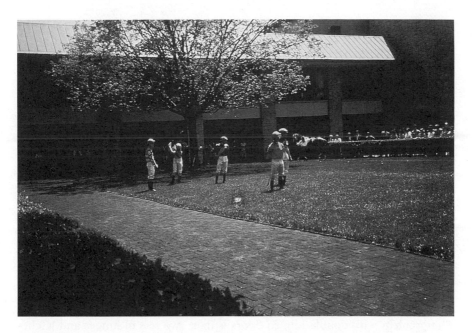

Figure 5.10 Interlocking rubber paving blocks in Keeneland Pre-race Parade Ring.

These bricks are attractive, safe, durable and have a non-slip surface. The cost of interlocking rubber paving bricks is approximately $US9.00 per square foot ($US100 per m²). An alternative synthetic flooring is fibre reinforced polyethylene interlocking blocks. This is a flooring material that possesses durability and good drainage and prevents horses from digging holes. The addition of stone dust, sand or native soil to the surface makes it easier on the horse's legs. The cost of this material is approximately $US3.30 per square foot ($US35 per m²). A new product is a flexible fibre grade of polypropylene. This is a tough yet flexible material designed for support, strength and chemical resistance and to allow drainage, with a non-skid surface. It has a good shock-absorbing surface that reduces moisture and is easy to clean. The cost of this material is approximately $US3.00 per square foot ($US32 per m^2). In recent years there has been considerable experimentation with different types of bedding for horses. Traditionally straw which is not dusty, is free of odour and faeces and of sufficient depth has been the bedding of choice. Alternative bedding materials include wood shavings, sawdust, paper, hay and peat moss; these are used for reasons of economy and availability and to reduce the prevalence of respiratory disease associated with the presence of pollens and moulds in dusty straw. Studies have shown that horses exhibit a strong individual preference for the type of bedding as measured by the amount of time they lie down.

Stall doors

There are many styles and designs of stall doors but the major consideration is that they contain the horse within the stall in a safe manner. The door must be opened and closed safely for both the horse and handler, and be strong and simple to operate. The stall door should be 120 × 240 cm (4 × 8 ft) with 120 cm the minimum width. For safety and ease of operation, the sliding door is the most suitable. When selecting a sliding door it is important that it possesses a good track and rollers as well as a good latch. Doors with drop-down bars or latches that protrude and may injure a horse are not suitable. The sliding door may be made of wood or metal. The full wooden door is heavy and does not permit light or ventilation into the stall. A metal door with a mesh screen (Figure 5.11) allows maximum ventilation and light into the stall. This system is valuable in a foaling barn permitting the foal to receive plenty of fresh air. One-piece hinged doors are not ideal as the weight of the swinging door causes hinges and latches to sag, making them difficult to close. If doors open inward, the horse may kick resulting in an injury, or equipment on the horse may catch on the door causing the horse to jump and become frightened. The problem with double-hinged doors is their two sets of hinges and latches so when the doors sag they have to be reset. With two latches, there is a greater risk that one may not be closed. The advantage of double doors is that the top door can be left open, allowing the horse to stick its head outside and take an interest in its surroundings. However, a young horse or stallion may try to go over the top if they are nervous or excited.

Many horse trainers prefer stall guards made out of webbing (Figure 5.12) or chains, half metal doors with a neck yolk, or screen doors (Figure 5.13). Stall guards have the disadvantage of being relatively easy for a horse to push out, go over or break and escape from the stall. They are acceptable if there is a sliding door that can be closed when there is no one around to keep an eye on the horse. Stall guards are inexpensive but alone are the least desirable for containing the horse.

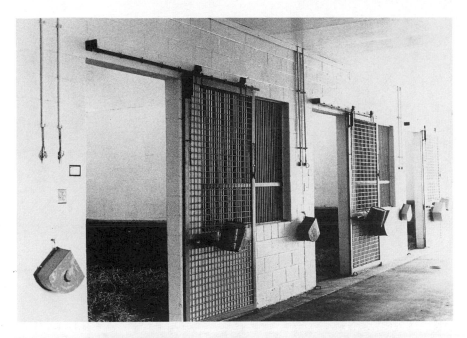

Figure 5.11 Sliding metal door.

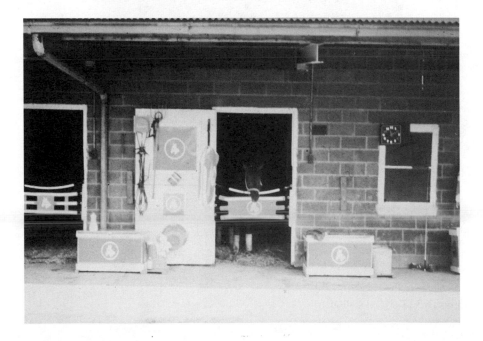

Figure 5.12 Stall guard.

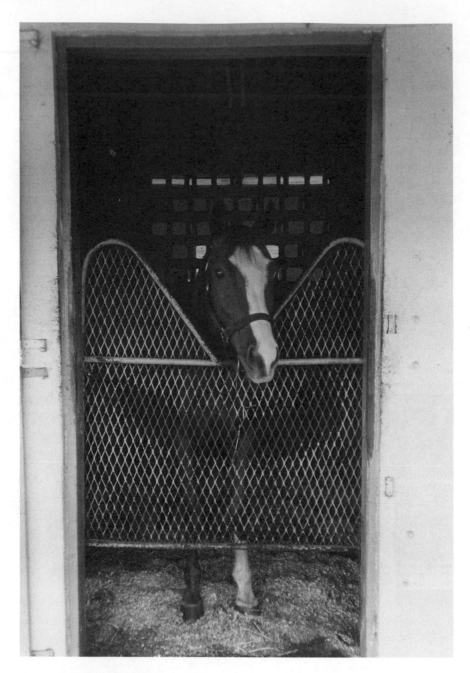

Figure 5.13 Metal stall guard.

Watering systems

If a farm has over 10 horses, there should be a separate water source from the residential supply so that in case of a breakdown the total water supply to the farm will not be cut off. The water supply in a barn should deliver 110–35 litres (25–30 gals) per minute, which can be supplied from a 12.5 cm (5 in) diameter well using a 3/4 hp (horse power) submergible pump. A well of this size should supply enough water to maintain 50–100 horses and also give adequate pressure for cleaning equipment. In areas which suffer a cold and prolonged winter, frost-free hydrants adequately located are essential. Inside the barn, water lines should be buried 60–90 cm (2–3 ft) below the ground surface and marked so they can be located. When selecting a watering system a frost-free hydrant, hose and bucket is perfectly suitable. The water hydrant should be recessed in the wall as shown in Figure 5.14 to eliminate any risk of a horse getting hurt or farm personnel hooking it with the wheel of a tractor or manure spreader. In the winter hoses attached to water hydrants should not be hung in an area where they can freeze when not in use. If horses are watered with a bucket it should be emptied at least once a day and washed every second or third day. If there is any type of illness in the barn, the bucket should be emptied and disinfected daily. Fresh water should be available for the sick horse at all times.

Many farms now use automatic waterers in order to save the labour of watering each horse twice or three times a day. Attention should be given to the design of the waterer and its location in the stall. Round waterers which need an angle brace for support are a hazard to a horse rolling in the stall, should it get its leg caught in the brace. Care is needed to ensure the manufacturer's recommendations are followed for installing waterers so the pipes do not freeze. Automatic waterers are best placed in the back corner of a stall so an overflow tube can be attached. If a valve sticks or the water freezes, the overflow will pass to the outside of the barn instead of the stall floor. Automatic waterers need to be cleaned regularly and all grain, manure and debris removed. Waterers should have a heating unit to prevent them from freezing. A properly installed automatic watering system is also an excellent addition for a pasture, especially if it contains a heating element to prevent water from freezing—a major problem with automatic watering systems. In most cold climates, the water feed pipe will need to be 120 cm (4 ft) or more below the surface of the ground and it is useful to check with the Soil Conservation Service, Weather Service or other advisory bodies to ascertain the depth of the frost in the area.

It is important to identify on the building plans where the water lines run and how far they lie underground so they can be located.

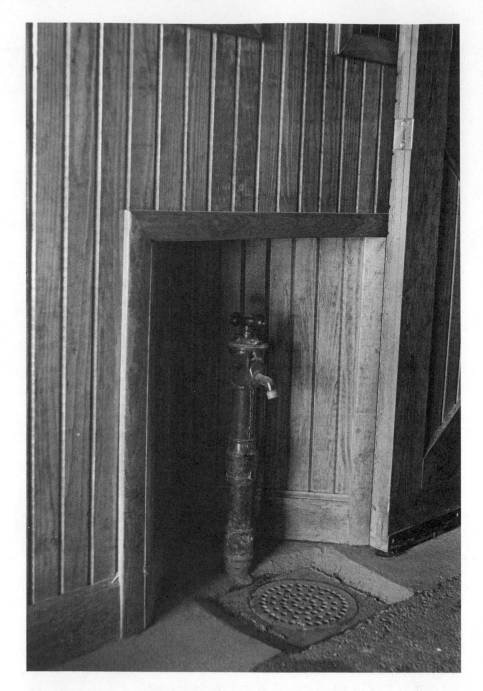

Figure 5.14 Recessed water hydrant.

Feed boxes and hay racks

There are many types of feeder made from a variety of materials, including reinforced rubber, plastic, fibreglass, wood and metal. They should be large enough to hold up to 7.5 kg (16 lb) of grain and be located so they are convenient and easy to clean. If they are positioned at the front of the stall the person responsible for feeding has the opportunity to look at the horse each time it is fed. Many aspects regarding the demeanour of the horse can be observed when it is fed. The grain feeder needs to be rugged and solidly attached to avoid destruction and excessive spilling of grain. Permanent feeders should be about two-thirds of the height of a horse from the floor, as indicated in Table 5.1. Hardwood such as oak and maple makes excellent

Table 5.1 Suggested feeder and hay rack height

Size of horse	Feeder height	Hay rack height
14 hands (142 cm = 56 in)	94 cm (37 in)	142 cm (56 in)
15 hands (152 cm = 60 in)	102 cm (40 in)	152 cm (60 in)
16 hands (162 cm = 64 in)	107 cm (42 in)	162 cm (64 in)
17 hands (172 cm = 68 in)	114 cm (45 in)	172 cm (68 in)
18 hands (183 cm = 72 in)	122 cm (48 in)	183 cm (72 in)

feeders for horses, is hard enough to discourage chewing and does not break or splinter. The one drawback of wooden feeders is that they are difficult to clean and disinfect. Softwood should not be used as horses will destroy it by cribbing or chewing. Steel, iron or aluminium feeders are more expensive but if cast with rounded edges and set in the corner of a stall are safe. They are more indestructible than other feeders and are easier to clean and disinfect. Horses will not crib on the edge of metal feeders and so they last a long time. Hard plastic or heavy rubber feeders are smooth and durable, easy to keep clean and disinfect. Rubber buckets and feeders require frequent cleaning, as they build up odours over a period of time. Rubber feeders will withstand abuse from the horse and are not damaged at freezing temperatures. Both plastic and rubber feeders yield to pressure without harming the horse. If plastic corner feeders are used, a 5 × 15 cm (2 × 6 in) board across the corner in front of the feeder will protect it from abuse. Plastic corner feeders with replaceable lips are useful should the horse be a cribber.

Hay racks

Hay racks in a stall are of questionable value. It is recommended that the hay is fed on the floor in a corner of the stall. Racks or nets should have a capacity of

9–14 kg (20–30 lb) of hay and may be located in a corner or on a wall where they are easy to fill. Care must be taken to make sure racks are not located too high as dust and chaff can fall in a horse's face, leading to eye or respiratory problems. When racks are placed too low they are a hazard to horses, which may catch their feet in them. If hay racks are to be used, the bottom of the rack should be level with the withers of the horse, as indicated in Table 5.1.

Lighting of horse barns and arenas

Most equine facilities have inadequate lighting, with little thought given to their appropriate placement. When lights are put in stalls, they should be recessed or have unbreakable covers. Electric wires should be in conduits so the horse cannot chew or rub against them. Stalls and alleyways should be well lit with at least 320–430 lux (30–40 foot candles) of light output. Riding rings should be lit with a uniform light pattern that eliminates dark spots and shadows. Good lighting is a combination of quality, quantity and colour. Minimum lighting requirements for different locations are provided in Table 5.2. Quality of light requires freedom of glare, control of shadows and the

Table 5.2 Minimum lighting requirements

Location	Requirements
Barn office	750 lux (70 ftc) Incandescent or fluorescent.
Rest room	320–430 lux (30–40 ftc) Incandescent or fluorescent.
Tack room	320 lux (30 ftc) Incandescent or fluorescent.
Feed room	270–320 lux (25–30 ftc) Incandescent or fluorescent.
Stalls and alleys	320–430 lux (30–40 ftc) Fluorescent in alleys if at least 300–360 cm (10–12 ft) high. Incandescent if recessed or with a protective cover in stalls, or fluorescent in stalls with 275 cm (9 ft) high ceilings.
Veterinary or farrier area	430–540 lux (40–50 ftc) Fluorescent with protective cover.
Wash rack	320–430 lux (30–40 ftc) Incandescent or fluorescent with protective cover.
Arena	320–430 lux (30–40 ftc) High intensity, cold weather, ballast fluorescent light with protective cover.

absence of sharp differences between light objects and their background. Glare causes discomfort which can be reduced by shading the light source or placing well above eye level. Many of the newer mercury or quartz lights provide more light than the older types. If the electrical circuit is broken they require a start-up time, which should be taken into account if the barn or riding arena is used as a public facility at night. A barn which contains 10 or more horses requires a

200 amp supply to provide an adequate number of lights and additional circuits.

A common mistake in many horse barns is not to provide enough power points. There should be at least one double outlet for every two stalls. A double outlet should be located in a barn so that a 30 m (100 ft) cord can reach any location in the barn. Feed and tack rooms should have an outlet positioned every 3.5 m (12 ft) along the wall.

The most satisfactory type of lighting is the fluorescent tube with a high-intensity cold weather ballast for quick start-up in cold weather. A protective covering over the tube can be obtained to make fluorescent bulbs safer for use in stall areas or feed rooms. If a tube breaks the glass particles are retained inside the plastic cover surrounding the bulb.

Wash stall

A central area to wash horses is a considerable practical asset in the barn as it can also be used for other purposes, including clipping, shoeing, bandaging and veterinary examinations. It should be a minimum of 300 cm (10 ft) wide and 365 cm (12 ft) deep with adequate head room. A solid non-slip floor should be provided, with a slight incline to a drain preferably positioned against the outside wall, and the sides must be smooth and easy to clean. A recessed hydrant providing hot and cold water should be available. An adequate light source is necessary with both the switch and source protected against water contact. Wall ties should be positioned in the side walls.

Arena and indoor training facilities

Arenas and indoor training facilities are basically clear span structures that will be part of, attached to or close to the main horse barn. They will be a minimum width of 11–15 m (35–50 ft), which can be used for exercising and training horses, but this is too limited for riding and too narrow to drive a horse. Clear span structures 15–30 m (50–100 ft) wide are necessary for exercise, training and riding arenas. Buildings with a width of 18–30 m (60–100 ft) are best for group riding or driving horses.

The ceiling height needs to be a minimum of 4.25–4.8 m (14–16 ft) for the horse's and rider's safety. The higher the ceiling, the better lit the arena or training area will need to be, with a minimum amount of shadows. A 4.8 m ceiling will allow the training of hunter/jumper horses with ample head room for the rider.

Parent materials on which the building is placed provide the footing as well as fill used to level the arena. Fill is made up of a mixture of sand and clay that will provide a firm footing. Added materials include sand, sawdust, woodchips, bark, tan bark, rubber shavings and wood fibre. Sand floors for arenas and training rings are relatively inexpensive, but their cohesive properties are poor and vary greatly with the amount of water that is applied. They have a tendency to be dusty and need constant attention to maintain them. Sawdust over a solid footing is a good material. It is relatively inexpensive and easy to obtain and maintain but can be very dusty. Sawdust needs to be 7.5–13 cm (3–5 in) deep to provide a good surface and must be 'topped up' continuously. Woodchips are a good surface material which last longer than sawdust, but the initial cost is higher. It is difficult to drag an arena of woodchips and obtain a uniform appearance. A drag made out of chain link fence is best for this purpose. Over a period, woodchips will break down and create a dusty atmosphere and will need to be replaced. In some locations, tree bark is available and is cheaper than woodchips. Bark has the disadvantage of being uneven until used for a period of time, and it is hard to dress the surface so that it remains even; but it requires a minimum of dust control. Rubber shavings to a depth of 5 cm (2 in) provide a good surface that has some give to it and is not slippery. It is easy to maintain because it does not require much raking and looks bright and black after watering. Some insurance companies do not permit the use of rubber shavings inside buildings as they are considered a fire hazard.

Dormit wood fibre is laid in an interwoven fashion that provides a solid surface with a good cushion. It is a good material that maintains a uniform surface that will not freeze and provides a useful surface on which to exercise horses. However, it is expensive and will break down over a period of time under constant use. A recently introduced track surface Equitrack (En-Tout-Cas) is composed of sand coated with a non-toxic, waterproof chemical polymer. The polymer-coated sand granules bind together to provide the advantages of a solid surface including uniformity, weather resistance and durability yet the surface retains a great deal of 'give' which reduces the incidence of leg injuries and breakdowns.

Of all the materials that have been discussed sand, sawdust and woodchips can be a particular problem as far as dust is concerned. The most often used and cheapest way to control dust is to apply water at regular intervals, which is effective but time consuming.

Some farms use chlorinated water to control dust, but this dries out the horse's hoof and causes foot problems. Old oil can be used, but is irritant to horses that work on the surface every day. It is also a dirty material that is hard to keep out of clothes or equipment. An alternative is vegetable oil, which is mixed with water and applied to the surface. It washes out of clothes and equipment, is non-toxic, inexpensive and has a long residual effect.

Manure disposal

As we become more environmentally conscious, the handling of manure becomes an increasing problem especially as the location of many horse operations is close to urban areas. The one advantage of horse manure is that there is less odour compared to other livestock manure. A 500 kg horse produces approximately 10 tonnes of manure per year comprising faecal material, urine and contaminated bedding. If liquids are absorbed by bedding or drain away the manure and bedding can be handled as solids. Manure disposal must be planned so there is no contamination of surface or underground waters, minimum impact of odours and unsightliness, and a reasonable labour requirement. The amount of water in the digestive tract and faeces depends on the horse's diet: high-grain diets result in less water than hay diets, and oats contain only 50% water. Local planning officials and pollution control agencies should be consulted when designing facilities for waste disposal. Stable drains should flow to an adequate disposal area which may include a septic or local sewage system as required by local regulations.

Manure should be stored at a site convenient to the stable but as remote from dwelling houses as practical. Good all-weather access should be provided for disposal vehicles and farm personnel. Manure should be stored away from stable walls, as ammonia and other compounds damage foundations and sidings. It attracts flies and contains parasites and other pathogens eliminated by horses so it should not be stored on pasture. Locate the manure heap away from water sources and drainage channels to avoid contaminating surface or underground waters. Manure runoff should drain away to approved disposal facilities. In the winter, fly control is not a problem so manure can be stockpiled, but in the summer it should be removed twice a week, especially during the fly breeding season, which starts when spring temperatures get above 18 °C (65 °F) and ends at the first frost in the autumn.

A manure pit is usually the least objectionable form of storage, as it confines manure to a small area, is out of view, and can be covered. A perforated cover keeps the pit out of sight, prevents children and animals from access, and allows composting fumes to escape. One side can be at ground level for emptying with a front-end loader. The usual method of storage is a manure heap. A wood or masonry backboard or three-sided structure aids in containing a pile and in scraping or loading manure.

The Appendix to this chapter is a checklist to consider before building a new barn or renovating an old barn. If positive answers can be given to the questions on the checklist, many major mistakes can be eliminated from the building programme.

Further reading

Ambrosiano N, Harcourt M (1989) *Horse barns big and small*. Breakthrough Publications, 310 N. Highland Avenue, Ossining NY, 10562.

Clarke A F (1987) Stable environment in relation to the control of respiratory disease. In Hickman J (ed) *Horse Management*. Academic Press, London, pp 125–74.

Farmstead Planning Handbook (1974) Midwest Plan Series Handbook, MWPS-18. Midwest Plan Service, Iowa State University, Ames, Iowa 50010.

Horse Handbook: Housing and Equipment (1971) Midwest Plan Series Handbook, MWPS-15. Midwest Plan Service, Iowa State University, Ames, Iowa 50010.

Livestock Waste Facilities Handbook (1975) Midwest Plan Series Handbook. Midwest Plan Service, Iowa State University, Ames, Iowa 50010.

Sainsbury D W B (1981) Ventilation and environment in relation to equine respiratory diseases. *Equine Veterinary Journal* **13**: 167–70.

Sainsbury D W B (1987) Housing the horse. In Hickman J (ed) *Horse Management*. Academic Press, London, pp 97–123.

Appendix 5.1

Building checklist

Old barn renovation

Is the building in a desirable location (with at least a 5% slope)?

Is there enough land around the barn for a desirable traffic flow pattern?

Is the structure sound?
    Is the foundation or footer straight and sound?
    Are floor joists and support structures sound?
    Are the rafters and roof sound?
    Are walls straight and sound?

Can you get adequate electricity and water to the site?

Ventilation:
    Is the paint peeling?
    Are there vents in roof overhangs, and are they working?
    Are there ridge or peak ventilators of at least 15 cm (6 in)?
    Can mechanical ventilators be added if necessary?

New barns and buildings

Have zoning laws and planning permission been checked and obtained?
    Is there an adequate area of land?
    Is there a minimum distance from the boundary line?
    Is there a minimum distance required from dwellings?
    Is a zoning variance needed and if necessary can one be obtained?

Has a detailed drawing been made of the barn and paddocks?

Have water lines, septic and electric lines been located on the map?

Is the barn orientated so that there is maximum utilization of air flow and odour control?

Has the cost of different building materials been checked?

Have at least three estimates on building the barn or renovating an old barn been obtained?

Is the architect familiar with livestock buildings and construction?

Is a ridge vent of at least 15 cm (6 in) planned?

Is there at least a 30 cm (1 ft) vented overhang planned?

Are peak end ventilators to be included?

Is barn ventilation designed so that there are at least 6–8 air changes per hour?

Barn essentials

Have barns with different building designs been looked at?

Are stalls planned at least 300 × 360 cm (10 × 12 ft) or larger?

Is there at least a 240 cm (8 ft) ceiling in the stalls?

Is the ceiling height in the alley and riding area known?

Are tack rooms and feed rooms placed in a suitable location?

If hay storage is planned overhead, have provisions for ventilation been made in the stall area?

Barn material selection

Have barns made of different materials been visited and investigated?

Has particular attention been given to insulation of the underside of the roof?

Has stall material been selected that leaves 30 cm (1 ft) of space above stall partitions for ventilation?

Stall floors

Have different floor materials been investigated and checked for desirable and undesirable qualities, including sand and clay, clay, limestone, wood, asphalt, cement and rubber mats?

Stall door design

Have different stall door designs been examined, including sliding or swinging doors, full or ½ doors and screen doors?

Watering systems

Have different systems for watering been investigated including bucket, in-stall automatic waterer, and corner automatic waterer?

Are water hydrants located in alleyways recessed into the walls?

Feeders and hay racks

Have different feeders been evaluated for ease of installation, sanitizing and safety?

Will the feeder hold 7.25 kg (16 lb) of grain and possess a lip or edge to reduce food wastage?

Has the proper height of the feeder and its placement been determined?

If hay racks are to be installed, where will they be positioned and at what height?

Lighting

Are stalls adequately lit? If stall lighting is used, is it recessed or covered with an unbreakable cover?

Do stalls and alleyways have 320–430 lux (30–40 candle foot) of light?

Does the light have a uniform pattern without dark spots or shadows?

Do all lights have safety covers?

Do lights in feed rooms and wash racks have dust- and moisture-proof covers?

Do the barn plans provide for a 200 amp supply?

If you can give a positive answer to these questions, and have viewed several establishments, you are ready to build your equine facility.

6 REPRODUCTIVE MANAGEMENT ON THE HORSE FARM
WALTER W. ZENT, DVM

Summary

Reproductive efficiency of an equine breeding operation is a cooperative effort between farm management and the attending veterinarian. The objective is to produce the maximum number of healthy foals, at the least expense, year after year. The means by which this can be achieved are discussed, emphasizing the basic principles of management, record keeping and veterinary skills.

Management is the most important factor in the establishment and running of an efficient broodmare operation. This chapter discusses the management of the broodmare herd and the veterinarian's role in the operation. The objective is to produce a high percentage of live foals as early in the breeding season as possible with the least amount of labour and expense. For the Thoroughbred it is important to make efficient use of the calendar bearing in mind the short duration of the breeding season. In the northern hemisphere this officially commences on 15 February and continues until 15 July, and foals should be born as soon after 1 January as possible, since this is their annual birth date. The southern hemisphere Thoroughbred mating season is even shorter, starting 1 August and ending on 25 December. As mares carry their foals for approximately 11 months they should conceive within 30 days of foaling if time is not to be lost. If mares fail to conceive within 30 days their foaling date moves progressively closer to the end of the mating season. When the oestrous cycles of barren, maiden and early foaling mares are synchronized so they come into season and are mated at approximately the same time foaling will occur within a limited time frame. This allows a greater number of mares to be examined during each visit by the veterinarian, thus saving time and money. When mares are managed in this manner the stallion can also be used more effectively. Maiden and barren mares will be mated in the early part of the season before foaling mares, and a popular stallion can be mated to more mares than would otherwise be possible. It is important when managing a stallion's book to spread the mares evenly throughout the mating season to prevent overworking the horse at any one period. With a popular stallion it is better to add mares in the latter half of the season than to overwork the horse in the middle. Over-breeding the stallion will reduce his fertility and lead to a reduction in the total number of pregnant mares by the end of the season.

The reproductive potential of a band of broodmares can be predicted by examining their age. As mares age their reproductive performance decreases and so a group whose average age is increasing should not be expected to perform as well as a group in which young mares are being introduced to replace poorly performing mares. Mares foaling late in the breeding season are less likely to become pregnant compared to mares foaling earlier in the season due to the limited number of times they can be mated. If the brood mare band has a high number foaling late in the year it is unrealistic to expect that a large percentage will be in foal at the end of the season. If these factors along with the reproductive histories of mares are considered the projected performance for a group of mares can be assessed without leading to false expectations. More importantly this will allow owners and managers to make rational decisions and to operate their mating operation in a business-like fashion.

Design of buildings

Properly designed housing has a part to play in making the broodmare operation more efficient and improving the health of the herd. Stable construction has been discussed in detail in Chapter 5 so only a brief comment with respect to its effect on reproductive performance will be considered. Thought given to planning a horse farm with an eye to efficient operation will pay great dividends in saving time and labour. The most important factor in the construction of a broodmare barn is ventilation, with windows and doors positioned so that fresh air is available at ground level. The head of the foal is closer to the floor than is the head of the handler or the mare. If air movement is limited to the upper part of the stall, the foal is forced to breath stale air laden with ammonia which is an irritant to the respiratory system. One of the most effective ways to increase ventilation is to provide doors made of materials through which air can pass as illustrated in Chapter 5. The openings should be small enough so that foals cannot get their feet caught. In many barns, doors are positioned on the outside wall to act as ventilators, comprising an inner and outer door, the latter of which can be closed during inclement weather. Windows placed in the outer wall can also be used for ventilation and light and should open in a manner that will permit air movement but prevent entry of rain and snow. Lofts if present should be built over the central alleyway and not obstruct the flow of air from the stall to the roof. If foals are born early in the year and heated stalls are necessary it should be possible to enclose one or two stalls as needed.

Barns should have as much natural light as possible as they are more pleasant to work in and farm personnel tend to keep them clean as accumulations of dirt and debris are more readily observed. Artificial light should be provided so that the mare and foal can always be seen and examined with ease. There should be sufficient artificial light so that mares can be placed on a lighting programme to regulate oestrus. In a 365 × 425 cm (12 × 14 ft) stall this will require the presence of a clean 200 watt bulb under the control of a timing mechanism.

Tack or warm rooms should be positioned so that several stalls can be observed. Slatted stall doors, mentioned above, have the added advantage of increasing visibility of the foal and the foaling mare especially when lying down. The easier it is to observe animals the less is the risk they will be overlooked. The less time taken by farm staff in moving mares and foals allows more time for other activities. Barns surrounded by paddocks and fields are more convenient than barns built on the perimeter of the land. The inside of barns should have few protrusions so that foals cannot be injured when they are following their mother. Doors should be positioned in the centre of the stall because if they are in a corner it is more difficult to catch mares. Barns should have alleyways that are wide enough for the teaser to be moved from stall to stall with ease. If the mares are to be teased at a bar or board it should be positioned centrally so mares will be moved the minimum necessary.

Oestrous cycle of the mare

Responding to fluctuations in hormone production the mare's reproductive cycle goes through fertility cycles that last on average 21 days. Two distinct phases comprise the continuous cycle: oestrus, when the mare is 'in heat' or 'in season', i.e. the receptive period lasting 5–7 days; and dioestrus, the period between successive oestrus periods, which lasts 14–16 days. Stimulated by increasing daylight a non-pregnant mare will start to cycle in the early spring after a period of inactivity or anoestrus. This transitional phase may be brief or persist for weeks and is characterized by erratic cycles during which the mare may or may not be fertile. After the first ovulation the oestrous cycles become regular until the autumn when the mare returns to anoestrus.

Mating must be timed precisely in order for conception to occur, regardless of whether it is done by natural or artificial means. The timing of insemination or mating is determined by a prediction of ovulation—the release of an egg from an ovary into the oviduct. The egg remains viable (i.e. capable of being fertilized) for only a short period, less than 12 hours. If it is not fertilized it will not pass to the uterus and gradually degenerates. The spermatozoa released by the stallion during ejaculation are propelled rapidly by contractions of the uterus into the oviduct, reaching the oviduct within 2 hours. Spermatozoa can survive on average for 2 days but their viability varies considerably from only a few hours to 6–7 days depending on the individual stallion and the uterine environment. Bearing in mind these various factors the optimal time to mate the mare is from 6 to 24 hours before ovulation occurs.

Hormonal control of the oestrous cycle

An increasing amount of light perceived by the retina of the eye, as occurs in spring, inhibits secretion of the hormone melatonin by the pineal gland in the brain. Removal of the inhibitory effect of melatonin allows the hypothalamus in the brain to release gonadotrophin-releasing hormone (GnRH). This hormone in turn stimulates the pituitary gland to secrete follicle-stimulating hormone (FSH). FSH stimulates the growth of one or more ovarian follicles, the structures within the ovary that contain the eggs or ova. As these follicles develop oestrogen is secreted, which acts on behavioural centres in the brain to stimulate oestrous behaviour in the mare. Oestrogen also causes relaxation of the cervix which facilitates passage of spermatozoa into the uterus and contractions of the smooth muscle of the reproductive tract. Finally oestrogen inhibits the secretion of FSH and stimulates the release of a second gonadotrophic hormone, luteinizing hormone (LH), from the pituitary gland. LH causes the ovarian follicle to mature and induces ovulation. After ovulation the follicle is replaced by the corpus luteum. This secretes progesterone, which initiates a period of unreceptiveness to the stallion. After 12–14 days, if pregnancy has not occurred, the uterus secretes the hormone prostaglandin ($PGF_{2\alpha}$) causing regression of the corpus luteum and a decline in the production of progesterone. The reduction in serum progesterone allows the mare to return to oestrus and the cycle to be repeated.

The fertilized egg enters the mare's uterus 4–5 days after ovulation. In order for pregnancy to continue the mare must recognize she is pregnant and continue secretion of progesterone. Recognition of pregnancy occurs 14–16 days after ovulation following signals from the embryo and suppression of prostaglandin secretion by the uterus. Around day 35 cells of the developing placenta invade the lining of the uterus to form the endometrial cups. The cups secrete pregnant mare serum gonadotrophin (PMSG), which stimulates secondary corpora lutea to secrete progesterone from 40 to 150 days of pregnancy. After that period the placenta becomes the sole source of progesterone.

Foaling

The foaling event and its proper management can greatly influence the future reproductive performance of the mare. If the mare has had her vulva sutured it should be opened prior to foaling. When a mare is ready to foal, it is advantageous to have an attendant present but in most foalings very little assistance is needed or advisable. As foaling commences, the attendant should examine the mare to make sure the foal is presented with the nose and front feet being palpable in the pelvic canal. If the presentation is normal the mare should be allowed to have the foal unassisted. When assistance is given very gentle traction or simply holding the feet and letting the mare push is usually sufficient. By allowing the mare to take her time the cervix is allowed to dilate and there is less trauma to the mare and foal than if traction is vigorously applied. Abnormal presentations, such as legs or head not being presented, are reasons for immediate intervention and it is better to call for veterinary assistance even if it subsequently turns out to be unnecessary. Foaling alarm systems and closed-circuit TV surveillance systems (e.g. Foal Alert Inc., USA) are helpful on farms with limited availability of personnel. One of the most satisfactory alarm systems is a small radio transmitter sutured to the mare's vulva containing a pin that becomes extracted when the foetal membranes are pushed through the vulva. When this happens the alarm is set off or the attendant's pager is activated. These systems are helpful but they are only adjuncts to good management and observation.

Teasing

Teasing is one of the most important operations undertaken on the broodmare farm. Without an efficient teasing programme the ability of mares to conceive is severely compromised. Most mares in season display or 'show' signs which include lifting the tail to one side, squealing, arching the back and squatting, 'winking' the vulva and urinating (Figure 6.1(a)). In contrast the mare in anoestrus or dioestrus will express behaviour ranging from passive disinterest to extreme displeasure. Many mares will strike violently when first presented to the teaser but will accept his attention after a period. Each mare is usually remarkably consistent in behaviour from one cycle to the next so keen observation, patience and meticulous record keeping are very important. Ideally the same person should handle the teaser and observe the mare throughout the breeding season.

A good teaser stallion possesses a strong libido but is easy to handle. He will vocalize, expose his upper incisors and gums, nuzzle, nip and lick the mare to sniff out her state of oestrus. To keep the teaser fresh and interested he may be allowed to mate occasionally. Record keeping and teasing should be done in an orderly and regular manner allowing ample opportunity for farm personnel to observe mares that are being or have been teased. Teasing methods vary depending on the facilities and farm personnel available. Mares may be teased in their own stall or a stall in the barn specifically designed for the purpose. The mare teased in her own stall is held and exposed to the stallion at both her head and hind quarters (Figure 6.1(b)). If the mare is teased in a specifically designed stall the teaser is usually held in the adjoining stall with a hole cut in the wall so he can put his head into the stall with the mare. This is a common method on both the broodmare farm and in the breeding shed and has the advantage of allowing teasing to be undertaken inside the barn. Teasing bars are also used to test mares. A teasing bar is a short wooden wall constructed outside the barn or at the side of a catch pen. The mare is taken to one side of the bar and the teaser stands on the other side. This procedure provides the teaser and the handler protection from an unwilling mare and is often used to test mares in fields or paddocks.

Some farm managers like to test mares by taking the teaser into a field with a group of mares. This can be a dangerous procedure if not done by a competent person. The opportunity for injury to a horse or handler is greater, particularly when mares have foals by their side. It is also difficult to keep accurate records when there are several mares in the field gathered around the teaser. Another method is to place the teaser in a field of mares but confined to a small pen. It is designed so that mares approach the pen and the teaser can reach through an opening and make contact. This is a useful procedure for mares that do not show well in the barn or at the bar because they are protecting their foal or do not adapt to the teasing procedure. The disadvantage is mares must be observed throughout the day. If an aggressive mare is in the field and keeps other mares from the teaser she must be removed so that timid mares will approach the teaser.

The frequency a mare is teased depends on the intensity of the breeding

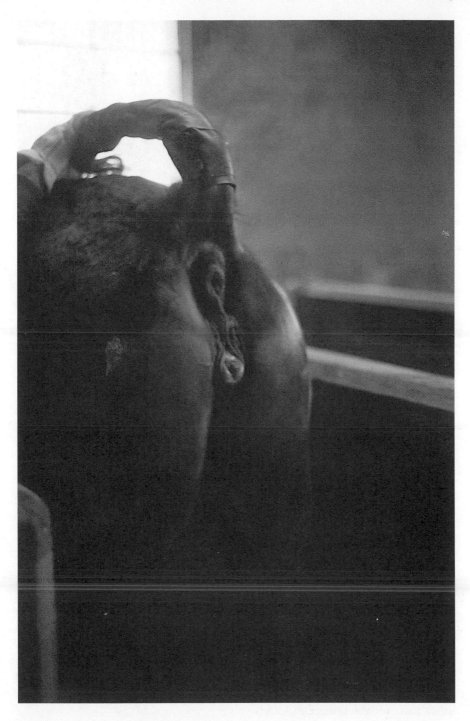

Figure 6.1 (a) A mare 'showing' in season.

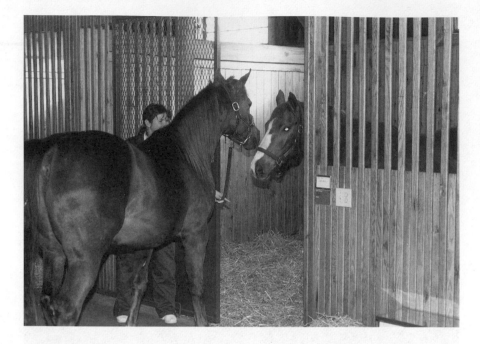

Figure 6.1 (b) A mare being teased inside her own stall.

programme and the stage of the mare's cycle. A mare to be mated to a stallion which stands on the farm could be teased every other day. Mares being mated at other farms by busy stallions may need to be teased daily, particularly when they are close to oestrus. Mares that are difficult may need to be teased more than once a day especially when close to the beginning of oestrus. Every mare should be tested immediately before she goes to the breeding shed even if she has been teased just a few hours previously. Mares should also be teased at the breeding shed particularly if it is on a different farm from the one on which the mare resides.

Demonstrative mares do not have to be teased as hard as mares that do not readily show signs of oestrus. It is less important to tease vigorously when the mare is between heat periods and not expected to be in season. When mares are teased in the stall with their foals they may not show signs of oestrus as they are preoccupied with protecting their foal. These mares should be taken away from their foals when they are tested. Placing a twitch on the mare may also take her mind off the foal. Some mares although they are in season will not show signs when teased. Such mares should be 'jumped', allowing the teaser on their back before they are sent to the breeding shed. This procedure should apply to all maiden mares when they are first sent to be mated, as well as any other mare of which there is doubt.

Record keeping

Records are an integral part of an efficient broodmare operation but should be simple and easy to access. Teasing records on all mares should be recorded on a single sheet of paper as illustrated in Figure 6.2 and kept in the broodmare

WEEKLY PALPATING CHART   WEEK OF _____

Mare:	To Stallion	Sun	Mon	Tues	Wed	Thurs	Fri	Sat
Amelia Knight	FS		C⁄C		N⁄20			(N 40⁄hCG)
Brassy Yankee	NP			30⁄N	(40⁄N hCG)			
Lady Belle	NP		40⁄30	40⁄40	◯	HAS⁄HAS		
Outrigger	NP	5	6 SUTURE	7 POOLING URINE	8 20⁄N	9 PASS	10 TREAT	11
Sassy Somolli	Ab		40⁄N	40⁄N	(hCG)	HAS		

Key:

HAS = Has ovulated

N⁄30 = Nothing significant on left ovary; 30 mm follicle on right ovary

C⁄C = Cluster of follicles on both ovaries

◯ = Mated

(hCG) = Mated and given hCG (human chorionic gonadotrophin to induce ovulation).

Small numbers in upper left of block indicate number of days since foaling or prostaglandin treatment. When a mare is checked on a Monday and the veterinarian wants to check her again on Wednesday, a diagonal line is drawn in the square for that day to act as a reminder.

Figure 6.2 Weekly palpating chart.

barn. They should be available when the veterinarian is present to examine the mares. Teasing records should identify how well the mare is showing 'in season' as compared to how she has shown in the past, when the mare was last mated and when she last went out of season. This information, as illustrated in Figure 6.3, should be kept in the barn with detailed records of the individual mare's teasing chart kept in the farm office. Palpation records of mares should also be available in the barn and should include details such as follicle location and size, the day the mare needs to be mated and whether or not the mare ovulated. Information noted on the individual mare's record should include the results and date of bacterial examination of the genital tract, hormone assay results and biopsy or cytology results as well as other procedures performed. The particular requirements of the individual farm on which the stallion resides should be available so that the appropriate documentation will accompany the mare and the required procedures completed before the mare is sent to be mated. The number of times and dates on which a mare has been mated during the year should be kept on one record containing information on several mares with easy updating for barn use.

Artificial lighting programmes

One management procedure that, if properly implemented, will improve the performance of the mare herd is the use of lights. Mares are seasonally poly-oestrous and their breeding cycles are influenced by increasing periods of daylight. If mares are exposed to increased day length by the use of artificial light they can be encouraged to come into season earlier than normal for the time of year. All types of mares benefit from being placed on a lighting programme, which should be initiated 60 days before the effect is required. Mares can be exposed to a lighting regime that increases in weekly increments or to a constant 16 hours of light for the entire 60 days. Unless electricity is very expensive the constant 16-hour day is the easiest to implement. There must be a period of darkness during the 24-hour period as the exposure to constant light will not have the desired effect. The greatest benefits using artificial light occur with maiden and barren mares. In the northern hemisphere they should be put under lights commencing 1 December. The lights can be placed in either stalls or sheds. If placed in a shed the mares should not be crowded and artificial light must be evenly distributed. This is the most economical method but if not done properly the results are disappointing. When mares are put on a programme in their stalls a single 200 watt bulb per stall is sufficient. The bulb should be kept clean and located so it is not hidden behind beams or other obstructions. Mares appear to respond better in stalls

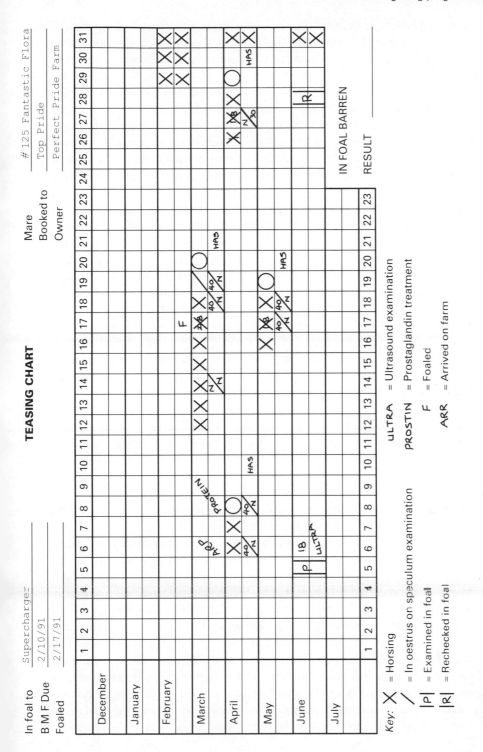

Figure 6.3 Individual mare teasing chart.

than in sheds possibly because they receive greater attention. If the climate is suitable and insufficient stalls are available, a shed or pen system can be constructed. The mares are turned out to pasture when the lights are switched off.

As already mentioned mares are seasonally polyoestrous, which means that regular oestrous cycles resulting in the production of follicles and ovulation are limited to a certain period of the year. In the northern hemisphere this occurs from mid-March to mid-November and in the southern hemisphere from mid-September to mid-May. This cyclical pattern is controlled more by the amount of light the mare is exposed to than by the ambient temperature or the level of nutrition. When mares start to cycle at the beginning of the season oestrus may last for 30 days or more. The mare will show all the outward signs of oestrus but though she will accept the stallion she will not ovulate. By the use of a lighting regime a mare will pass through the non-ovulatory period before the start of the breeding season. When the breeding season commences these mares will be cycling normally and can be mated when they come into oestrus.

The advantage of using a lighting programme, particularly for barren and maiden mares, is that it encourages them to cycle early in the breeding season. At the beginning of the breeding season stallions are mated to fewer mares so the mare in season can be mated at the optimum time. Mares that become pregnant will foal earlier the following year and consequently have an excellent opportunity to become pregnant again. The veterinarian's time will also be used more efficiently as the mares examined will be cycling and in a position to be bred.

There are some disadvantages to the use of a lighting programme. One is expense—it costs more in labour and feed to confine mares for a large part of the day and night. If early foals are a part of the farm programme this expense is justified but if there is no demand for early foals because the breed does not perform until they are adults the expense may not be justified. There is also a disadvantage in colder climates as foals born in the winter months require more care than foals born during the spring.

Artificial lighting can also be used to improve the productivity of foaling mares. It is particularly useful for mares that are due to foal early in the breeding season. The length of time foaling mares are exposed to artificial light is similar to the regime for barren mares. When foaling mares are exposed to artificially increased day length they foal approximately 10 days earlier than the average 342 days for mares not exposed to artificial light. The procedure should not therefore be used on mares if there is a chance they would foal before 1 January. The shortening of the gestation length may not be significant when only one mare is involved but among a group of mares it can provide a significant saving in allowing them to be mated earlier. Of even more value is that exposure to increased day length helps decrease the incidence of post-foaling or lactational anoestrus. Some mares have a foal heat at 9 days and if they do not conceive fail to return to oestrus 20 or so days later. Other mares may never come into oestrus, a condition referred to as lactational anoestrus. The ovaries of these mares are small and inactive and frequently 90–120 days will elapse before they begin to cycle. Many different types of therapy have been tried, mostly without success. Most post-foaling anoestrus occurring in mares that foal early in the season is associated with the lack of stimulus of increasing day length. By exposing foaling mares to artificially longer days the incidence of this problem can be reduced.

Hormone therapy

Hormonal manipulation of barren, maiden and foaling mares when associated with careful management can significantly improve the reproductive performance. Progesterone, progestogens, oestradiol, prostaglandins and gonadotrophin-releasing hormone (GnRH) are all used with varying degrees of success.

The orally administered synthetic progestogen, altrenogest (Regumate, Hoechst-Roussel) is used for oestrus synchronization and to delay the onset of oestrus in cycling mares. It is given for 10 days and then withdrawn allowing ovulation to occur 2–10 days later. The administration of altrenogest to a group of mares will concentrate oestrus into a smaller time frame than would occur under natural conditions. When the drug is withdrawn, however, mares will ovulate at varying times making it an imprecise method of oestrus control. A mixture of 150 mg progesterone and 10 mg oestradiol injected daily will also prevent ovulation and follicular development. When this combination is given for 10 days and withdrawn, ovaries develop follicles and ovulate at about the same time. Most mares come in season at about 7 days and ovulate between days 9 and 11 post-treatment. This technique can be used to synchronize mares for shipment to stallions some distance away, and reduces the number of examinations undertaken by the veterinarian. Where artificial insemination is being used it maximizes the use of the stallion as it allows mares to be organized into groups to be covered at one insemination.

Oestrus in the foaling mare can also be manipulated. Mares that conceive on the foal heat have the minimum time between foaling and conception. The heat period occurs from 7 to 14 days after foaling and the most important factor determining fertility is the length of time from foaling to ovulation. The longer this period the greater the chance the mare will conceive. Mares that ovulate before 9 days postpartum have little chance of conceiving whereas mares that ovulate 10 days or later conceive at a rate of 50% or higher with fertility increasing as the time from foaling lengthens. There are several methods by which this interval can be increased. Foal heat can be delayed for as many days as desired by giving the mare daily injections of progesterone and oestradiol commencing within 12 hours of foaling. If the treatment is given for 4 days a mare that would normally ovulate on the tenth day will ovulate on the fourteenth day postpartum. Another approach is to allow the mare to go through her foal heat, particularly if she ovulates early, and give an injection of prostaglandin to lyse the corpus luteum causing the mare to return to oestrus early. When the corpus luteum is lysed the serum progesterone level drops and the mare will return to oestrus earlier than normal. This method may not be appropriate for mares that ovulated 10 days or later after foaling but it can be applied to mares that ovulate early or mares that cannot be mated on their foal heat due to problems at foaling or because the stallion's book is full.

Hormone therapy can be utilized in the management of barren and foaling mares at other times during the breeding season. Prostaglandin is used to short cycle mares not mated when in season either because the stallion was not available or the time of ovulation was misjudged. Prostaglandin is also used to return a mare to oestrus when the corpus luteum has not lysed and conception has not occurred. Those mares that retain their corpus luteum have a high level of serum progesterone and their behaviour is similar to that of a pregnant mare. When they are examined for pregnancy there is no evidence of an embryo by palpation or ultrasound. An injection of prostaglandin will lyse the corpus luteum and cause the serum progesterone level to drop and the mare to return to oestrus. It is of the utmost importance that a mare is examined rectally before prostaglandin or any other therapy is given.

Progesterone and oestrogen therapy is of use when mares develop several small follicles which are not likely to ovulate. The condition occurs in foaling mares and to a lesser extent in barren mares. Mares will show minimal or incomplete signs of oestrus, but on rectal palpation do not have a follicle that is likely to ovulate. When these mares are given progesterone and oestrogen the entire cluster of follicles will usually regress and a single follicle develops.

With any treatment used on mares in the management of their reproductive cycle it is imperative that the stage of the mare's cycle is foremost in mind. If therapy is not designed to correct a particular condition but used with no particular criteria in mind the results are frequently disappointing. The reproductive state of the mare prior to treatment should be determined by a thorough veterinary examination.

The reproductive examination of the mare

Most reproductive examinations can be carried out in a stall or using the entrance to the stall as illustrated in Figure 6.4, to provide some degree of protection for the veterinarian and other personnel. The mare should be kept with her foal; as if they are separated the mare will become irritated and make examination difficult. It is helpful if more than one person is available to assist the examiner so that the tail can be held aside and other assistance provided. If a speculum or ultrasound examination is to be made, it is important to have the mare out of the sunlight so the operator can see. Most examinations are currently performed using disposable equipment so the spread of disease from mare to mare is no longer a factor. Mares must be washed to remove dirt and faecal material from the vulva prior to an examination. The examination of a mare's vagina, vestibule, and cervix with a speculum is an important step in determining the mare's reproductive state. Before the speculum is introduced the conformation of the mare's vulva should be determined. Poor vulva conformation allows aspiration of air and faecal material into the mare's vagina. The vulva should be upright and the lips have sufficient tone to keep the opening closed. A mare with thin vulva lips, or one that is flat rumped or possesses an anus that retracts anteriorly causing the vulva to tip forward is also prone to aspirate air leading to faecal contamination of the vagina. When these conditions occur, the lips of the vulva can be closed by scarifying the edges and suturing the vulva closed to the level of the brim of the pelvis.

With the aid of the speculum the presence of blood and lacerations on the vaginal wall and cervix as a consequence of foaling can be visualized as well as the presence of urine on the floor of the vagina. The degree of relaxation of the cervix can be determined, which is of assistance in evaluating the stage of the oestrous cycle.

Rectal palpation

When rectal palpation is combined with an efficient teasing programme the information obtained is extremely useful. It is important to know when palpating a mare whether or not the mare is in heat, the intensity of signs, and when she was last mated and ovulated. Rectal palpation can determine if a mare has a normal or abnormal uterus and ovaries. Ovarian cysts and tumours, postpartum haemorrhage, uterine adhesions and other abdominal structures can be diagnosed by careful rectal palpation. More definitive diagnosis of these conditions is possible by hormone assays and ultrasound examination but skilled rectal palpation can make a reasonably accurate diagnosis. Careful palpation can pinpoint the time mating should take place and reduce the number of matings required for conception. This is particularly important when mares are mated to busy stallions or stallions not residing on the same property as the mare. The mare should be palpated so development of the follicle can be charted allowing the mating schedule to be predicted 48 hours in advance. The number of palpations necessary will depend on the speed at which the follicle is developing and how accurate the forecast of ovulation needs to be for a particular stallion—the less fertile the stallion the more accurate the prediction of ovulation in the mare must be to compensate for the reduction in the longevity of the sperm. The palpater should note the number of follicles present on the ovaries and the number that actually ovulate. This information will help the scheduling of ultrasound examinations and the management of twin embryos should they be present.

The other value of rectal palpation is for pregnancy diagnosis. With the routine use of ultrasound careful palpation for early pregnancy has lost some of its importance. Skilled rectal palpaters can make an accurate diagnosis of pregnancy as early as 25 or 26 days post-ovulation and in the young maiden mare even earlier. Before the use of ultrasound, pregnancy diagnosis by palpation was performed at days 28, 35 and 45 and every 30 days subsequently until the end of the breeding season. Ultrasound has been substituted for the 28-day examination but otherwise rectal palpation is still relied upon to confirm pregnancy. Rectal palpation is by far the most frequently used diagnostic technique for the veterinarian in broodmare practice.

Ultrasound examination

As new medical technologies have developed they have been adapted to equine reproductive practice. Mares are biopsied to examine the cellular structure of their uterus. The flexible endoscope has made it possible to visually examine the lumen and lining of the mare's uterus, and laboratory tests have allowed cytological and bacteriological evaluation of the reproductive tract. But the technology which has made the largest contribution to enhancing reproductive performance of broodmares is ultrasound (see Figure 6.4). Ultrasonography uses the ability of tissues and fluid-filled structures to either reflect or propagate sound waves. A sound beam is emitted from a transducer or probe and that proportion of the beam which is reflected back to the probe is converted to electrical impulses and displayed on screen as a moving image. Liquid-filled structures do not reflect sound waves and appear black whereas dense tissues such as bone reflect more of the beam and appear white. Other tissues are seen as various shades of grey depending on their ability to reflect sound. Ultrasonic examination of the mare's reproductive tract has made the diagnosis of pregnancy, the management of twins and the diagnosis of uterine and ovarian abnormalities easier and more accurate. The initial use of ultrasound for pregnancy diagnosis of the mare was performed during the late 1970s and has become a routine procedure in all major horse breeding areas of the world. The first ultrasound machines were large and difficult to manage and because of the size of the rectal probe had the possibility of causing a rectal tear. Today ultrasound machines are the size of a briefcase, are portable and the probes are

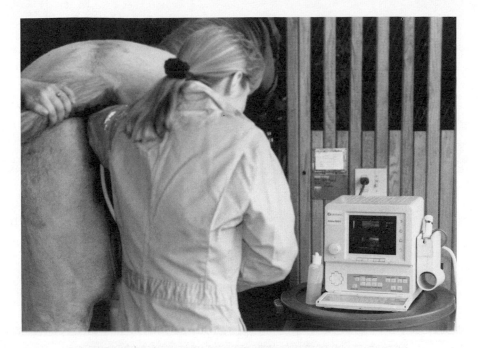

Figure 6.4 Performing an ultrasound examination.

the size of a small flash light. The image produced has greater definition than earlier machines so small defects and early pregnancies can be readily visualized. Veterinary ultrasound machines are continually being modified to incorporate a variety of options including video capabilities, built-in computers and calipers for taking measurements, and changes of frequency to enhance the image. When used judiciously ultrasound is an economical and useful tool, but should be used in conjunction with a complete reproductive management programme and not as a substitute for other routine procedures such as teasing.

The most modern ultrasound machines allow the diagnosis of pregnancy as early as 11 days following ovulation when the embryo or vesicle is about 9 mm in diameter and it is very mobile. Around 16 days post-ovulation the embryo becomes fixed in one of the horns of the uterus and has grown to about 20 mm. The developing embryo at days 17, 32 and 45 as observed by ultrasound is illustrated in Figures 6.5a, b, and c. The size of the embryo varies depending on the size of the lumen of the uterus. When high-quality ultrasound imaging is available the embryo and heartbeat are initially visualized at 22 days post-ovulation and by 26 or 27 days are very visible. When determining the time that ultrasonic examinations are to be carried out it is particularly important to calculate the days from ovulation and not days from mating as the embryo

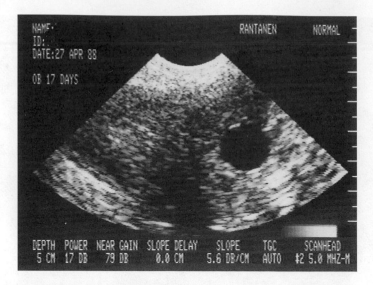

Figure 6.5 (a) Ultrasound photograph: day 17.

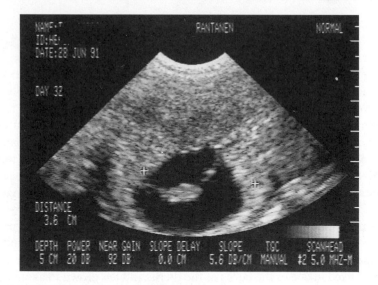

Figure 6.5 (b) Ultrasound photograph: day 32.

starts to develop after ovulation and fertilization have occurred. A mare can ovulate several days after she has been mated and still become pregnant so if the mating date is used rather than the ovulation date apparent discrepancies in the size of the embryo may be misinterpreted.

The times for pregnancy diagnosis will vary from farm to farm depending on

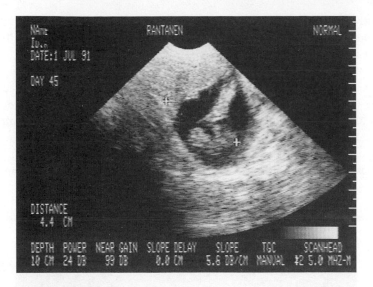

Figure 6.5 (**c**) Ultrasound photograph: day 45.

the intensity of management, the value of the mare and stallion fee, and availability of the veterinarian. The protocol on many broodmare farms requires a minimum of two ultrasound examinations, the timing of which depends on the number of rectal palpations performed. If a mare has ovulated one follicle and is a good teasing mare that shows 'in season' she will be given an ultrasound examination around 18 days post-ovulation. This provides sufficient time for the mare to return to oestrus if she is not pregnant so that an ultrasound examination is then unnecessary. It is also early enough in the cycle to enable the mare not showing normal oestrus and found not to be pregnant to be treated and mated again.

Ultrasound is used during the later stages of gestation to confirm pregnancy and evaluate the viability of the foetus. When mares have a large uterus with poor muscle tone the embryo may be difficult to palpate even in the more advanced stages of gestation. On these occasions ultrasound will confirm whether a mare is pregnant. If mares show signs of foetal distress, such as vaginal discharge and udder development, ultrasound can evaluate foetal viability. Using a large probe the foetus can be monitored through the abdominal wall to observe movement, heart rate, fluids and the placenta providing an excellent guide to the health of the foetus and the time of impending parturition or premature birth.

Sex determination of the foetus is another technique which has been made possible with the advent of ultrasound. There are specific times during gestation when sex determination is relatively easy to perform: at 60 days using a rectal probe and later using an abdominal probe. Sexing of embryos is not presently undertaken on a routine basis but with advances in reproductive technologies such as embryo transfer and *in vitro* fertilization it is likely to become more widely practised.

The management of twin pregnancies has been greatly improved by the use of ultrasound. Prior to its introduction, many mares were not mated when double follicles were palpated during oestrus. If mares were mated it was before the second follicle had ovulated, which required careful palpation. Using ultrasound, mares with double follicles are routinely mated, with the mare examined 14–16 days post-ovulation; if twin embryos are present (Figure 6.6) there are several options. One of the embryos can be ruptured manually,

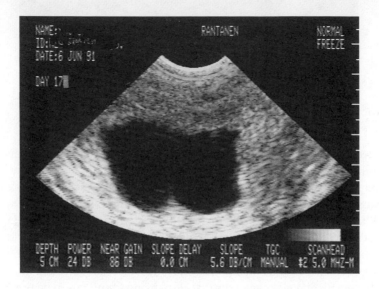

Figure 6.6 Ultrasound photograph of twin embryos at 17 days.

which is not difficult when they are in separate horns of the uterus as there is no danger to the remaining embryo in the other horn. Frequently, however, two embryos will be located in the same horn and in contact with each other. If the ultrasound examination is performed before 16 days the embryos will not be fixed. They can be separated by manipulation and one embryo ruptured— this requires considerable skill by the veterinarian. If both embryos rupture prostaglandin can be administered causing the mare to return to oestrus. Whenever manual reduction is performed it is important to perform an ultrasound scan on the mare within 4–72 hours to be sure the remaining embryo is progressing normally.

When twin pregnancies are not diagnosed early but are found at a later stage of pregnancy their management becomes more difficult. Manual rupture of an embryo can be performed up to 30 days post-ovulation but the survival rate of the remaining embryo is reduced. If the diagnosis is not made until after 30 days it is wiser to wait and re-examine the mare at about 115 days of gestation. Frequently one of the foetuses will die and become resorbed without any intervention. If this has not occurred, one foetus can be destroyed by injection of potassium chloride, allowing the other foetus to develop normally. If no intervention occurs, a large percentage of twins are likely to be aborted. Twins born alive are usually smaller than a single foal and their viability is poor. The mare is frequently more difficult to get in foal after she has delivered twins.

Pathological and abnormal conditions of the uterus can also be diagnosed with ultrasound. The most frequently observed uterine pathology is the presence of endometrial cysts. Cysts are present throughout the uterus but are usually observed to the right or the left of the uterine bifurcation. Although not a welcome finding they are compatible with pregnancy and cause few problems unless they are large and multiple, when they interfere with development of the embryo. They make diagnosis of pregnancy and twin detection difficult as small cysts look very similar to twin pregnancies. Large multiple cysts make the diagnosis of early pregnancy impossible. As the definition of high-quality ultrasound improves the differentiation between cysts and embryos becomes easier but the images may still be confusing. Cysts can be removed manually although a decision to do so should be based on the mare's reproductive history and the number and size of the cysts. Prior to the use of ultrasound the presence of cysts was diagnosed by palpation and consequently they had to be large before they were recognized.

It is now possible to determine the amount and consistency of fluid in a mare's uterus with the aid of ultrasound. As any appreciable amount of fluid is abnormal its presence is important in judging the suitability of a mare for breeding. When fluid is visualized an assessment can also be made of the type of fluid present. Blood, urine or exudate will show grey echogenic particles while normal transudate will be clear. The uterine musculature is also easily visualized during ultrasound examination. A haematoma in the musculature of the uterus can be recognized as well as the occasional tumour. These are not common but when present they have an adverse influence on the mare's fertility. When relying on palpation alone it is difficult to determine what exactly the enlargements are, and ultrasound has provided a non-invasive way to make a definitive diagnosis.

Structures palpated on a mare's ovaries can be evaluated by ultrasound. Follicles and corpora lutea can be visualized, counted, and ovulation sites confirmed. Anovulatory follicles can be differentiated from haematomas of the ovary, retained corpora lutea can be diagnosed, and tumours and cystic ovaries differentiated.

Laboratory aids to improve reproductive performance

Bacteriological examination

The most common procedure undertaken to evaluate a mare's reproductive state is the swabbing of the cervix, uterus and clitoral sinuses to identify the presence of bacterial pathogens (Figures 6.7 and 6.8). Uterine swabs are taken through a vaginal speculum when the mare is in heat and the cervix open. If a mare has an inflamed cervix with the presence of exudate a swab taken from the uterus should reveal the presence of pathogenic bacteria. The most common bacterium isolated is *Streptococcus zooepidemicus* followed by *Escherichia coli*, *Pseudomonas* and *Klebsiella*. Other bacteria, yeasts and fungi are isolated much less frequently. A swab taken under these conditions that does not reveal the presence of a pathogen should be repeated and the mare re-examined. By the same token if a mare appears normal on speculum examination and a swab reveals the presence of a bacterial organism the mare should be recultured before antibiotic therapy is initiated. This is particularly true if the bacteria isolated are not ones normally associated with uterine pathology.

Cytology

Cytology can be helpful in determining the status of the mare's uterus. A sample is taken by placing 60 ml of saline solution in the mare's uterus and withdrawing as much as possible. It is then centrifuged to concentrate the cells and examined under the microscope. The presence of inflammatory cells will assist in confirming results obtained by bacteriological examination.

Biopsy

Biopsies taken from the mare's uterus are more invasive than procedures discussed so far. They are obtained by passing a biopsy forceps through the cervix and pressing part of the wall of the uterus into the jaws of the forceps and taking a sample, which is then examined under the microscope. The procedure is performed to evaluate the state of a barren mare's uterus and predict the chances of a mare conceiving. Biopsies are graded from 1 to 3 depending on the extent of pathological lesions observed. Mares that are barren for no apparent reason should be biopsied before the next breeding season so if a problem is identified it can be treated prior to the start of the season. The diagnosis of uterine fibrosis can only be made by taking a biopsy. The presence of neutrophils in the wall of the uterus signals the presence of an inflammatory process even if no bacteria are cultured from the uterine swab.

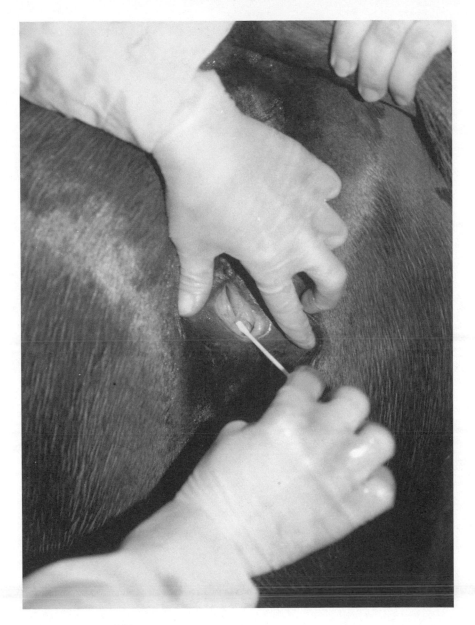

Figure 6.7 Swabbing the clitoral sinuses of a mare.

Endoscopic examination

Endoscopic examination of the reproductive tract is performed after the mare has been examined by other available methods which have proved inconclusive. The flexible endoscope has made direct visualization of the lumen of the

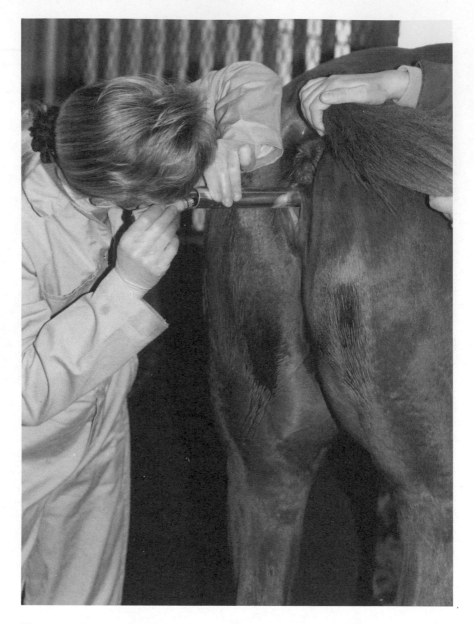

Figure 6.8 Examination of the mare's cervix.

mare's uterus possible. Endoscopic examination allows the operator to visualize and evaluate cysts, uterine fluid, tumours, adhesions and foreign bodies in the uterus. Cysts, fluid and tumours can in most instances be diagnosed by ultrasound examination so their presence will be known prior to the use of the endoscope. However, uterine adhesions, which cause serious infertility problems, are difficult if not impossible to diagnose by ultrasound but are easily visualized with the endoscope. Foreign bodies such as staples left after suturing a mare's vulva and the tips of swabs have been found with the aid of the endoscope; these would not have been identified by any other method.

Hormone assays

Many commercial test kits are available to determine levels of progesterone, testosterone, and oestradiol. The interpretation of the results is in several instances difficult as sufficient information regarding the range of normal values has yet to be established. Progesterone produced by the corpus luteum is one of the primary hormones responsible for the maintenance of pregnancy. Because of the cyclic nature of its production blood levels are difficult to interpret and the levels necessary to maintain pregnancy appear to vary considerably. In many instances progesterone therapy is given as a protection or insurance rather than to treat a specific deficiency. Corpus luteum malfunction with low levels of progesterone as a cause of reproductive failure is suspected but not proven. When progesterone is given to mares that have a history of abortion many will retain their pregnancy although this may be due entirely to chance. Progesterone blood levels are very useful in the non-pregnant mare as a diagnostic tool to identify the 'non-cycling' mare or the mare that is not showing signs of oestrus. The presence of even low levels of progesterone will override the oestradiol necessary to initiate oestrus and prevent the mare from showing signs. The source of progesterone in these cases is the corpus luteum which is still active and has not regressed, or a corpus luteum that was the result of an ovulation which was not detected. When progesterone is present in the non-cycling mare treatment with prostaglandin will destroy the corpus luteum and the mare will begin cycling. Not all mares which fail to show oestrus have a retained corpus luteum; some may be anoestrous. The anoestrous mare is not cycling because her ovaries are not functioning, no follicles are being produced and there is no oestradiol or progesterone production. Such mares must be differentiated from the cases described above since prostaglandin will not help these mares. Progesterone assay has made the differentiation of these two conditions possible and consequently therapy is more effective.

Oestradiol is produced by the ovarian follicle and foetus and assays are used to assess foetal health in the pregnant mare. In the later stages of pregnancy it can be used to predict the health of the foetus in cases of placental infection or systemic disease of the mare.

Pregnant mare's serum gonadotrophin (PMSG) produced by the endometrial cups stimulates production of progesterone by the ovaries until the cups regress. If the cups have formed and are producing PMSG the mare will not return to oestrus for 150 days whether she remains pregnant or not. Consequently foetal loss that occurs after the formation of the endometrial cups is likely to result in a mare not being mated again before the end of the breeding season. PMSG assays are a method of pregnancy diagnosis and although a useful test, can give a positive result after pregnancy loss has occurred. The assay is helpful in determining that a mare is no longer pregnant. Mares with detectable levels of PMSG in the blood are difficult to return to oestrus after pregnancy loss even following intensive therapy. If PMSG is not found in the pregnant mare it is likely that the endometrial cups have not formed and the likelihood of abortion is increased due to lack of secondary corpora luteal formation. In these instances progesterone therapy for the maintenance of pregnancy may be warranted.

Assays for luteinizing hormone are useful for the diagnosis of the non-cycling mare. It is important to know if LH is being secreted because by using GnRH therapy LH secretion can be stimulated. The same therapy would be counterproductive if sufficient LH were present and the inability to cycle was due to other factors.

Stallion management

Equally important to the success of a breeding operation is the effective management of the stallion. Stallion management has developed significantly following the introduction of techniques for artificial insemination and the transportation and use of chilled and frozen semen. The equine industry has not reached the same levels of sophistication in the handling of stallion semen that the cattle industry has with bull semen but there have been many advances in recent years. Several breed associations involved in the registration of their horses have placed restrictions on the use of artificial insemination but the development of these techniques has greatly enhanced our understanding of the physiology of equine semen and helped in the evaluation and handling of problem stallions.

Stallions are handled as individuals so it is the practice to tailor the feeding and exercise of the horse to its particular needs. The stallion should be in good physical condition and not allowed to become overweight. This is difficult if the horse has unlimited access to high-quality pasture but should be controlled. If the stallion is allowed to become overweight he will perform poorly; exercise programmes including regular walking or riding are very beneficial.

When a new stallion arrives at the farm, particularly if he has been in training, it is important to give him a chance to acclimatize before he is put to work as a breeding animal and before his fertility is evaluated. Stallions introduced to the breeding shed for the first time should be evaluated by collecting semen in an artificial vagina and examining a sample in the laboratory. In addition to semen evaluation the stallion's physical condition should be assessed. His testicles should be palpated and measured as testicular size and consistency is a good gauge of potential fertility. If the testicles are small and of poor consistency the chances of good semen quality are reduced. Whereas if the testicles are large and have a firm resilient consistency the chances of acceptable semen quality are increased. Semen evaluation should be performed by an experienced examiner as if improperly performed the results are of little relevance. Semen is adversely affected by temperature and by residues left in the artificial vagina so it must be handled correctly to obtain results which are accurate and repeatable.

Young stallions which are to be collected using an artificial vagina are often allowed to mate naturally at first until they have confidence in mating a mare. When the young stallion is introduced to the artificial vagina care must be taken that it is large enough and does not pinch the penis (Figure 6.9). It is critical that the water temperature of the artificial vagina is between 37.8 and 38.9 °C (100–102 °F) at the time of collection (Figure 6.10). An inappropriate temperature is one of the major reasons for failure to collect. If the stallion will not ejaculate into the vagina and becomes frustrated it is better not to continue than allow him to become upset.

Stallions should be easy to handle in the breeding shed and disciplined to eliminate unruly behavioural problems. Time taken in educating the stallion to the routine of the breeding shed will be of considerable benefit, especially when he is mated to difficult mares. Stallions that are taught not to rush mares and take their time are less likely to injure themselves, the mares and their handlers. The breeding shed or covering area should be large enough to accommodate the personnel needed to assist with mating. A minimum of three people are needed: one to hold the mare's head, one the tail, and the stallion's handler. The stallion should be allowed to approach the mare and mount only after he has developed a proper erection. If he has not been allowed to mate for days or weeks it is advisable to clean smegma from his penis and sheath with a mild soap and rinse with water. After mating, the penis should also be washed with water. Too much washing with disinfectant solutions is counterproductive as it will kill the normal bacterial flora on the penis and allow pathogenic bacteria to multiply. As with the stallion, it is appropriate to wash the mares with clean water and mild soap, rinse well and bandage the tail before breeding (Figure 6.11). Any mare showing signs of illness should not be taken to the breeding shed as it is an ideal environment to spread contagious or other infectious disease among a herd and the entire equine community.

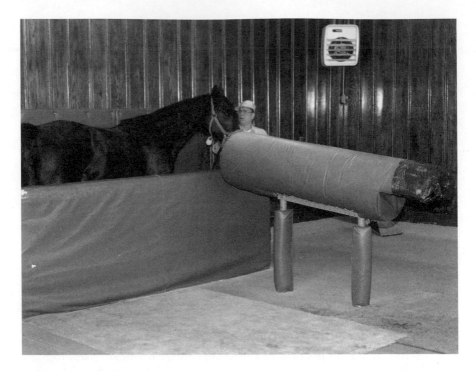

Figure 6.9 Dummy mare for stallion to mount during semen collection.

Stallion managers should not book too many mares to a young stallion until his fertility is known. If a young horse covers a group of fertile mares early in the season his fertility can be assessed and other mares added as the season progresses. When a stallion is over-booked and he has to mate mares three or four times a day, his fertility and libido become reduced. When a stallion's semen reserves are depleted by frequent breeding his daily sperm output becomes reduced. This applies particularly to horses with a small testicular size and they should be regularly evaluated by the examination of semen samples.

Older mature stallions are easier to manage because they have an established pattern of reproductive performance. Their physical condition and semen quality should be examined at the beginning of the year and changes in semen quality or testicular consistency noted. Stallions with reduced fertility the previous season should be evaluated and if necessary an adjustment made in the number of mares to be mated. If a stallion is so popular that mares can be selected from a pool of applicants it is wise to select mares on their reproductive history as well as their pedigree. As the breeding season progresses mares should be monitored to ensure they are not returning to oestrus or coming back into oestrus under 17 days. If the return rate on mares is higher

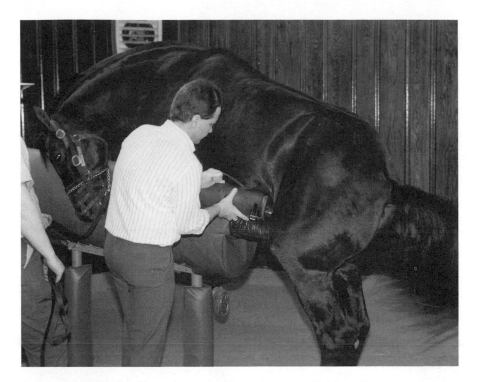

Figure 6.10 Collecting semen from a stallion using an artificial vagina.

than 50% a semen evaluation and general examination should be performed to determine if there has been a decline in the stallion's fertility. The stallion should be observed during mating to be sure he is ejaculating properly. Some stallions develop behavioural traits which cause them to appear to have ejaculated when they have not. If mares mated by the stallion are under the control of the stallion manager and his veterinarian they should be examined, particularly for evidence of infectious disease. However, if mares come from several farms it is often more difficult to establish the pattern of infection as it is not immediately evident that a problem in one mare is common to other mares mated by the same stallion. When this situation arises it is essential to enlist the co-operation of all farms sending mares to the stallion so a diagnosis can be reached quickly.

In major horse breeding centres around the world the stallion is the focal point of the breeding operation. Mares from a wide geographical area are mated and return home or reside permanently on the farm throughout the breeding season. When mares are sent from many different farms to be mated the risk of the spread of disease, including venereal disease, is high. The stallion manager should be constantly aware of this situation and ever vigilant. Experience has demonstrated that a little over-reaction early in a disease

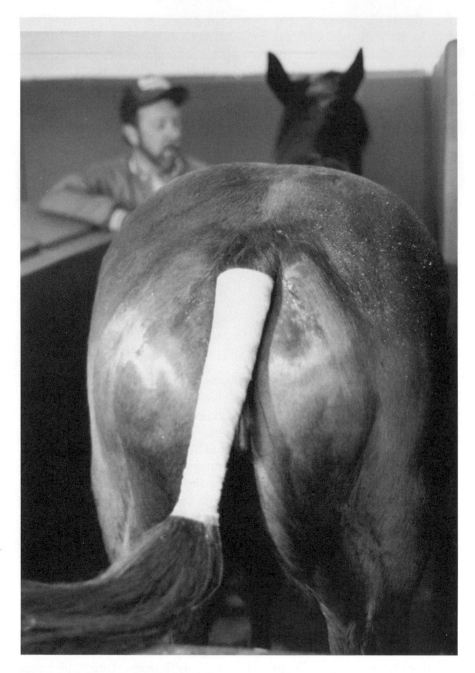

Figure 6.11 Bandaging the mare's tail prior to mating.

outbreak can save time and money. Respiratory disease caused by influenza, strangles and venereal diseases including equine viral arteritis, contagious equine metritis, coital exanthema, *Pseudomonas* and *Klebsiella* infections can all be spread in the breeding shed.

Stallions with reduced fertility of non-infectious cause can sometimes be helped with hormone therapy if the condition has been accurately diagnosed. Of particular current interest is the use of GnRH, and although the number of horses treated is small the results are encouraging. GnRH stimulates testosterone production and appears to improve sperm motility and libido. The most practical way to administer GnRH at the present time is by a pump that gives regular injections several times a day. When a stallion's infertility is due to low number or poor viability of sperm he should be managed to maximize the opportunity of getting mares to conceive. If the problem is the lack of sufficient numbers of sperm his book should be reduced so there is sufficient sperm production between each ejaculation to result in fertilization. If sperm viability is the problem then mares must be examined frequently so they are mated as close to ovulation as possible to maximize the chance of conception.

The management of broodmares and stallions is a complicated mix of horsemanship, veterinary skills, and record keeping which when working in harmony can produce successful and spectacular results.

Further reading

Ginther O J (1992) *Reproductive biology of the mare: basic and applied aspects* 2nd edn. Equiservices, Cross Plains, WI.

Ginther O J (1986) *Ultrasonic imaging and reproductive events in the mare*. Equiservices, Cross Plains, WI.

Morrow D A (1986) *Current therapy in theriogenology 2*. W B Saunders, Philadelphia.

Pickett B W, Amann R P, McKinnon A O, Squires E L, Voss J L (1989) *Management of the stallion for maximum reproductive efficiency. II*. Animal Reproduction Laboratory Bulletin No. 05. Colorado State University, Fort Collins.

Pickett B W, Squires E L, McKinnon A O (1987) *Procedures for collection, evaluation and utilization of stallion semen for artificial insemination*. Animal Reproduction Laboratory Bulletin No. 03. Colorado State University, Fort Collins.

Robinson N E (1992) *Current therapy in equine medicine 3*. W B Saunders, Philadelphia.

Rossdale P D, Ricketts S W (1980) *Equine studfarm medicine* 2nd edn. Baillière Tindall, London.

Van Camp S D (1988) *Reproduction*. The Veterinary Clinics of North America, Equine Practice, W B Saunders, Philadelphia.

Varner D D, Schumacher J, Blanchard T L, Johnson L (1991) *Diseases and management of breeding stallions*. American Veterinary Publications, Goleta, CA.

INTERNAL PARASITES AND THEIR CONTROL

J. HAROLD DRUDGE, DVM, ScD; and EUGENE T. LYONS, PhD

Summary

The vitality and well-being of horses of all ages are threatened by a variety of internal parasites, and the use of control measures ensures vigour and best performance. The occurrence, developmental cycles, clinical signs and control methods for infections of the five most important internal parasites are discussed. These parasitic infections include large strongyles, small strongyles, ascarids, pinworms and bots. Additionally, less important infections of tapeworms, lungworms and the intestinal threadworm (*Strongyloides*) are described briefly.

Horses, ponies, and other equids are hosts for a large number of internal parasites. Five types occur commonly and are generally regarded as the most harmful. This chapter will focus on four helminth worm infections (large and small strongyles, ascarids and pinworms) and one insect (bots). All of these parasites undergo direct development in their life cycle (Figure 7.1) and no intermediate host is required.

Nearly every horse is infected with one or more of these internal parasites at any given time, except for newborn foals, which are born free of parasites. However, foals are quite susceptible and usually start 'picking up' worm infections (ascarids, strongyles and pinworms) when initially turned out during the first two weeks of life. The amount of contact, either direct or indirect, between foals and their dams and other mature or adolescent horses determines the intensity of the parasite burden acquired by foals.

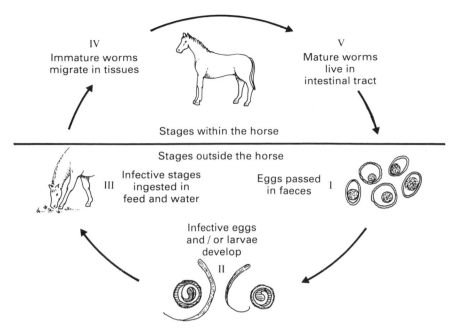

Figure 7.1 Life cycle illustrating direct development, i.e. without an intermediate host, typical of strongyles, ascarids and pinworms in equids.

Several other factors affect these parasitic infections. Season and climatic conditions are influential to varying degrees. Bot infection produces only a single generation per year. Therefore, the activity of the adult botfly and the occurrence of the larvae (bots) in the horse are seasonal. Pasture herbage functions as the vehicle for transmission of strongyle larvae. Spread is favoured by warm, moist climatic conditions. On the other extreme, ascarid eggs are exceptionally resistant to environmental conditions, and once contaminated, soil in stables, paddocks and pastures may remain a potential source of infection for several years on a year-round basis.

Development of each of these parasites within the horse follows a distinctive pattern. Migrations of some helminths, e.g. small strongyles, are limited to the superficial intestinal tissues, infections tend to be benign, and development to maturity takes only 6–12 weeks. In contrast, large strongyles undergo extensive migration in the visceral tissues and organs and cause severe and even fatal damage. They require a long time period of 6–11 months to develop into adult worms. Age relationships are also a feature of these parasitic infections. Young equids, especially suckling and weanling foals, are usually infected with ascarids. Exposure during early development stimulates an immune response which renders the infections self-limiting, as a result of which adult ascarids are not found in mature equids. In contrast other parasites, bots and small strongyles do not elicit a significant immune response even with repeated exposures, and infections recur throughout the life of the horse. Large strongyles are intermediate between the two foregoing extremes. Foals are especially susceptible and are prone to suffer the acute effects of redworm (bloodworm) infection (*Strongylus vulgaris*). Adolescent and mature horses remain vulnerable to infection but the effects tend to be chronic and recurrent episodes of colic are a typical sign.

Parasite control continues to be an important element in the preventive health care of horses. Infections of one or more parasites are an everyday problem, as opposed to bacterial or viral infections, which tend to be sporadic. Accordingly, successful strategies for parasite control are continuous long-term undertakings rather than short–term measures such as antibiotic therapy to control bacterial infection.

The design of a parasite control programme depends upon several factors and demands recognition of the biological aspects of the infections. The variables noted previously are compounded by the presence of concurrent infections of two or more types of parasites. Farm factors such as number, type and age of horses present, type and amount of grazing available, management practices, etc. must be taken into account. Ideally, the design of a programme for a given farm should be a co-operative venture between the farm owner/ manager and the veterinarian.

Considerable progress has been made over the last 50 years in the control of internal parasites using anthelmintics and other drugs. Commencing in 1940 with the compounds phenothiazine and carbon disulphide, there are now over 25 compounds or mixtures from eight different chemical classes of drugs currently available. Thus, for many years, there have been effective methods to control all of the important gastrointestinal parasites of the horse. Whilst considerable reliance has been placed on these anthelmintics, good sanitary and management practices are recognized as an important adjunct and are used to supplement the antiparasitic drugs. Presently, there is no means of biological control and no antiparasitic equine vaccine has been developed. The five important parasites will be discussed separately because each has distinctive aspects of development, types of infections and control requirements. Several parasites of lesser importance including tapeworms, lungworms and the intestinal threadworm (*Strongyloides*) are discussed briefly in a separate section. Dosages for compounds or products mentioned herein are not detailed because of changing formulations, conditions or individual preferences and because the label and package inserts should be read and understood completely before any product is used.

Information presented in this chapter is derived from a number of sources in the scientific literature and from the authors' personal experience. These are not specifically cited in the text, but those seeking more information on the subject matter are referred to the works cited under 'Further Reading'.

Large strongyles

These roundworms, also known as 'redworms' or 'bloodworms', are the most dangerous of all of the parasites that infect the horse. Their life-threatening potential results from the extensive and prolonged migrations of the invading larval stages in several abdominal or visceral organs and tissues. Severe, often fatal, tissue damage may be caused by a seemingly small number (500) of larvae. The adult or sexually mature large strongyles damage the gut lining where they attach and suck blood.

The large strongyle group contains three species—*Strongylus vulgaris*, *Strongylus edentatus* and *Strongylus equinus*. The first two are prevalent in equids world-wide; the third is less common and sporadic in occurrence.

Development

Strongyles complete their developmental cycles directly, as illustrated in Figure 7.1, without an intermediate host. The free-living or extrinsic phase of development takes place outside the host on pastures and paddocks. Eggs laid by mature strongyles inhabiting the large intestine pass to the outside in the faeces. With favourable temperature and moisture conditions the eggs develop to third stage or infective larvae in about 1 week. Infective larvae do not feed but are quite active on pasture herbage (Figure 7.2). Their development is dependent upon being swallowed by grazing horses. Horses also ingest strongyle larvae from pond water and bedding. Cold weather and short periods of rainfall slow larval development. Infective larvae can survive winter or drought because they are enclosed in a protective sheath. However, longevity of larvae is limited because depletion of their stored food supply is certain to occur—a matter of weeks or months during warm seasons in temperate climates.

Following ingestion by the horse, infective larvae undergo further development. Large strongyle larvae penetrate the intestinal wall and migrate extensively in abdominal tissues or organs before reaching maturity in the large intestine. Larvae of *S. vulgaris* are the most notorious because their migrations damage the inner lining of the anterior mesenteric artery and its branches, resulting in aneurysms, thrombi and embolisms (Figure 7.3). Larvae of *S. edentatus* and *S. equinus* follow different routes of migration in the abdominal organs and tissues and may be found under the peritoneal lining of the abdomen, in the liver, pancreas and intestinal walls. They are not involved in aneurysms of the mesenteric arteries. The migration of immature large strongyles is prolonged and development to sexual maturity requires about 6 months for *S. vulgaris*, 9 months for *S. equinus*, and 11 months for *S. edentatus*. Adult worms attach themselves to the inner lining of the caecum and colon

(Figure 7.4), causing damage to the mucosa as they suck blood. Mixed infections of large strongyles with small strongyles are very common.

Clinical signs

Signs of large strongyle infections are related to arterial lesions produced by migrating larvae of the true bloodworm, *S. vulgaris*, of which colic is the most common sign. Bouts of colic tend to recur, and prior to the advent of modern anthelmintics to control strongyle infections, the vast majority of colics were caused by migrating *S. vulgaris*. Fatal infections may occur in suckling and weanling foals if several hundred larvae of *S. vulgaris* are ingested over a short period of time and there is blockage of the mesenteric arteries. Intermittent episodes of colic in older horses and the sudden acute attacks of abdominal distress in foals indicate the need to review and upgrade the parasite control practices.

Faecal consistency may be affected by strongyle infections, of which diarrhoea is the most common sign. It is frequently associated with arterial lesions caused by *S. vulgaris* larvae, but a persistent diarrhoea is also related to hepatic damage due to larvae of *S. edentatus*.

Changes in blood cell and serum protein components are also related to infections of large strongyles. Anaemia, as noted by paleness of mucous membranes or reduced red blood cell values following haematological examination, is a common finding. An increase in white blood cells, especially granulocytes and eosinophils, is regarded by some as a specific marker of arterial infections of *S. vulgaris*. The increase of eosinophils may also be caused by *S. edentatus* and small strongyles as well as other non-verminous allergic-type agents. Biochemical tests may reveal changes in serum proteins and other chemical components. Increases in total serum protein, coupled with a decrease in the ratio of the albumin/globulin fractions are indicative of early strongyle infections.

Other less definitive clinical signs of large strongyle and other parasitic infections include unthriftiness, dull or roughened hair coat, and impaired performance even when there is an adequate level of nutrition.

Control

Large strongyles should be the focal point of the internal parasite control programme among groups of horses. Measures applied to suppress the continuous presence of strongyles will also be helpful in curbing infections of other parasites. Control measures should include the following.

Sanitation

Care of stables, drylots (small pens devoid of vegetation) and paddocks should ensure clean, dry bedding plus protection of feed troughs, hay racks and waterers from faecal matter. Manure and soiled bedding should be composted or spread on arable fields to avoid contamination of areas grazed by horses. The daily removal of manure deposits from pastures is theoretically sound, but is usually found to be incomplete, time-consuming and unfeasible in practice.

Pasture rotation

Movement of horses to clean, uncontaminated pastures is helpful, but often limited by stable and fencing restrictions. Young foals and yearlings should be given preferential consideration for grazing locations.

Stocking rate

Population density should be held within reasonable limits, because strongyle infection risks increase geometrically; i.e. doubling the horses/hectare quadruples the exposure.

Rotation of animal species

Sequential grazing of pastures with horses and ruminants serves to reduce parasitic infections in both species because cross-transmission of internal parasites does not occur except for one species of stomach worm, *Trichostrongylus axei*, of minor importance in horses.

Chain harrowing and clipping (topping) of pastures

These are good agronomic practices and also make microclimatic conditions in the pasture less favourable for the development and survival of strongyle eggs and larvae.

Treatment with anthelmintics

Contemporary control programmes for strongyles as well as other internal parasites rely heavily on the administration at regular 6–8 week intervals of therapeutic doses of antiparasitic agents as listed in Table 7.1. This approach removes adult, egg-bearing strongyles and other parasites from the intestinal tract, which in turn results in reduced pasture contamination with eggs and larvae. A large number of compounds or mixtures have been developed and are currently used for internal parasite control. Most of these compounds,

Table 7.1. Antiparasitic compounds for major internal parasites of horses available in the USA.

Class	Generic name	Tradename	Manufacturer	Method of administration[3]
Avermectins	Ivermectin[1]	Eqvalan	Merck	P,T
Benzimidazoles (BZ)	Fenbendazole (FBZ)[1]	Panacur	Hoechst	T,F,P
	Mebendazole (MBZ)[1]	Telmin	Pitman-Moore, Janssen	T,F,P
	MBZ + TCF	Telmin B	Pitman-Moore	T,F,P
	Oxfendazole (OFZ)[1]	Benzelmin	Syntex	T,F,P
	OFZ + TCF	Benzelmin Plus	Syntex	P
	Oxibendazole (OBZ)[1]	Anthelcide EQ	SmithKline Beecham	T,F,P
	Oxibendazole (OBZ)[1]	Equipar	Coopers	T,F,P
	Thiabendazole (TBZ)[1]	Equizole	Merck	T,F
	TBZ + PPZ	Equizole A	Merck	T,F
Phenylguanidines (PRO − BZ)	Febantel (FBT)	Rintal	Haver	T,F,P
	FBT + TCF	Combotel	Haver	P
Organophosphates	Dichlorvos (DDVP)[1]	Equigard	Squibb	F
	Trichlorfon (TCF)	Combot	Haver	T,P
Piperazines	Piperazine (PPZ)[1]	Various	Various	T
	PPZ-CDS + PTZ	Parvex Plus[2]	Upjohn	T
	PPZ + PTZ + TCF	Dyrex T.F.	Ft. Dodge	T
Pyrimidines	Pyrantel (PRT)	Strongid T	Pfizer	T,F
	Pyrantel (PRT)[1]	Strongid Paste	Pfizer	P
	Pyrantel (PRT)	Strongid C	Pfizer	F (LL)
	Pyrantel (PRT)	Imathal Equine	SmithKline Beecham	T,F
Other	Phenothiazine (PTZ)	Various	Various	T,F
	Phenothiazine (PTZ)	Various	Various	F (LL)
	Carbon Disulphide (CDS)	Various	Various	T

[1] Available in UK.
[2] Not available currently.
[3] P = paste; T = stomach tube; F = feed; LL = low level.

including ivermectin, fenbendazole, mebendazole, oxfendazole, oxibendazole, thiabendazole, dichlorvos pellets, febantel and pyrantel, are efficacious against large strongyles as well as other internal parasites. Additionally, several products utilize mixtures of piperazine with phenothiazine or levamisole for effective activity against strongyles. Several of the newer compounds including ivermectin, fenbendazole and oxfendazole are active against migratory large strongyle larvae at regular dosages or in prescribed dosage regimens. This is important because control of strongyles is enhanced considerably whenever these compounds are used.

Several guidelines should be followed to obtain maximum benefit from the use of antiparasitic agents in a control programme:

(a) The advice of the farm's veterinarian should be sought in developing and implementing the control programme which should be designed on an individual farm basis.

(b) All equids on the farm should be included in the programme. Benefits are quickly lost by omitting treatment of a barren mare, teaser or pony, thereby allowing repeat contamination of pastures and paddocks.

(c) Temporary boarders and other new additions should be isolated and wormed before being turned out with resident horses.

(d) Laboratory examination of faecal samples should be undertaken periodically to monitor the effectiveness of the anthelmintics being used and the overall success of the control programme. Comparisons of post-treatment (2-week) worm egg counts (eggs per gram) with those obtained immediately before treatment provide an index of drug resistance—indicated if reduction of the count is less than the anticipated 90–100%.

(e) Rotation of anthelmintics. It is not advisable to use one compound or class of drugs exclusively. Prolonged use of a single product fosters the selection of drug-resistant parasites. This has not been demonstrated for large strongyles, but phenothiazine- and benzimidazole-resistant small strongyles have been recognized for a number of years. A variety of control programmes, calling for six or more treatments per year, can be devised from the large number of available products. Some rotation of products provides a complementary effect of different compounds, especially the larvicidal action of some of the newer products. Trade or brand names of products can be deceptive, and the unwary may unwittingly use the same class of chemicals or even the same compound repeatedly. Professional veterinary advice and assistance with the generic names of active ingredients will obviate any confusion on this aspect of product selection.

(f) Method of administration. Changes of dosage formulation have accompanied the development of compounds with higher levels of activity. Pastes, gels and feed premix formulations, as well as those containing piperazine for traditional stomach tube administration, are available. The activity of a given compound is the same irrespective of the product formulation or method of treatment, providing the intended therapeutic dose is successfully administered. In this regard the stomach tube, although requiring the expertise of the veterinarian, is most reliable. Administration via the feed should be monitored carefully to ensure complete consumption. Paste or gel formulations can be given quickly with minimum restraint of the horse and low risk of injury to personnel, and are a significant advance in the treatment of parasitic infections of the horse. Dosing with pastes or gels is handicapped by food or excess saliva in the mouth, which may enable the horse to spit out the drug. It is advisable to delay feeding until after attempting treatment with a paste or gel. Currently no injectable products are available.

(g) Labels and package inserts. These should be read and completely understood before a product is administered. Active ingredients are indicated along with dosage recommendations and special preparatory procedures. Precautions and contraindications on the label should be strictly adhered to.

Small strongyles

The small strongyle group is a large, heterogenous mixture of helminths found in the caecum and large colon of equids. Some workers currently refer to the largest portion of this group as 'cyathostomes', formerly known as 'trichonema'. The small strongyle designation includes 40 species of strongyles whose biological characteristics are similar to each other but different from large strongyles. Of all of the equine parasites small strongyles are the most common. Except for the newborn or very young foal, it is unusual for a horse to be completely free of small strongyles. Infections of small strongyles often number in the tens of thousands, in contrast to the several hundreds or fewer of large strongyles.

Development

The life cycle of small strongyles is direct, without an intermediate host, and their development outside the host is essentially the same as that outlined for large strongyles. Characteristics of development and survival of infective larvae on pasture herbage are also similar to those of large strongyles. Larvae of both large and small strongyles commingle and occupy the same sites on pastures.

The major difference between large and small strongyles occurs during development within the horse. Following ingestion, migration of the invading infective larvae of small strongyles is limited to the inner lining of the gut wall. For many species, the larvae locate superficially in the mucosa of the caecum and large colon and may not induce a noticeable tissue reaction as shown in Figures 7.5a and b. For other species, invading larvae encyst more deeply and may stimulate the formation of small nodules. After a period of development in the mucosa, small strongyle larvae emerge into the gut lumen as fourth stage larvae. These are commonly found with the fifth stage adult small strongyles in gut contents. Adult small strongyles tend to concentrate in the contents of the large intestine in proximity to the mucosa. This appears to be a favourable site for feeding because, with the exception of a few species as illustrated in Figure 7.6, small strongyles do not attach to the gut lining.

The time required for maturation of the invading larvae into sexually mature worms varies for the small strongyle species, but is about 6 to 12 weeks. Under natural conditions, development may be inhibited and time to reach maturation is extended. This process of inhibition, so-called 'hypobiosis', is not completely understood, but larvae are known to persist in the mucosa for 2–3 years. This inhibited or delayed developmental phase is very important to the understanding of small strongyle control.

Clinical signs

Signs of small strongyle infection are generally less noticeable than those associated with large strongyles. The damage caused by small strongyles results from the encystment of the larval stages in the gut mucosa. Heavy infections of the encysted larvae seriously impair the digestive function of the large intestine and cause intermittent spells of diarrhoea, constipation, and occasionally impaction. Sudden onset of diarrhoea in mature horses in the springtime has been associated with the massive emergence of large numbers of inhibited small strongyle larvae from the mucosa. Changes in blood parameters described for large strongyles have also been associated with small strongyle infections. Alterations in the serum proteins may be similar and changes in red and white cell components may also occur, but generally to a lower order of magnitude than from large strongyle infections. Less definitive systemic effects, such as unthriftiness, are also attributable to infections of small strongyles.

Control

All of the sanitary and hygienic measures plus pasture and management practices outlined for large strongyles, will assist with the control of small strongyles. Likewise, all the anthelmintics that are effective for large strongyles are more efficacious for removal of small strongyles, except for the drug-resistant populations.

The resistance of small strongyles to the chemical classes of compounds known as the benzimidazoles (BZ) and probenzimidazoles (PRO-BZ) including phenylguanidines has become widespread in recent years. Characteristically, a population of small strongyles in a group of horses that is resistant to one BZ-compound is refractory to other drugs in the class (e.g. thiabendazole, mebendazole, fenbendazole and oxfendazole) and the PRO-BZ, febantel, but not to oxibendazole. The reason for the exceptional effectiveness of oxibendazole against populations of BZ-resistant small strongyles is not understood. There is limited evidence it may be transitional and long-term intensive use will reduce oxibendazole's effectiveness. Recently, data indicated low-grade levels of resistance to piperazine and pyrantel for two populations of BZ-resistant small strongyles in Kentucky. Compounds from other classes of chemicals, including ivermectin, pyrantel, and dichlorvos, remain effective in curbing the build-up of BZ-resistant small strongyles in equine populations.

Options to combat BZ-resistant populations of small strongyles are provided by mixtures of compounds. These include piperazine mixed with thiabendazole or other benzimidazoles. The high efficacy of the BZ-component against large strongyles is retained and the piperazine acts against the BZ-resistant small strongyles. A variety of control programmes can be designed from the large number of anthelmintic products currently available.

Ascarids

The large roundworm (*Parascaris equorum*) is the largest parasite in the horse. Infections are very common, especially in suckling foals and weanlings and to a lesser extent in yearlings and 2-year-old horses. Immunity develops by exposure to infection during adolescence so mature horses are usually not infected with adult ascarids. Mature ascarids inhabit the anterior and midportions of the small intestine. In addition to their size—females can grow to 25 cm or more in length—large masses consisting of several hundred worms may be present.

Development

A simple direct life cycle is also a feature of the large roundworm. Female worms are prolific egg-layers, producing about 200 000 eggs/female/day. Eggs are passed to the outside in the faeces. Under favourable environmental conditions, eggs develop to the infective stage in 2 weeks. Ascarid eggs do not hatch outside the host; instead the infective larva is retained within the thick egg shell. This protective feature favours perpetuation of the species, as the thick-shelled eggs are resistant to adverse environmental conditions and survive for years in the soil of stables, paddocks and pastures.

Embryonated ascarid eggs are ingested by foals in contaminated feed or water. The eggs hatch in the intestine, releasing larvae that penetrate the intestinal wall. Thereafter, they migrate in the bloodstream via the portal circulation to the liver and thence to the lungs. The liver-lung migration takes about 2 weeks before the larvae penetrate the respiratory passages, are coughed up and swallowed a second time. Development to maturation takes place in the

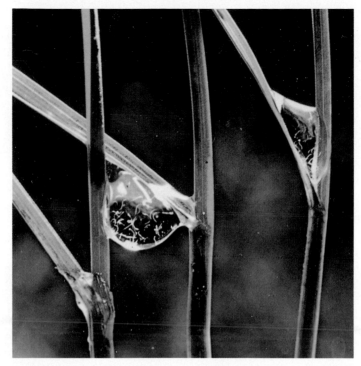

Figure 7.2 Infective larvae of strongyles present in droplets of water on blades of grass awaiting ingestion.

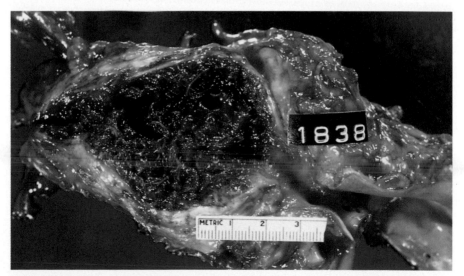

Figure 7.3 Aneurysm of the anterior mesenteric artery caused by migrating larvae of *Strongylus vulgaris*, showing large thrombus in the lumen of the enlarged artery.

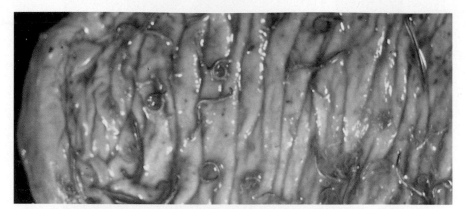

Figure 7.4 Mature, blood-engorged large strongyles attached to the mucosa of the large intestine.

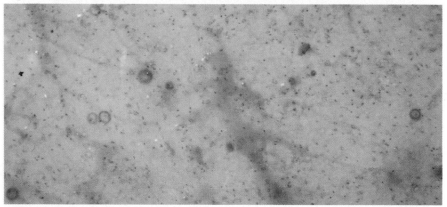

Figure 7.5 (a) Larvae of small strongyles embedded in the mucosa of the caecum and colon. Gross view showing range of sizes between large red signet-ring forms and the small black specks.

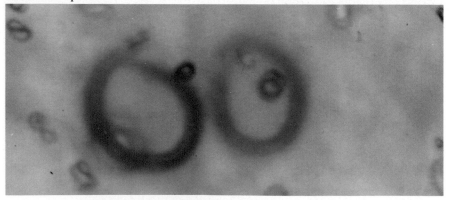

Figure 7.5 (b) Photomicrograph of small strongyle larvae embedded in mucosa revealing the form of the specks in Figure 5 (a).

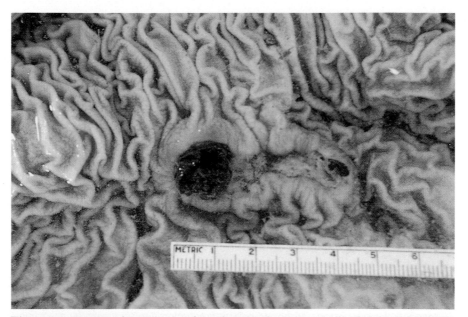

Figure 7.6 Mucosa of dorsal colon featuring a darkened crater-like lesion caused by a small strongyle (*Triodontophorus*).

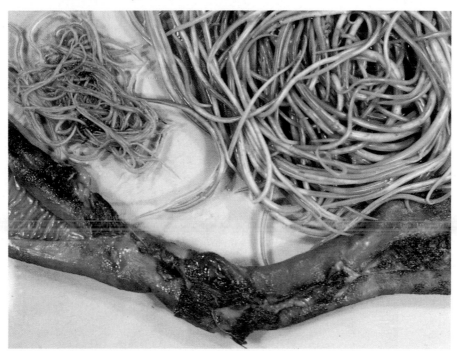

Figure 7.7 Masses of immature (left) and mature (right) ascarids (*Parascaris equorum*) near a rupture of the wall of the small intestine of a foal.

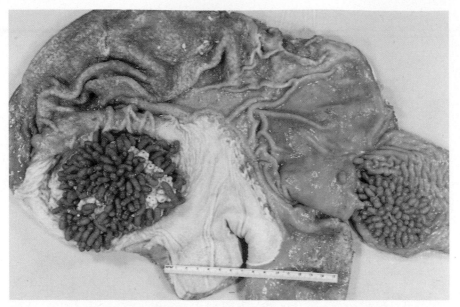

Figure 7.8 Typical clusters of the red-coloured common bot (*Gasterophilus intestinalis*) and the yellow-coloured throat bot (*G. nasalis*) attached to walls of stomach and duodenum, respectively.

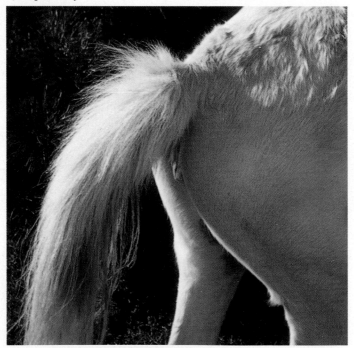

Figure 7.9 Tailhead of horse with loss of hair and roughened appearance due to rubbing induced by pinworm infection (*Oxyuris equi*).

small intestine about 10 weeks after the infective eggs are ingested. The principal source of infection is soil contaminated with egg-laden faeces from foals of previous years. Patent or mature ascarid infections are first observed when foals are 10–12 weeks old.

Clinical signs

Respiratory signs including coughing and excess oral and nasal exudates have been associated with the lung migration of ascarid larvae. Naturally exposed foals usually do not ingest sufficient numbers of ascarid eggs to induce overt respiratory signs. Other agents including viruses and bacteria are more likely to induce coughs and nasal exudates among foals.

In the small intestine, low-grade ascarid infections are usually asymptomatic, but accumulations of worms may cause several manifestations. Colic may be a sign of an ascarid-induced hypermotility or telescoping of a segment of the small intestine. More severe abdominal distress, shock and death are seen when the small intestinal wall is ruptured and peritonitis develops. This primary danger stems from accumulations of masses of ascarids and it usually occurs in foals in late summer or fall (Figure 7.7). In recent years, however, the widespread use of piperazine and broad-spectrum anthelmintics has markedly reduced the prevalence of intestinal rupture by ascarids.

Systemic effects of ascarid infection in foals include unthriftiness, lassitude and loss of appetite. A 'pot-bellied appearance' of foals is regarded by some as typically indicative of ascarid infection.

Control

Sanitation and management, especially of stalls and paddocks, can be a significant aid in the control of ascarid infection. Successive crops of foals acquire their infections from the carry-over of ascarid eggs in the environment from year to year. This source of early infection in foals is potentiated by the practice on many farms to repeatedly use the same barn and associated paddocks for foaling and housing of mares and their young foals.

Preventive measures for reduction of ascarid egg infestation of stables and paddocks include proper manure disposal, protection of grain bunkers and waterers from faecal contamination, and rotational use of paddocks for young horses on a long-term basis rather than annually. Muzzling of foals for the turn-out periods during the first few weeks after birth has been used in the past to reduce exposure to ascarid infection.

Treatment of foals with anthelmintics is the most effective means of suppressing transmission and reducing the level of ascarid infections. It requires a sustained schedule of periodic treatments of succeeding crops of foals over a period of years. For nursery operations in central Kentucky, a routine treatment schedule for ascarid control is initiated when foals are about 8 weeks of age. This removes the earliest ascarid infections before they mature and eggs are shed. Subsequent treatments are administered at 8-week intervals to prevent maturation of later infections. These bimonthly treatments are continued until the foals become yearlings, when the emphasis is shifted to strongyle control. Most of the compounds used for strongyle control also remove ascarids. Continuation of periodic treatments for strongyles serves to remove ascarids, which occur in decreasing frequency in adolescent and mature horses.

Drug resistance of the equine ascarid to anthelmintics has not been reported. Piperazine has been the mainstay of ascarid control for over 30 years without apparent loss of activity. Shortcomings against ascarids are recognized for some of the modern-day anthelmintics although none of these has been attributed to acquired drug resistance.

Bots

Bots are usually found in the stomach. They are the larval stages of botflies, and are therefore quite different from the worm parasites. Bots have rivalled strongyles as being the most common of the parasitic infections. All ages of horses are infected and bots are found in stomachs at any time of the year. Two main species, the common bot (*Gasterophilus intestinalis*) and the throat bot (*G. nasalis*), have a world-wide distribution. Additional species (*G. pecorum* and *G. inermis*) infect equids in other countries, but the general biological features and control measures are similar to those of the common and throat bots.

Adult botflies are similar to honeybees in size and general appearance. Botflies do not bite or feed because their mouthparts are under-developed. In temperate zones, activity of adult flies is limited to the warm months from spring until frost in the autumn. The grub or larval stages in the stomach appear to be an adaptive mechanism for overwintering within the equine host.

Development

Female flies deposit eggs on the hairs of the horse. The tell-tale eggs of the common bot are distributed mainly on the forelimbs, chest, neck and mane. Eggs of the throat bot are laid obscurely in the short hairs of the skin on the cheeks and throat between the jawbones. Development of eggs to first instar or infective larvae takes about 1 week. Embryonated eggs of the throat bot hatch spontaneously. Eggs of the common bot require warmth and moisture provided by the horse's lips as they nuzzle or nibble at the egg-bearing areas. In either case the newly hatched larvae enter the mouth and invade oral tissues, mainly the tongue and gums. After 3–4 weeks of growth and development into second instars they emerge and pass to the stomach where they attach to the lining. Further growth and development over a 3 to 4-week period results in third instars. The larvae remain attached to the stomach wall for varying periods of time, at least 5 months before they detach and pass to the outside in faeces. Expelled bots burrow into the soil, undergo pupation, and adult flies emerge in about 1 month. Characteristically, female botflies dart around the forequarters and adjacent parts of the horse, depositing eggs on the hairs.

Clinical signs

Annoyance of the horse results from activities of the adult flies in their persistent efforts to deposit eggs. Even-tempered animals may react unexpectedly and endanger each other as well as riders or handlers. Invasion of bot larvae in oral tissues is irritating and deep-seated periodontal ulcers are produced. Such lesions result in poor mastication and improper feeding which contribute to unthriftiness and impaired growth of young horses.

Some adverse effects undoubtedly result from the deep pits produced by bots attached to the stomach wall (Figure 7.8). Obscure digestive disturbances, colics and obstructions have been ascribed to stomach bots, but definitive signs have not been verified. Occasionally a pit will perforate through the stomach wall resulting in a fatal peritonitis. Tearing and rupturing of the stomach wall, as well as ulceration, have been ascribed to bots.

Control

Grooming can be an aid in limiting infections of the common bot. Clipping or plucking of hairs with the attached bot egg cases has the advantage of removing all egg cases containing larvae as well as those already hatched so newly deposited eggs can be seen readily. Of less value is warm water sponging or rubbing of the forelimbs and other egg-bearing areas. Although this stimulates the hatching of eggs and destroys the larvae, it leaves the empty egg shells, which cannot be differentiated visually from newly deposited eggs. The foregoing grooming practices are not effective for the throat bot. Eggs tend to be buried in the short hairs of the cheeks, chin and throat and are not readily observed. Hatching of throat bot eggs occurs as soon as development is completed so induced hatching by warm water and massaging is not a useful practice for throat bot control.

Treatment of horses for removal of bot larvae usually supplants rather than supplements the above grooming practices. Removal of bots occurs following treatment with carbon disulphide, organophosphates, trichlorfon and dichlorvos, and ivermectin. Both the phosphates and ivermectin remove the young bot larvae in the mouth as well as those from the stomach. Carbon disulphide is not active against the oral-dwelling larvae and available formulations require administration by stomach tube. Treatment with bot-removing compounds has been traditionally undertaken in the late autumn or early winter in temperate zones. Administration of treatment about a month after the first frost, which stops fly activity, generally coincides with maximal accumulation of bots in the stomach. Coordination of treatment with the grooming procedures enhances control by eliminating the residual sources of infective larvae of the common bot. The use of broad-spectrum products, dichlorvos or ivermectin, at other times during the year for strongyle control provides the added benefit of bot removal. There have been indications in recent years that bot infection in horses is on the wane.

Pinworms

The common pinworm (*Oxyuris equi*) is a helminth parasite of the colon of equids. Adult pinworms are commonly found in young horses, but are relatively uncommon in mature horses. Immature oxyurids occur in all age groups of horses and heavy infections, numbering in the thousands, may be present.

Development

Adult pinworms live in the posterior portion of the digestive tract, the dorsal and small colons. Gravid female worms migrate to the rectum and anus to discharge their eggs. The process is unique in that the females are quite fragile and often rupture. Eggs and other irritating worm-derived products adhere to the skin in the anal and tailhead areas. Some mature female pinworms are voided intact in the faeces. They are white, like ascarids, but the adult females are only 5–8 cm long and have sharp, pointed tails.

Pinworm eggs stick to stable walls and fixtures, on bedding, fences and other objects. Development is rapid and the egg shells contain infective larvae in 3–5 days. They are consumed in contaminated feed and water or from other objects. Following ingestion by the horse, the infective pinworm eggs move through the digestive tract to the colon and develop in 3–10 days into fourth stage larvae without penetration of the gut wall. The immature phases of development are not completely understood. About 5 months elapse before sexually mature adult worms develop.

Clinical signs

The main sign of pinworm infection is the horse rubbing its tailseat and rear quarters on fences, walls or any available object. The irritation is caused by egg and other pinworm deposits on the skin. Rubbing results in loss of hair from the tail, giving it the characteristic 'rat-tail appearance' as illustrated in Figure 7.9.

Pinworm larvae also feed on the mucosa of the colon, but this has not been associated with clinical signs.

Control

Sanitation and management have more limited efficacy in curbing pinworms than other nematode infections because of the extent of contamination of animals, structures, objects and materials with the sticky eggs following tail-rubbing activities. Protection of feed troughs and waterers should be stressed in the application of hygienic measures. Thorough cleaning of stalls, followed by a period of disuse in coordination with treatment, has been advocated. In problem situations, egg deposits especially on the perianal region and udders of mares have been removed by washing with water.

Periodic treatment programmes designed primarily for strongyle and ascarid control also provide anti-pinworm activity because of the broad-spectrum activity of most of the compounds or mixtures. Pinworms are therefore not singled out for special attention except in problem situations. Vulnerability of this parasite to modern antiparasitic compounds has markedly reduced the prevalence of pinworms among horses on well-managed farms that utilize routine treatment regimens for internal parasites.

Tapeworms, lungworms and *Strongyloides*

Tapeworms

Three species of tapeworms occur in equids, but only the perfoliated species (*Anoplocephala perfoliata*) has been found commonly in Thoroughbreds in recent years. All ages of equids are infected and this tapeworm tends to aggregate in clusters at the ileo-caecal valve area in the bowel (Figure 7.10). Severe mucosal ulcerations, blockages of the lumen and telescoping of the ileum into the caecum may occur, but usually infections are asymptomatic. Horses pick up the infection while grazing, but a free-living mite on pastures is required for transmission. Only one of the anti-nematode products, pyrantel, is active in removing this tapeworm. In the past, veterinarians have used a double dose for treatment, but recent tests have revealed that the regular therapeutic dose is also efficacious.

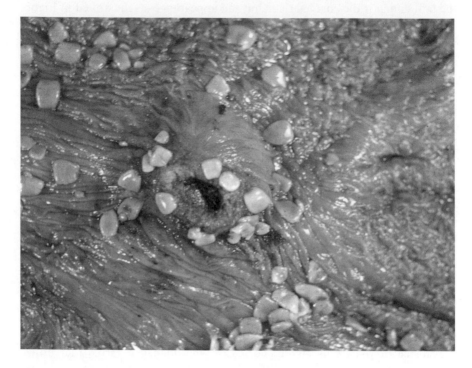

Figure 7.10 Tapeworms (*A. perfoliata*) attached to ileo-caecal valve area of caecum. Note ulceration of mucosa around orifice of the ileum.

Lungworms

This helminth parasite (*Dictyocaulus arnfieldi*) occurs in equids world-wide. Donkeys are the natural host as infections are well tolerated, whereas horses and ponies are abnormal hosts and severe pulmonary damage may develop. The life cycle is direct, similar to that outlined for strongyles, and takes 4–5 weeks to complete. Persistent coughing is the main sign in horses and ponies, while infection in donkeys is usually not evident. For control, complete segregation of donkeys from horses and ponies is mandatory. Ivermectin is currently the treatment of choice.

Strongyloides

This tiny nematode (*Strongyloides westeri*) is a common parasite of foals. It is usually the first parasitic infection of foals because it is acquired via the mare's milk. Development is rapid, within 2 weeks, and worms locate in the small intestine. Diarrhoea may occur, but this is not a constant or reliable sign. Control has relied heavily on anthelmintics. Two benzimidazoles, thiabendazole and oxibendazole, are effective at regular doses for removing the adult worms from the foal's intestine. Ivermectin at the therapeutic dose rate is active against the tissue stages in the mare and reduces transmission. It is also effective when given to the foal for the intestinal forms of *Strongyloides*.

Further reading

Arundel J H (1985) *Parasitic diseases of the horse*. Veterinary Review 28, Postgraduate Foundation in Veterinary Science. University of Sydney, Sydney, NSW.

Drudge J H, Lyons E T (1986; revised 1989) *Internal parasites of equids with emphasis on treatment and control*. Hoechst-Roussel Agri-Vet, Somerville, NJ.

Georgi J R, Georgi M E (1990) *Parasitology for veterinarians*, 5th edn. W B Saunders, Philadelphia.

Herd R P (1987) Diagnosis of internal parasites. In Robinson N E (ed.) *Internal parasites in current therapy in equine medicine 2*, W B Saunders, Philadelphia, pp 323–36.

Jacobs D E (1986) *A colour atlas of equine parasites*. Lea & Febiger, Philadelphia.

Levine N D (1968) *Nematode parasites of domestic animals and man*. Burgess, Minneapolis

Ogbourne C P, Duncan J L (1985) Strongylus vulgaris *in the horse: its biology and veterinary importance*, 2nd edn. Commonwealth Agricultural Bureaux, Wallingford, Oxon

Soulsby E J L (1982) *Helminths, arthropods and protozoa of domesticated animals*, 7th edn. Lea and Febiger, Philadelphia.

Yakstis J J, Johnstone C (1981) *Parasites of horses*. MSD-AGVET, Merck and Co., Rahway, NJ.

8 VACCINATION OF HORSES

DAVID G. POWELL, BVSc, FRCVS

Summary

There are more than a dozen bacterial and viral diseases of horses for which vaccines are presently available. This chapter provides a brief history of the development of vaccines and a short discussion of the immune response of horses to vaccination. Each disease for which a vaccine is available is considered separately providing information on its distribution and the recommended vaccination schedule. Consideration is also given to current developments in molecular biotechnology which will assist in the development of new and improved equine vaccines.

Brief history

Following the chapter on parasite control it is appropriate to discuss the vaccination of horses, which also plays an integral part in equine preventive medicine. Vaccination involves the administration of antigens, derived from viruses or bacteria, that provoke an immune response in the host. The immune response protects the horse from signs of disease when challenged by the infectious agent from which the antigen was derived. Immunity develops following stimulation of lymphocytes, phagocytes and other accessory cells present in the lymphoid organs, including the bone marrow, thymus, spleen and lymph nodes. These cells are also present in the blood circulation and the submucosa of the respiratory and intestinal tracts. By a complex series of events they produce antibodies which are capable of binding to viruses and bacteria so neutralizing or minimizing their pathological effects and eventually destroying them. In addition to protecting the individual horse vaccination is necessary to build up 'herd immunity' within a group of animals. In doing so the risk of an infectious agent being transmitted from an infected horse to a susceptible horse is progressively reduced consistent with the overall level of herd immunity. Vaccines to be effective must produce a prolonged immunity avoiding the necessity for frequent revaccination, be inexpensive and produce no adverse side-effects.

Two types of vaccine are available, referred to as live or attenuated, and killed or inactivated. A live vaccine contains viable organisms which have been altered or attenuated in such a way that they are no longer capable of causing disease but are still capable of multiplying once inoculated into the host. Attenuation of viruses was initially undertaken by repeated passage in laboratory animals including hamsters, mice and rabbits but is now achieved by serial passage in tissue culture. Live vaccines possess advantages over killed vaccines in that they stimulate a more prolonged and broader immune response. They do, however, have the potential for causing disease or reverting to their natural virulent state and must be properly stored to maintain their viability. Killed vaccines contain antigens which have been inactivated so they no longer have the ability to multiply and cause disease in the host. Inactivation is performed by exposure to irradiation, formalin, alcohol or β propriolactone. During inactivation it is important to preserve the molecular configuration of the antigen which is necessary for antibody production. Killed vaccines are relatively cheap to produce and easily stored without loss of efficacy. The majority of killed vaccines contain an adjuvant which serves to enhance the immune response. In the early days equine vaccines contained adjuvants which resulted in a high incidence of reactions at the site of injection. Over the years it has been possible to eliminate many components that contributed to local or systemic reactions by the identification and purification of protein subunit antigens of the virus or bacteria which are immunogenic and non-toxic.

The administration of antigen by vaccination results in the development of active immunity, which should be distinguished from passive immunity involving the transfer of antibodies. Passive immunity occurs under natural circumstances when the newborn foal suckles its dam and receives colostrum. Colostrum contains high levels of antibodies against a variety of antigens which are absorbed from the foal's small intestine into the circulation during the first 24 hours of life. An alternative method of providing passive immunity is to inject a concentrated source of antibody, as occurs with the use of tetanus antitoxin to treat wounds that may have become contaminated with the bacterium *Clostridium tetani*.

The earliest recorded attempt at vaccination in any species is credited to the Chinese who in the 10th century noted that individuals who recovered from smallpox were resistant to the disease and deliberately infected infants with smallpox to protect them. The practice continued and by the 19th century was referred to in Europe as 'variolation'. It was further refined toward the end of the 18th century by Edward Jenner, a physician from the west of England who utilized an observation by one of his patients that farm workers who handled cows did not develop smallpox. He inoculated patients with cowpox, which considerably reduced the serious consequences sometimes associated with 'variolation'. Whilst the details of this story have become distorted with time the technique pioneered by Jenner culminated in the world-wide eradication of smallpox by 1979. Jenner published his findings in 1798 and called the technique vaccination, derived from the Latin *vacca* meaning cow, and his work continues to have a profound effect on the development of vaccines for human and veterinary medicine. Live vaccines currently available for horses include those which protect against African horse sickness, equine viral arteritis and rhinopneumonitis. Toward the end of the 19th century the legendary French scientist Louis Pasteur and his colleagues developed the first vaccines against anthrax and rabies. The Pasteur Institute in France is credited with the initial use of horses to produce antisera after it was shown that serum from a horse hyperimmunized with *C. tetani* toxin injected into another horse made it temporarily resistant to tetanus. Horses are still used to produce a wide range of human and animal antisera and antitoxins.

The 1950s and 1960s saw the introduction in North America and Europe of equine vaccines against tetanus, influenza and virus abortion. These and African horse sickness vaccine developed during the 1930s in South Africa were not without their problems. Local reactions at the site of injection involving oedematous swellings, granulomas and abscesses were a feature of the first generation of equine vaccines. Many of the reactions were associated with the inclusion of Freund's adjuvant, which proved extremely irritant and is no longer incorporated in equine vaccines. The reactions resulted in many horse owners refusing to allow their horses to be revaccinated, an attitude which persisted for several years. Incidence of reactions with the present generation of vaccines has been significantly reduced so it no longer constitutes a reason for not vaccinating. Various systemic reactions giving rise to amyloidosis, serum sickness, serum hepatitis, purpura haemorrhagica, anaphylaxis and encephalitis were also noted following the initial introduction of equine vaccines. Equine serum hepatitis, a fatal disease, was initially reported in 1919 by Sir

Arnold Theiler in South Africa and was subsequently observed following the administration of vaccines against African horse sickness, anthrax and tetanus to horses. Fortunately these conditions are rarely observed with the current generation of equine vaccines due to the improved methods of manufacture, the strict standards of quality control and tests for safety imposed by the licensing authorities prior to commercial distribution of the vaccine.

The immune response

With the initiation of vaccination programmes against several equine diseases in the 1960s considerable emphasis was placed on measuring serum antibody levels following vaccination. It was considered that measurement of circulating antibody, i.e. the humoral response, provided a reliable assessment of protection afforded by vaccination. Nowadays with the considerable advances in immunology it is recognized that the cellular response also plays a role in protection and there is significant interaction between humoral and cell-mediated immunity. Cell-mediated immunity recognizes cells within the host that are foreign or have become modified following infection and is capable of eliminating them. It is not appropriate in this chapter to discuss the exceedingly complex details of humoral and cell-mediated immunity although basic principles which affect the success or failure of vaccination programmes will be considered.

The development of humoral immunity is a function of lymphocytes, whereas phagocytes, which include monocytes, macrophages and neutrophils, are primarily responsible for cell-mediated immunity. Phagocytes are distributed throughout the body, especially in the respiratory and intestinal tracts, and it is their function to engulf invading pathogens and assist in their breakdown. Macrophages transport antigens to the nearest lymph node or lymphoid tissue where they become bound to antibody which is secreted by lymphocytes. The antigen bound to antibody is then engulfed by phagocytes, digested by enzyme action, and destroyed.

Lymphocytes are the predominant cell type found in lymph nodes, spleen and submucosal areas of the respiratory and intestinal tract. The two organs which regulate the production and differentiation of lymphocytes are the thymus and bursa of Fabricius. The latter is present only in birds, its function in mammals having been taken over by the bone marrow. Lymphocytes develop in the embryo from the yolk sac, foetal liver and bone marrow and differentiate into two groups identified as B- or T-cells depending on whether they originate from the bursa (B) or thymus (T). B-lymphocytes produce immunoglobulins (Ig), i.e. the antibodies, and constitute the humoral component of the immune system. When initially exposed to an antigen B-cells multiply and differentiate into two cell types, plasma cells which secrete IgM antibody and memory cells which produce IgG antibody. T-cells undergo considerable proliferation and differentiation in the thymus giving rise to several subpopulations which are distributed via the blood and lymphatic circulation to the various lymphoid tissues. The subpopulations of T-cells undertake a multitude of activities not all of which are currently understood. They include assisting B-cells in the production of antibody and helping phagocytic cells in the cell-mediated response. T-helper (Th) cells enable B-cells to switch from IgM to IgG production, which is essential for the secondary immune response. T-cells also release a variety of substances collectively known as lymphokines, including interferons that activate macrophages and other phagocytic cells. Another subgroup, cytotoxic T (Tc)-cells are capable of destroying virus-infected cells. T-cells produce memory cells and also play a role in controlling the overall immune response through suppressor (Ts) cells.

Antibodies

Antibodies are serum proteins or immunoglobulins (Ig) produced by lymphocytes following contact with antigen and are split into four classes: IgG, IgM, IgA and IgE. IgG is present in the greatest concentration and is composed of several subclasses. Under the electron microscope IgG has a Y-shaped configuration. The two ends of the Y are referred to as the Fab fragments, are identical and possess the ability to bind antigen. The tail or Fc fragment does not bind antigen. Because of its small molecular size IgG can escape from blood vessels and participate in the immune response within tissue spaces and body surfaces. IgM has the second highest concentration in serum and because of its large molecular size does not perfuse from blood vessels and so plays little part in the body's defences outside the blood circulation. IgA is the major immunoglobulin present in secretions and protects the mucous membranes of the respiratory and intestinal tract and is also present in colostrum and milk. In domestic animals including the horse IgE is present in only very small amounts and is associated with the immune response to parasitic infection. Both IgG and IgM antibodies are capable of neutralizing the effects of viruses and bacteria. Their antiviral activity involves direct lysis or death of the virus, preventing virus from attaching to cell surfaces and causing aggregation of virus particles so they are easily phagocytosed. Their activity against bacteria results in death of the organism, neutralization of toxins and enzymes released by bacteria, and the promotion of phagocytosis. Antibodies are helped by complement, a series of proteins produced by the liver, intestinal epithelium and macrophages and present in the globulin fraction of serum. The various components of complement are identified by the prefix C and labelled numerically C1, C2, C3, etc. Complement activity is triggered by antigen-antibody interaction causing a cascade effect culminating in destruction of cell membranes leading to the death of cells and pathogenic organisms. Destruction of bacteria by antibody is also facilitated by the enzyme lysozyme, which is present in neutrophils. IgA antibodies prevent binding of antigen to the mucosal surface but do not elicit complement or phagocytic activity.

Following the administration of vaccine by injection there is an antibody response which is specific to the antigen present in the vaccine. Antibody develops within 7 days and reaches a peak by 10–14 days before declining rapidly. This is known as the primary response and is composed of IgM antibody. If a second dose of antigen is administered after an interval of 14–28 days, the antibody level rises to a peak within 2–3 days and then falls away slowly. This is known as the secondary response and is composed primarily of IgG antibody. The secondary response is specific in that it is only induced by the same antigen that provoked the primary response. It can be invoked months or years following the primary response although the magnitude of the secondary response declines as the duration of the interval increases. The secondary response occurs even though the primary response was so weak as to be undetectable. A third injection of antigen known as a booster will provoke a further rise and more prolonged antibody response. It is the repeated administration of the same antigen at regular but not too frequent intervals that forms the basis of vaccination programmes. If the second dose of antigen is given too quickly following the first it will bind with antibody produced by the primary response so diminishing the secondary response. Multiple injections of antigen do not lead to successively higher levels of antibody.

Colostrum as a source of antibodies

Foals are born with no antibodies because they have not been exposed to antigen *in utero*. The placenta of the mare is composed of six layers and does not permit large molecules, including IgG, to perfuse between the adult and foetal circulations. The newborn foal derives passive immunity from colostrum, which is an accumulation of secretions from mammary tissue and protein transferred from the mare's circulation. Colostrum is an extremely rich source of IgG, IgA and IgM but is composed primarily of IgG which is 5–10 times more concentrated than the IgG in maternal sera. The multitude of antibodies produced by the dam's immune system are concentrated in colostrum, which is available to the foal when it suckles during the first 24 hours of life. The ability of the dam to concentrate antibodies in colostrum is enhanced by vaccination of the dam during the last month of pregnancy. The first 24 hours in the life of the foal are critical for the passive transfer of immunity as it is only during this brief period that surface cells of the small intestine are capable of absorbing large IgG molecules which are transferred to the foal's circulation. After 24 hours the surface cells of the small intestine are replaced by more mature cells that do not allow passage of large molecules, so passive transfer is no longer possible. The process of transfer is assisted by enzyme inhibitors in colostrum which prevent the breakdown of large protein molecules in the intestine. Foal serum immunoglobulin levels peak within 12–24 hours of birth providing the foal has had ample opportunity to suckle. Immunoglobulin levels decline and reach a low by 1 month although passive antibodies may persist for 5–6 months. Between 1 and 3 months of age the foal begins to produce its own IgM, IgG and IgA following primary and secondary responses to various antigens to which it is naturally exposed. By 4 months the levels of immunoglobulins are equivalent to those present in the adult. Whilst the presence of passive immunity provides immediate protection it does have an inhibiting effect on the development of active immunity by the foal. Thus vaccination of foals during the first 3 months of life is unlikely to stimulate a satisfactory level of humoral immunity, especially if the dam has been administered a vaccine containing the same antigens during the last month of pregnancy.

The concentration of IgG in the mammary secretions declines significantly within 24–36 hours of parturition coinciding with the transition from colostrum to milk production. The fall in IgA is less so it becomes the predominant immunoglobulin in milk and persists throughout lactation. IgA antibodies derived from milk remain in the intestine of the young foal and provide local protection against a variety of intestinal pathogens. By acting as an immunological barrier in the intestine IgA antibodies prevent the attachment of viruses and bacteria to the epithelial cells of the intestine. During pregnancy and lactation antigen-sensitized plasma cells migrate from the intestine to the mammary gland where they secrete large amounts of IgA.

The role of adjuvants

The word 'adjuvant'—derived from the Latin *adjuvere*, to help—refers to a substance which when mixed and administered with an inactivated antigen enhances the immune response. The first adjuvant to be used in equine vaccines was Freund's which is composed of a mineral oil, killed *Mycobacterium bovis* organisms and an emulsifying agent. Freund's adjuvant was included in equine influenza vaccines during the 1960s and stimulated an excellent antibody response but resulted in a very severe reaction at the site of injection. These vaccines were quickly withdrawn and Freund's adjuvant is no longer used in vaccines administered to horses. Several different types of adjuvants are currently used including mineral and vegetable oil emulsions with the antigen concentrated in the soluble water phase. Mineral salts including alum, aluminium hydroxide and aluminium phosphate are commonly used. Various saponins including Quill A, a glycoside from the bark of a South American tree, referred to as ISCOM (immune stimulating complex), are also used as adjuvants.

Adjuvants slow down the rate of antigen breakdown at the site of injection by forming a depot where antigen is concentrated and released over a prolonged period so extending the duration of the immune response. The presence of adjuvant stimulates an inflammatory reaction resulting in the formation of a granuloma which increases interaction between the antigen and T-cells. A phenomenon known as lymphocyte trapping also occurs whereby the reaction between antigen and macrophages stimulates the release of lymphokines which attracts lymphocytes to the site of vaccine administration.

Storage and administration of vaccines

Irrespective of whether the vaccine is live or killed it should be stored at refrigerator temperatures, i.e. 2–7 °C (35–45 °F) but not frozen. All equine vaccines possess a batch number and an expiry date which should be recorded at the time of use. The majority of vaccines have a shelf life of at least 12 months and it is inadvisable that they should be used after the date of expiration. Killed vaccines are available in liquid form either in pre-filled syringes sufficient for one dose or in sterile containers which contain multiple doses. Vaccine is injected as 1 or 2 ml doses and the entire contents should be used once a multidose container is opened. Any remaining should be discarded. Live vaccines are prepared as freeze-dried preparations in sealed vials which immediately prior to use should be aseptically rehydrated using sterile diluent supplied with the vaccine. The entire contents should be used and any remaining discarded. Both live and killed vaccines contain an antibiotic and a fungistat to reduce the possibility of contamination at the time of administration.

Vaccines are administered by deep intramuscular injection into the muscle

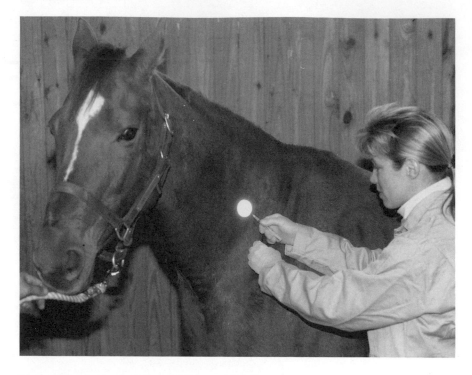

Figure 8.1 (a) Site for intramuscular vaccination.

of the neck or hind quarters as shown in Figure 8.1a and b and occasionally into muscle of the upper forelimb as in Figure 8.1c. If pre-filled syringes and needles are not supplied 1 or 2 ml disposable syringes and a 1 or 1½-in 20 gauge disposable needle should be used. On no account should syringes and needles be re-used. Prior to injection it is imperative that the vaccine should be shaken vigorously to ensure even dispersal of the contents. This applies equally to killed vaccines, to disperse the adjuvant, and to live vaccines to disperse antigens in the diluent. The site of inoculation should be carefully wiped with an alcohol swab to reduce contamination from organisms and dirt on the skin surface. It is not advisable to mix different vaccines in the same syringe and administer them together.

Licensing of vaccines

The production of all vaccines is strictly controlled by the responsible government authorities who have the right to license establishments where vaccine is

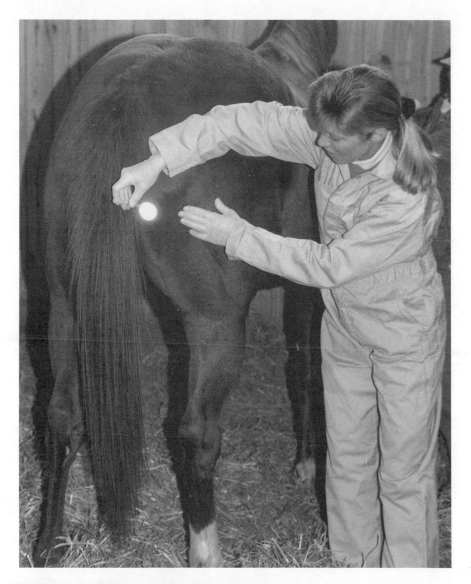

Figure 8.1 (b) Site for intramuscular vaccination.

produced. The licensing authorities are responsible for inspecting the premises to ensure facilities are appropriate, the methods employed are satisfactory and that minimum standards of hygiene, security and quality control are fulfilled. These criteria also apply to vaccines produced in a country different from the one in which the vaccine is to be used. All vaccines are checked for safety and potency and include tests to confirm the identity of the antigen and ensure the vaccine is free of contaminating organisms. Prior to a licence being granted the

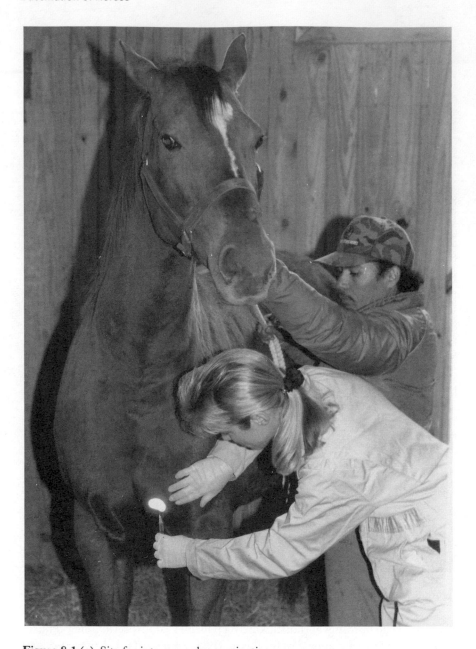

Figure 8.1 (c) Site for intramuscular vaccination.

vaccine must be field tested on several hundred horses to ensure it is safe and does not cause adverse reactions following its administration.

Vaccination schedules

There are more than a dozen equine bacterial and viral diseases for which vaccines are available. Vaccines produced against bacteria are referred to as bacterins or toxoids. A bacterin contains whole killed bacterial antigen whereas toxoid contains treated antigen derived from toxins released by bacteria. A particular vaccine is used depending on the disease prevalence in the equine population and whether it is approved by the licensing authorities of the country. In most countries vaccines are available against tetanus, influenza and rhinopneumonitis. An exception is Australia and New Zealand which have remained free of equine influenza and where horses are not vaccinated against the disease. Australia currently does not permit vaccination against rhinopneumonitis. In North America a wide range of vaccines are available to immunize the equine population reflecting the prevalence of respiratory viral infections and vector-borne viral diseases. The number of equine vaccines licensed in Europe is less, reflecting the absence of vector-borne viral diseases. In the United Kingdom and Ireland the absence of rabies also precludes the use of vaccine against this disease. To avoid repeated inoculations antigens against a variety of pathogens have been incorporated in a number of combined vaccines. These are used extensively in North America where there are a variety of vaccine products containing permutations of antigens to tetanus, influenza, rhinopneumonitis and viral encephalitides. A suggested vaccination schedule against several major equine diseases is contained in Table 8.1. Vaccines against all these diseases are licensed in the USA but not necessarily in other countries.

Vaccines are also available against equine diseases which are exotic to North America and most parts of Europe, including African horse sickness, Japanese encephalitis and Getah virus. When devising a vaccination programme several factors should be considered. The disease distribution in a country or on a regional basis will influence whether vaccines against the viral encephalitides, rabies, botulism, Potomac horse fever, equine viral arteritis and to a more limited extent African horse sickness and Getah virus are available and if so whether they should be incorporated in the programme. If horses are to be transported to another country or region they need to be vaccinated against diseases to which they might be exposed. The disease history on any particular premises will dictate the validity of a vaccination programme against strangles.

Table 8.1. Vaccination schedule for major equine diseases in the USA.

Vaccine	Initial series	Booster
Botulism	3 injections, 1 month apart	Annual booster for broodmares within 1 month prior to foaling in endemic areas
Encephalitis Eastern/Western	3 injections at 3, 4 and 6 months of age	Annual booster for broodmares within 1 month prior to foaling. In endemic areas a booster every 6 months
Venezuelan	Only needed when threat of outbreak exists	
Equine viral arteritis	1 injection	Mares and stallions 3 weeks prior to breeding
Influenza	2 injections 3–4 weeks apart	Annual booster or every 3–6 months for horses at risk of exposure
Potomac horse fever	2 injections, 1 month apart	Annual booster during May/June in endemic areas
Rabies	1 injection	Annually
Rhinopneumonitis	2 injections, 3–4 weeks apart	Every 3–6 months for horses at risk of exposure; pregnant mares at 5, 7, and 9 months gestation
Strangles	2–3 injections, 1 month apart	Annually or prior to possible exposure
Tetanus toxoid	2 injections, 3–4 weeks apart	Annually or at time of injury, surgery

Vaccination against tetanus, influenza and equine rhinopneumonitis should be standard procedure except for horses in Australasia. In establishing a programme that incorporates the appropriate vaccines given at the correct intervals and utilizing available vaccine combinations the advice of the veterinarian responsible for the horses should be sought.

Each disease for which vaccine is available will be discussed separately indicating its geographical distribution and recommended vaccination schedule.

African horse sickness

African horse sickness is one of the most serious viral infections of equidae because of the high mortality, over 75% following infection. Horses are most susceptible, with donkeys, mules and zebras being less so. The disease is endemic to the continent of Africa south of the Sahara desert but epidemics have occurred in Europe and the Middle East within the last 100 years resulting in the death of thousands of horses. Most recently African horse sickness occurred during 1987 in Spain following the importation of zebras from Namibia in southwest Africa. Cases have recurred each summer through 1990 with the disease spreading to Portugal and Morocco and the death of over a 1000 horses. African horse sickness is caused by an RNA orbivirus, of which there are nine distinct serotypes, and it is transmitted by the biting midge of the *Culicoides* species. Epidemics occur during hot wet months when adult female midges transmit virus from infected to susceptible horses when the midges take a blood meal.

A live attenuated vaccine prepared in mice was developed against individual serotypes in South Africa during the 1930s. Since then the virus has been adapted to grow in tissue culture and additional serotypes have been identified which have been incorporated in the vaccine. The live vaccine is currently manufactured only in South Africa and is available against a single serotype as a monovalent vaccine or as a polyvalent vaccine containing several serotypes. Its use is restricted to those countries in which African horse sickness has been diagnosed. Polyvalent vaccine is used annually in South Africa where the disease is not endemic except for the northern provinces of the Transvaal and Natal. Horses are vaccinated to create an immune barrier in these northern provinces to prevent the disease from tracking south during the summer months. It is not possible to include all the serotypes in a single dose of vaccine so it is administered as two injections, 3–4 weeks apart, each containing four serotypes. Protection against all serotypes using the polyvalent vaccine is only achieved after the third or fourth injection. In an epidemic situation as occurred recently in Spain, Portugal and Morocco a monovalent vaccine against the serotype responsible for the outbreak, type 4 was used as it provides a superior level of protection compared to the polyvalent vaccine. Whilst earlier inactivated vaccines were not successful a recent experimental study using an inactivated vaccine against the type 4 serotype has given encouraging results.

Botulism

Botulism results from the presence of the extremely potent toxin released by the Gram-positive sporing bacterium, *Clostridium botulinum*. The organism is widely distributed in soil where it survives indefinitely. Horses develop clinical signs following the ingestion of pre-formed toxin or ingestion of spores which release toxin in the intestinal tract. The toxin is rapidly absorbed and causes neuromuscular paralysis by interfering or binding with the release of acetylcholine at neuromuscular junctions. In adult horses the clinical signs are referred to as 'forage poisoning' whereas in the foal under 6 months of age it is known as 'shaker foal syndrome'. *C. botulinum* releases several different toxins; type B toxin has been implicated in foal mortality in the eastern USA and type C with mortality of horses of all ages in California and Europe. Horses are particularly susceptible when they ingest forage in which the conditions of storage have allowed the production of toxin. Very tightly packed bales of hay and silage, wrapped in polythene, containing soil or animal remains contaminated with *C. botulinum* provide an ideal anaerobic environment for multiplication of the organism and release of toxin. Foals in the USA born in areas including central Kentucky and New York with a known history of botulism caused by type B toxin can be protected by vaccination of the mare during pregnancy. A series of three injections of type B toxoid is given at monthly intervals during the last third of gestation. During subsequent pregnancies a single injection during the last month is recommended. A licensed type B toxoid is available in the USA but there is no cross-protection between the different toxins.

Endotoxaemia caused by Gram-negative bacteria

A variety of Gram-negative bacteria including *Salmonella* spp., *Escherichia coli* and less frequently *Pseudomonas*, *Actinobacillus* and *Klebsiella* cause septicaemia in the horse, producing clinical signs and mortality. Septicaemia is defined as the presence of bacteria and their endotoxins in the blood circulation. Septicaemia may occur among foals during the first weeks of life following infection of the umbilical cord or as a result of enteritis. In older horses it is a possible consequence of colic, retained placenta, mastitis and enteritis. Endotoxin is a lipopolysaccharide component of the cell wall of Gram-negative bacteria which is responsible for the antigenic and toxic properties of the bacteria. This cell wall component comprises three units: O-specific polysaccharide, which is unique to each species of bacteria and imparts antigenic properties and serological specificity to the organism; lipid A, which confers the toxic properties of the endotoxin; and the core antigen, which is common to most Gram-negative endotoxins, so that antibodies to this antigen are cross-protective. The intestinal flora of horses contains a stable population of Gram-negative bacteria which release endotoxins into the lumen of the intestine. In the healthy horse the intestinal mucosal barrier and the phagocytic cells of the liver combine to prevent bacteria and their endotoxins from entering the systemic circulation. Signs of septicaemia develop when these defences are overwhelmed giving rise to endotoxaemia. The several mechanisms by which endotoxin elicits signs of septicaemia include the release of prostaglandins, activation of complement to promote blood coagulation and a direct toxic effect on endothelial cells, platelets and leucocytes. Clinical signs develop rapidly and include fever, depression, increased heart and respiration rate, diffuse haemorrhages and diarrhoea.

Initial attempts to prevent the effects of endotoxaemia included the use of autogenous vaccines derived from specific bacteria, usually a *Salmonella* sp., isolated from a horse with signs of septicaemia. These whole cell bacterins inactivated by formalin were of limited efficacy as they stimulated antibody against the O antigen which was type-specific and so did not protect against other Gram-negative organisms. Three injections were given at intervals of 7 days but there was a high risk of local and systemic reactions.

More recently R-mutants of *Salmonella* spp. or *E. coli* have been used as antigens in an attempt to improve the degree of cross-protection. R-mutants are 'rough' appearing cell colonies of either *Salmonella* or *E. coli* from which the O antigen is partially or completely missing. Removal of the O antigen by mutation allows the core antigen of the cell wall to be exposed thereby stimulating antibody which is cross-protective against the majority of Gram-negative bacteria that cause septicaemia. A vaccine (Endovac-Equi™; Immvac, Inc.) containing an R-mutant of *Salmonella typhimurium* has recently been developed in the USA but its efficacy and safety under field conditions have yet to be proven. The radiation-inactivated bacterin contains an adjuvant and detoxified endotoxin (endotoxoid) which is administered as two injections at an interval of 2–3 weeks followed by an annual booster injection. Endotoxoid can also be given to mares in the last month of pregnancy to passively protect foals via colostrum. The majority of vaccinated horses develop a local reaction and it is recommended they should be vaccinated in the muscles of the hind quarters and given moderate exercise for several days following vaccination. A high titre antiserum prepared from R-mutant *S. typhimurium* is also available to treat clinical cases of Gram-negative endotoxaemia.

Equine encephalitides

There are several arthropod or insect borne viral infections which result in signs of equine encephalitis or encephalomyelitis: Eastern equine encephalitis (EEE), Venezuelan equine encephalitis (VEE) and Western equine encephalitis (WEE), which are found in the Americas, and Japanese encephalitis (JE), which occurs in the Far East. The pathogenic viruses also cause encephalitis among humans and are therefore of zoonotic importance. The viruses of EEE, VEE and WEE are classified as alphaviruses in the family Togaviridae and prior to their identification were collectively referred to as the cause of 'sleeping sickness'. Different species of mosquitoes act as vectors of the four viruses. The seasonal and irregular epidemic pattern of their disease incidence is primarily accounted for by climatic factors, especially temperature and rainfall, which influence the dynamics of the vector population. Epidemics of VEE are maintained by a mosquito/horse cycle whereas EEE, JE and WEE are maintained by a bird/mosquito cycle.

Eastern equine encephalitis

As its name implies EEE is a cause of disease in humans and horses primarily in the Atlantic and Gulf Coast states of North America although equine cases have been reported in more inland states. The disease is also present in the Caribbean, Mexico, Panama and countries of northern South America. Equine cases usually occur during August and September in coastal marshes and swamplands with a mortality in the region of 75%. The highest incidence of equine cases in the USA occurs in Florida where the disease is diagnosed throughout the year. A considerable variety of birds, particularly those that inhabit marshes and swamplands, act as the reservoir hosts. The endemic arthropod vector is the mosquito *Culiseta melanura*, although other mosquito species including *Aedes sollicitans* and *A. vexans*, as indicated in Figure 8.2, are involved in the epidemic cycle when infection spills over into the equine and human population.

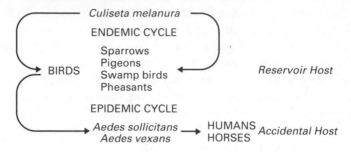

Figure 8.2 Natural history of Eastern equine encephalitis infection.

Vaccination of horses in North America is undertaken using formalin-inactivated vaccines which contain antigens to both EEE and WEE virus grown in chicken cells. The antigens are also included in vaccine products which protect against VEE, tetanus and influenza. Two initial injections given 3–4 weeks apart followed by an annual booster injection is the minimum recommended schedule. Recently the programme has been modified based on observations in Florida that foals and yearlings despite being vaccinated succumb to EEE infection. The modified programme recommends vaccination of foals at 3, 4 and 6 months of age followed by a booster vaccination every 6 months. Pregnant mares should be vaccinated within 1 month of foaling.

Japanese encephalitis

Japanese encephalitis (JE) is a mosquito-transmitted viral infection causing disease in humans, horses and pigs. The virus is a member of the family Flaviviridae producing seasonal epidemic disease in the western maritime Pacific countries from Siberia in the north to Taiwan in the south. It is endemic in South and South East Asia where the incidence of subclinical disease is high in humans and domestic animals including the horse. Formalin-inactivated vaccines using antigens grown in mouse brain, pig or chicken cell cultures are available in Japan. It is recommended that two injections 1–4 weeks apart should be given to horses in known areas of JE activity.

Venezuelan equine encephalitis

There are at least four subtypes of VEE virus not all of which are pathogenic for horses. Within subtype 1 there are several antigenic variants which are highly virulent for horses and are referred to as the epidemic strains. Other less virulent viruses are referred to as the endemic strains. The epidemic strains are found in northern South America, including Colombia, Ecuador, Guyana and Venezuela where disease in horses occurs at irregular and unpredictable inter-vals. The last major epidemic occurred from 1969 to 1972 and gradually spread north from South to Central and North America entering Texas from Mexico in 1971. By the time the epidemic reached Texas it was estimated that several hundred people and 50 000 horses had died. The signs in the horse range from a mild febrile response to a fatal encephalitis with mortality in the region of 80%. Horses, donkeys and mules develop a viraemia which lasts for several days during which time transmission of the virus by a variety of blood-feeding mosquitoes can occur from horse to horse and horse to human. How VEE epidemic virus strains survive during the inter-epidemic period remains unknown. Endemic VEE virus strains are present in tropical and subtropical areas of the Americas including Florida, Central America and northern parts of South America. The reservoir hosts of these endemic strains are small rodents and marsupials with transmission occurring by mosquito vectors.

During the epidemic of the late 1960s and 1970s an attenuated live vaccine prepared for use in humans to protect against the possibility of biological warfare was administered to approximately 3 million horses in the southern half of the USA. Outside the period of an epidemic vaccination of horses in the USA is not recommended although some horses along the border with Mexico are vaccinated as a precautionary measure. An adjuvanted inactivated vaccine is now available containing antigens to EEE, VEE and WEE. VEE antigen is derived from virus grown in tissue culture and inactivated with formalin. The vaccination programme requires two injections at intervals of 3–4 weeks followed by an annual booster or when an epidemic is threatened.

Western equine encephalitis

There are several antigenic variants of WEE present in the western USA, Canada and central and eastern South America. Wild birds are the reservoir hosts and the mosquito *Culex tarsalis* is the primary insect vector. The disease in the horse is the least severe of the three viral encephalitides occurring in the Americas, causing a mild febrile response with only occasional signs of encephalitis and mortality around 25%. Particular foci of the disease in the USA include the Central Valley of California, eastern Colorado and the plains of Texas. Cases among horses occur during midsummer when *C. tarsalis* switches its feeding pattern from birds to various mammalian species including humans and horses.

Inactivated vaccines which incorporate both EEE and WEE antigens as already discussed are used extensively in the USA to immunize the equine population.

Equine rhinopneumonitis

Equine rhinopneumonitis is the name given to disease resulting from infection with either equid herpesvirus type 1 (equine abortion virus, EHV-1) or equid herpesvirus type 4 (respiratory infection virus, EHV-4). EHV-1 is the cause of several different clinical entities. It is a cause of abortion in the mare, occasional perinatal mortality, sporadic occurrences of paralysis in horses of all ages and respiratory disease. EHV-4 is a common cause of respiratory disease especially among foals and yearlings and has been reported as an occasional cause of abortion. Abortion attributable to EHV-1 infection was of considerable concern to the horse breeding industry of North America during the 1950s and 1960s. Following the introduction of an inactivated vaccine during the late 1970s the incidence of abortion due to EHV-1 has fallen significantly particularly the number of 'abortion storms' with multiple abortions occurring on a single farm. However abortion attributable to EHV-1 continues to be a problem in major horse breeding populations throughout the world. EHV-1 and EHV-4 were previously referred to as EHV-1 subtypes 1 and 2 respectively but in this chapter the recently accepted classification will be adhered to. Equine herpesviruses are widely distributed among equine populations throughout the world and the majority of horses become infected early in life following aerosol infection of the respiratory tract. Natural infection results in a short, 3–5-month immunity as a consequence of which horses are constantly reinfected. Like other herpesviruses that infect humans and other animals it is now recognized that EHV-1 and EHV-4 have the ability to cause latent infection which is activated under conditions of stress. Examples of stress include transportation by road or air, the addition of new horses into a group thereby altering the 'peck order', and procedures such as weaning, breaking, castration and even vaccination.

Live and killed equine rhinopneumonitis vaccines are licensed for use in most countries although Australia is a current exception. Their efficacy is limited as they stimulate a short duration of immunity and until very recently the vaccines contained antigens derived only from EHV-1 strains and therefore were limited in the degree of cross-protection which they provided. Both live and killed vaccines stimulate a degree of humoral antibody production but it is increasingly recognized that immunity against herpesvirus infection is dependent on a combination of humoral and cell-mediated immunity. In order to overcome the short duration of immunity vaccination at frequent intervals is necessary. The killed vaccine (Pneumabort®-K and the more recently introduced Pneumabort® K + 1b (Fort Dodge Laboratories) is recommended for use in pregnant mares to prevent abortion and is administered during the 5th, 7th and 9th months of pregnancy. The 1b strain of EHV-1 was recently incorporated in the vaccine as it was identified as a significant cause of abortion during the 1980s in both North America and Europe. Groups of pregnant mares which are vaccinated annually are protected but occasionally an individual mare will abort from EHV-1 infection during the last third of pregnancy. This might occur as a result of reactivation of a latent infection or because immunity becomes overwhelmed by EHV-1 infection. Not mixing mares during the later stages of pregnancy and maintaining pregnant mares as a closed herd is critical in preventing introduction of infection. It is recommended that foals between 3 and 6 months of age should be given two doses of vaccine 3–4 weeks apart followed by booster injections at intervals of 6 months. Despite vaccination foals and yearlings are susceptible to respiratory infection caused by EHV-4, but as they get older a combination of natural infection and vaccination helps build a level of immunity which virtually eliminates signs of respiratory disease. Inactivated vaccines containing EHV-4 antigens introduced in the USA during 1991 were Fluvac® EHV-4 (Fort Dodge Laboratories) and Prestige™ (Haver/Mobay Animal Health), which contains EHV-1 and EHV-4.

The live EHV-1 vaccine (Rhinomune®; SmithKline Beecham) is recommended to prevent respiratory disease but is also given to pregnant mares. The vaccination schedule requires two injections at an interval of 4–8 weeks commencing at 3 months of age followed by regular boosters at 3–6 month intervals. The prevention of equine rhinopneumonitis requires adherence to a regular programme of vaccination coupled to judicious management designed to reduce the introduction of infection and alleviation of stress to minimize the recrudescence of latent infection. The incidence of EHV-1 abortion and the pregnant Thoroughbred mare population in Kentucky over a 30-year period is shown in Figure 8.3. Despite a significant increase in the population during the late 1970s and 1980s the level of abortion has fallen dramatically emphasizing the significant role that vaccination has played.

Equine viral arteritis

Prior to the isolation of equine arteritis virus (EAV) from an outbreak of abortion on a Standardbred farm in Bucyrus Ohio in 1953 the clinical signs of

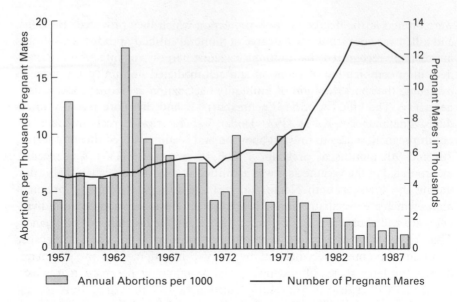

Figure 8.3 The incidence of EHV-1 abortion and the population of Thoroughbred mares in Kentucky, 1957–1988. From Ostlund E N, Powell D, Bryans J T (1990) *Equine herpesvirus 1: A review. Proceedings of the 36th Annual Convention of the American Association of Equine Practitioners, Lexington*, pp 387–95.

the disease had frequently been confused with equine influenza or rhinopneumonitis. The severity of equine viral arteritis disease (EVA) is extremely variable and many cases develop no clinical signs at all. Signs when observed include fever, depression, oedema of the limbs and abdomen, skin rashes, nasal discharge and abortion among pregnant mares. The virus is readily transmitted by the respiratory and venereal routes with persistently infected 'carrier' stallions acting as the focus of venereal transmission within the equine population. EAV is widely distributed in the equine population around the world although the prevalence of infection varies considerably from one breed to another. In the USA serological studies have demonstrated a very low prevalence in the Thoroughbred population but a much higher prevalence of EAV antibody in the Standardbred population. Despite its distribution, outbreaks of disease attributable to EVA have been infrequent and sporadic. During 1984 an outbreak of EVA in Kentucky marked the first occasion that the disease had been reported in the Thoroughbred population of North America. The outbreak demonstrated that a high percentage of infected stallions became chronic carriers and remained persistent shedders of virus in their semen. During the 1960s an attenuated live vaccine derived from the Bucyrus strain was developed by repeated passage in tissue culture. Following the 1984 outbreak this vaccine virus was adapted to grow in an equine dermal cell culture and was licensed in the USA and Canada (Arvac™; Fort Dodge

Laboratories). At present live or dead vaccines against EVA are not licensed for use anywhere else in the world. The primary role of the vaccine has been to immunize stallions to ensure they do not become infected and hence shedders of EAV in their semen. In the state of Kentucky it is currently mandatory that all Thoroughbred stallions which are not shedders of the virus are vaccinated at least 3 weeks before the commencement of each breeding season. Mares served by shedding stallions should be vaccinated 3 weeks before they are mated to ensure they do not develop clinical signs following venereal transmission. If an outbreak of EVA occurs then it is possible to control the spread of the disease by vaccinating all in-contact horses. Various concerns were expressed that the use of a live EVA vaccine might have certain adverse effects in the stallion or mare. Extensive field observations and experimental studies have shown these concerns to be groundless and the vaccine has proved to be safe and effective. Vaccination of the stallion does result in a brief febrile response and a temporary reduction in the number of normal sperm. Whilst it is possible to vaccinate pregnant mares it is recommended that mares in the last 2 months of pregnancy should not be vaccinated.

Getah virus

Getah virus first came to prominence in 1978 when it was implicated as the cause of an acute febrile illness among racehorses in Japan. Other signs include oedema of the limbs, nasal discharge, urticarial rashes on the body and enlarged lymph nodes of the head. Affected horses make an uneventful recovery within a week of the onset of signs. The virus has been isolated from horses and pigs in South East Asia and Australia. It is transmitted by mosquitoes but aerosol transmission from horse to horse may occur. Horses in Japan are protected against Getah virus by an inactivated vaccine.

Influenza

Influenza in horses is manifest as epidemics of acute respiratory disease characterized by a short incubation period of several days and pronounced coughing. The disease spreads rapidly by aerosol droplets among groups of susceptible horses. Only horses which are in the acute or early stage of the disease are capable of transmission and recovered horses are no longer a source of infection to other horses. Clinical signs include an elevated temperature, coughing and a mucopurulent nasal discharge due to secondary bacterial infection. In recent years the incidence of outbreaks of influenza has increased due to the international movement of horses by air transportation. Because of the short incubation period infected horses showing no apparent signs at embarkation are capable on arrival at their destination of transmitting virus to other horses.

Two strains of equine influenza virus are recognized: equine influenza virus A subtype 1, first isolated from horses in Czechoslovakia in 1959 and sometimes referred to as the Prague strain, and equine influenza virus A subtype 2 or Miami strain, first isolated in 1963 from horses in Miami that had been recently imported from South America. Epidemics of subtype 2 continue to occur throughout the world, major ones occurring in South Africa during 1986–87 and Europe and China in 1989. The last reported outbreak of subtype 1 occurred among horses in Malaya and Singapore in 1977 following the importation of horses from England and Ireland. There is a possibility that subtype 1 virus is no longer circulating in the equine population although at present all influenza vaccines contain antigen against subtype 1 virus. The occurrence of recent epidemics of equine influenza is shown in Figure 8.4.

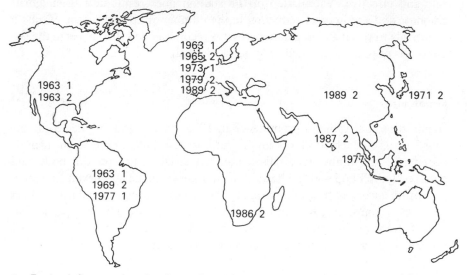

1 = Equine influenza virus A subtype 1   2 = Equine influenza virus A subtype 2

Figure 8.4 Recent epidemics of equine influenza.

Equine influenza viruses possess the ability to undergo antigenic change through alteration in the configuration of their surface glycoproteins, the hae-magglutinin (H) and neuraminidase (N). It is by means of these surface proteins that the various types of influenza are identified and a change of their antigenic configuration can lead to emergence of a new strain. A major change or 'antigenic shift' occurred in 1963 with the emergence of subtype 2 (H_3N_8) which was antigenically distinct from subtype 1 (H_7N_7). Within both subtypes minor changes referred to as 'antigenic drift' have occurred from one epidemic to the next. These minor changes do not alter the antigenic designation of the haemagglutinin and neuraminidase. The emergence of new or altered strains has a considerable impact on the efficacy of influenza vaccines. Equine vaccines which contain only the prototype Prague and Miami antigens do not stimulate such an effective immunity against recently isolated strains. In the absence of subtype 1 outbreaks it has not been necessary to update antigen to this subtype. Current vaccines contain antigens Kentucky 1981 or Fontainebleau 1979 derived from subtype 2 influenza outbreaks which occurred during those years, in addition to Miami 1963 antigen.

Inactivated influenza vaccines containing subtypes 1 and 2 are used extensively as a single vaccine or as a variety of combined vaccines which include tetanus, equine herpesvirus and viral encephalitides antigens. Influenza vaccines contain either whole or subunit viral antigens combined with an adjuvant and are administered by intramuscular injection. The traditional schedule requires two injections given 2–12 weeks apart followed by a booster at 6 months and thereafter at intervals of 12 months. Recognizing that cases of influenza can occur among vaccinated horses a more frequent booster vaccination programme has been advocated and is routinely undertaken in North America. Field studies have established that the level of circulating antibody falls 3–4 months after primary or booster vaccination, especially among young horses, and does not prevent clinical signs. Frequent booster vaccination of racehorses, show and competition animals is therefore recommended every 3–4 months. Booster vaccination stimulates an immediate secondary response within several days and is recommended for previously vaccinated horses at risk during an outbreak. Influenza vaccine may be administered to horses of all ages commencing with foals at 3 months of age.

Horses in the UK, France and Ireland which race and compete under Jockey Club rules must undergo a mandatory programme of influenza vaccination, details of which are entered on the horse's passport and endorsed by a veterinarian. The rules stipulate that a horse must have received two injections given no less than 21 days apart and no more than 92 days apart. Following this series of injections a horse foaled after 1 January 1980 must have received a booster injection no less than 150 days and no more than 215 days after the second injection. Subsequently the horse must have received booster injections not more than a year apart. None of the above should be given within 7 days of a horse entering racecourse property. Horses competing under Federation Equestre Internationale (FEI) rules, the organization responsible for international equestrian competition, are also required to be vaccinated against influenza. They should have received a similar course of two initial injections followed by booster injections within each succeeding 12 months. None of the injections should have been given within 10 days of the horse entering a competition stable. It is important that the name and batch number of the vaccine as well as the correct date are entered on the horse's passport at the time of vaccination.

Potomac horse fever

Potomac horse fever, sometimes referred to as equine monocytic ehrlichiosis, is a newly recognized disease of horses in North America and has recently been reported as infecting horses in Western Australia. It occurs during the summer months producing a variety of signs including fever, depression, colic, mild to profuse diarrhoea and laminitis. The disease was first described towards the end of the 1970s among horses pastured close to the Potomac River in the state of Maryland. The causal agent was identified in 1984 as a previously unrecognized rickettsia of the genus *Ehrlichia* present in the monocyte fraction of white blood cells and was named *Ehrlichia risticci*. The mode of transmission is still not recognized but it is suspected that blood-feeding insects are the vectors. The disease is restricted to endemic localities with the majority of cases occurring as single isolated episodes. Premises on which cases have occurred are likely to report further cases in subsequent years. Inactivated vaccines against the disease are available in the USA. The initial series of two injections is given at an interval of 3–4 weeks followed by an annual booster. The vaccine should be administered to horses during the spring or early summer in those areas where there is endemic disease and especially to horses on premises where cases of the disease have been confirmed.

Rabies

In the USA on average 55 cases of equine rabies were reported annually during the 1980s. The disease in the horse presents very variable clinical signs which include behavioural change, low grade fever and convulsions. The signs progress rapidly over several days culminating in recumbency and death. Wildlife, particularly skunks and raccoons in North America and foxes in Europe, are the primary source of infection to horses. Cases of equine rabies in North America frequently occur during the first few months of the year which coincides with the mating season of the skunk when they are active and roaming pastures. Horses, particularly foals and yearlings because of their curiosity, will pursue wildlife in a pasture and expose themselves to a bite on the nostril or lips. The incubation period in the horse is usually short, from 2 to 9 weeks. The closer the bite is to the brain the shorter the incubation period as the virus travels along nerves and enters the brain. Vaccination of horses in areas where the incidence of rabies in wildlife is high is strongly recommended. Inactivated vaccines are available which are given as a single injection commencing with foals at 3 months of age followed by an annual booster. The modern generation of rabies vaccines do not cause the degree of reaction that some of the earlier vaccines produced and are safe and provide protection against the disease. In those countries which are free of rabies, notably the UK, Ireland, Australia and New Zealand, vaccination of the domestic animal population including horses is not necessary and is prohibited.

Strangles

Strangles is a highly contagious disease of the horse caused by the Gram-positive bacterium *Streptococcus equi*. It invades the mucosal surface of the upper respiratory tract resulting in abscess formation of lymph nodes of the head and neck. Occasionally *Strep. equi* causes abscess formation throughout the body which is referred to as 'bastard strangles'. The classical signs of strangles include fever, loss of appetite, a profuse mucopurulent nasal discharge and enlargement of the submandibular and parotid lymph nodes. These characteristic signs were frequently observed at the beginning of this century among the large stables of horses kept for various types of transportation. As the population of horses gradually fell so did outbreaks of strangles, to be replaced by a milder form which is frequently misdiagnosed as influenza or rhinopneumonitis. Strangles is still widespread, occurring in equine populations throughout the world although the enlarged nodes rarely burst to drain the thick creamy pus which was a feature of the typical outbreaks in previous years. A possible reason is that many cases are treated with antibiotics which reduce the severity of signs but do not eliminate *Strep. equi* from the infected nodes. Once antibiotic therapy is removed the organism continues to multiply, resulting in the horse being a continual source of infection. As well as persisting in the horse indefinitely *Strep. equi* survives in the environment, especially when protected within the copious discharge that readily contaminates mangers, water troughs and other equipment.

Because of the serious and contagious nature of the disease attempts to immunize horses against *Strep. equi* have been tried for the past 50 years without much success. Killed vaccines derived from the whole organism or from extracts of the bacteria are available in many countries where strangles is a problem. The vaccines stimulate a poor immune response of limited duration and have been associated with a higher than normal incidence of local and systemic reactions.

Strangles bacterin is prepared by treating whole suspensions of *Strep. equi* with either β propriolactone or formalin and suspending the killed antigen in an adjuvant such as aluminium hydroxide. A second type of strangles vaccine contains M protein antigen, an inactivated extract of *Strep. equi*. Because this vaccine does not contain several antigens present in the whole cell bacterin it is less likely to cause adverse reactions.

The initial vaccination programme requires three injections given at intervals of 3 weeks followed by an annual booster. Reactions associated with *Strep. equi* vaccines include muscle soreness and abscess formation at the site of injection as well as the occasional systemic reaction and purpura haemorrhagica. The latter is observed in horses that have recently been sensitized to *Strep. equi* antigen and possess high levels of antibody as a result of natural exposure or vaccination. Signs of purpura develop within 2–3 weeks and include fever, depression, oedema of the body and small haemorrhages on the mucosal surface. They are the result of damage to the walls of blood vessels allowing the leakage of blood cells and fluid into surrounding tissue.

Whilst the use of strangles vaccines is of value in reducing the incidence on premises which have a chronic history of the disease the poor level of protection and incidence of reactions limit their usefulness. Considerable attention should be given to eliminating the organism from the environment by disinfection and cleaning as well as strict isolation of known infected horses.

Tetanus

Tetanus was one of the first infectious diseases of man and animals against which a programme of active and passive protection was devised. Tetanus develops following contamination of a deep penetrating wound with *Clostridium tetani*, a Gram-positive sporing bacterium which releases extremely potent neurotoxins under anaerobic conditions. The types of wound which pose a risk of contamination include a puncture wound in the sole of the hoof from a nail or sharp object or following a bone fracture, castration, umbilical cord infection and obstetrical complications. *C. tetani* is a normal inhabitant of soil and is often found in the intestinal contents and faeces of domestic animals. Its ability to form a spore protects it from the effects of heat and light and allows the organism to survive indefinitely in the outside environment. *C. tetani* is infectious without being contagious so the organism is seldom, if ever, transmitted from one animal to another. Infection occurs when the organism present in soil or faeces penetrates a deep wound. In the presence of dead tissue and the absence of oxygen the organism changes from its vegetative sporing state and multiplies, releasing neurotoxin into the surrounding tissues. The toxin enters the blood circulation and tracks along nerves of the peripheral nervous system diffusing into the central nervous system, at which time the classical signs of tetanus are observed. They include spasms of various groups of muscles, including those of the face, giving rise to the term 'lock jaw'; this prevents the horse from drinking and eating and causes the horse to regurgitate via the nostrils. Prolapse of the third eyelid or nictitating membrane and rigid extension of all four limbs are also characteristic. Death is likely to occur within 5–7 days.

Tetanus toxoid is one of the most effective equine vaccines. Toxin is incubated with formalin until the toxicity is destroyed but retains its antigenic properties. The adjuvanted toxoid is incorporated in several combined vaccines or as a single vaccine. Foals receive two injections of toxoid 4–8 weeks apart commencing at 3 months of age followed by an annual booster injection. Mares should receive a toxoid booster during the last month of pregnancy in order that colostral levels of antibody will protect foals during the early weeks of life.

Horses with an unknown or no history of vaccination against tetanus which receive accidental or surgical wounds should be given immediate passive protection by administration of 1500 units of tetanus antitoxin. Horses in the early stages of tetanus will also benefit from the administration of antitoxin but at much higher doses, up to 100 000 units. It has been reported that some horses receiving tetanus antitoxin are at a risk of developing serum hepatitis but in recent years very few cases have been recorded. Horses with a history of tetanus vaccination during the previous 12 months that develop a wound should be given a booster injection of tetanus toxoid.

Failure of vaccination

It is generally accepted but not always understood why vaccination against a specific disease does not guarantee 100% protection. There are several different reasons for apparent vaccine failures which relate to deficiencies of the vaccine or failure of the horse to develop a protective immune response following vaccination. The most common cause is unrelated to either and occurs when a horse develops clinical signs mistakenly attributed to infection against which the horse has been vaccinated. This particularly applies to signs of respiratory disease caused by a variety of different viral or bacterial pathogens, only a few of which is it possible to vaccinate against.

If a horse is vaccinated against a specific disease and is incubating infection to the disease at the time, the vaccine will not protect against the onset of clinical signs. This can occur when horses are vaccinated in the face of an epidemic such as influenza. The majority of horses at risk in this situation when given a booster vaccination will develop a rapid immune response which should protect against the onset of clinical signs. Vaccination can constitute a stress reaction causing recrudescence of latent infection. Killed vaccines, through the irritant effect of antigens and adjuvants, and live vaccines, which induce a brief period of viraemia, may activate latent equine herpesvirus infection. It is inadvisable to vaccinate horses during or just prior to recognized periods of stress when the ability of the horse to mount an effective immune response may be reduced. Examples of stress include weaning, the mixing of horses, long road or air journeys and the presence of other diseases especially those of a chronic debilitating nature such as parasitism. Following vaccination it is recommended that a horse should be put on the 'easy list' for several days and not given serious exercise. The horse may be walked to help alleviate soreness that might occur at the site of injection.

The presence of maternal antibody derived from colostrum in foals up to 3 months of age will combine with antigen in the vaccine to block the development of an active immune response. It is therefore inadvisable to vaccinate foals prior to this period particularly if the dams have been vaccinated with the particular antigen during the last month of gestation. Within a large population the response to vaccination will vary considerably, with some horses developing a better immune response than others. Those that develop a poor response may not be protected against natural infection. An example is the small number of pregnant mares that despite regular and frequent EHV-1 vaccination abort following EHV-1 infection. Influenza virus subtype 2 has been isolated from horses showing mild signs of respiratory disease, a slightly elevated temperature and an infrequent cough. Many such animals have a history of influenza vaccination within the previous 12 months, which emphasizes that despite vaccination horses still become infected and develop signs. Such horses are capable of transmitting influenza virus to other horses. The short duration of immunity that develops following exposure to certain viral antigens, particularly influenza and equine herpesvirus, necessitates that horses must receive frequent booster vaccinations. Too frequent vaccination may also have a deleterious effect in that peak levels of antibody gradually diminish with successive booster injections. This phenomenon has been observed following repeated influenza vaccination and the practice of monthly vaccination cannot be recommended. When a pathogen such as *Strep. equi* invades the mucosal surface of the upper respiratory tract local secretory IgA antibody is essential to provide protection against the onset of clinical signs. Whilst conventional vaccination programmes are designed to stimulate circulating IgG antibodies the poor protection that results following strangles vaccination is in part related to inadequate levels of secretory IgA. Vaccine failure may also be caused by an inappropriate strain being used as the source of antigen. This applies to influenza where antigenic change among field strains requires updating of the vaccine antigens. Epidemics of influenza due to subtype 2 which occurred during the late 1970s and early 1980s showed little evidence of antigenic change but continuous surveillance is necessary to identify possible new strains. Finally, inadequate storage of live vaccines can lead to loss of viability so it is imperative that they are kept refrigerated prior to use.

Adverse reactions following vaccination

As discussed in the introduction to this chapter the incidence of reactions following the administration of the present generation of equine vaccines is much lower than was experienced in earlier years. When severe reactions, either local or systemic, do arise the circumstances should be recorded and reported to the vaccine manufacturers and the licensing authority. Local reactions involving an oedematous swelling at the site of injection persisting for 2–3 days, as shown in Figure 8.5, are not uncommon and need not be reported.

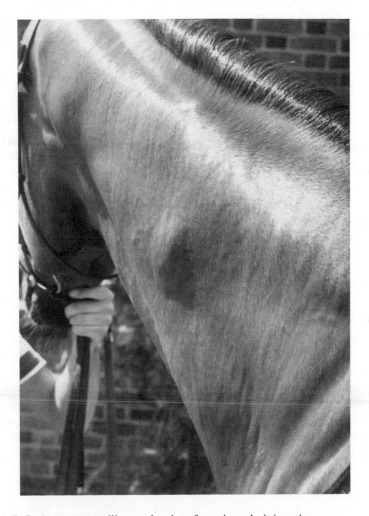

Figure 8.5 Oedematous swelling at the site of vaccine administration.

Occasionally an abscess may develop at the site of injection from which a variety of bacteria, most commonly *Streptococcus zooepidemicus*, is isolated. This is usually caused by contamination of the injection site by bacteria present on the skin surface. It may also occur if the same needle or syringe is used to vaccinate more than one animal or if vaccine is drawn from a partially used multidose container which has been contaminated.

A systemic reaction is rare but may occur as a hypersensitive or exaggerated abnormal immune response following inoculation of vaccine. These reactions are classified as one of several types according to the speed of the response and the immune mechanism involved. A Type I reaction is an immediate response which resembles allergic asthma or hay fever and develops within minutes of vaccination. It follows activation of mast cells and other mediators of the acute inflammatory response. The signs are those of an anaphylactoid reaction with a fall in blood pressure and increased permeability of blood vessels resulting in oedema. Type I sensitivity usually occurs following multiple injections of a killed vaccine and is not necessarily in response to the vaccine antigen. It can occur in response to other constituents of the vaccine such as egg albumin or tissue culture components which are used to prepare vaccine antigen. The present generation of vaccines have had many of these 'impurities' removed so the risk of anaphylaxis is greatly reduced. If a Type I reaction does develop it may be necessary to treat the horse with adrenaline (epinephrine) to reverse the clinical effects. The Type III, immune complex-mediated or Arthus reaction is rarely observed but encompasses a variety of syndromes referred to as serum sickness, amyloidosis, serum hepatitis and purpura haemorrhagica. A Type III reaction involves the deposition of antibody/antigen complexes in various organs particularly the liver, kidneys and blood vessels, causing increased permeability leading to haemorrhage and oedema. Serum sickness was associated with the use of the very first equine vaccines and resulted in a massive antibody response to non-equine serum. Type III reactions involving the development of purpura haemorrhagica have been reported following the use of strangles vaccines. A Type III granulomatous reaction was observed in the early days of equine vaccine production associated with the inclusion of Freund's adjuvant. The adjuvant stimulated the production of antigen-sensitive T-cells which attracted macrophages resulting in the development of a large granulomatous lesion.

Post-vaccinal neurological disease was associated with the use of a particular live EHV-1 vaccine in the USA during the 1970s. Cases varied from mild hindlimb paralysis to complete paralysis as a consequence of which the vaccine was withdrawn from the market.

Future developments in equine vaccines

The market for equine vaccines is small compared to the demand for vaccines in food animals and companion animals. The cost of developing, testing and licensing a vaccine is the same whatever the market size, consequently many pharmaceutical companies are loath to embark on developing new equine vaccines. Rather they prefer to use technologies developed for vaccines in other species and adapt them to similar products for the horse. The merging of international pharmaceutical companies involved in the manufacture of veterinary biological products has resulted in fewer organizations being prepared to develop new products for the small equine market.

In an era when molecular biology and genetic engineering have made tremendous strides in our understanding of the basic immunological events which accompany infection and disease, a number of innovative alternatives to conventional vaccination programmes have been proposed. The majority of these are still in the development or experimental phase and have yet to be subjected to field trials. Most are concerned with developing new or improved vaccines against a variety of human diseases including AIDS, influenza, hepatitis, rabies and herpes. Several of the new technologies have been adapted to the possible control of equine diseases including influenza, equine herpes and strangles. The studies which are underway have concentrated on identifying more specifically the antigenic determinants within the virus or bacteria that are responsible for stimulating the immune response. By incorporating those antigens in a more concentrated and purified form it will be possible to elicit an immune response which is protective whilst at the same time eliminating antigens that are non-immunogenic and toxic.

There is considerable interest in developing a live influenza vaccine which would overcome the deficiencies of the present killed vaccines such as the short duration of immunity and lack of protection at the mucosal surface of the upper respiratory tract. One approach has used DNA recombinant technology to produce a temperature sensitive (*ts*) mutant of influenza which has the ability to replicate only at a temperature of 37–38 °C. When this *ts* virus is administered as an aerosol it multiplies in the cooler temperature of the upper respiratory system stimulating a local immune response. It does not replicate in the higher temperature of the lower respiratory tract where influenza infection causes typical signs of disease. A *ts* mutant for equine influenza virus has been genetically engineered by fusing *ts* human influenza with equine influenza through a process known as genetic reassortment. The resulting recombinant virus is temperature sensitive and contains the genetic code for the surface glycoproteins haemagglutinin and neuraminidase, the major antigens responsible for eliciting the protective immune response to influenza virus.

Another approach, referred to as recombinant technology, is to use viruses and bacteria as vehicles or vectors by which to administer antigens against which it is desired to stimulate an immune response. Vaccinia virus has been used extensively as a vector because it is relatively harmless and it is easy to insert the genetic material from other viruses into its viral genome. The resulting vaccinia recombinant retains the ability to replicate and causes no adverse effects or signs of disease when administered to the host. A recombinant containing the genes responsible for haemagglutinin and neuraminidase of equine influenza has been developed but has yet to be tested under natural conditions. A possible limitation of vaccinia recombinants is that if booster vaccination is necessary the horse will possess antibodies to vaccinia antigens as a result of which the recombinant virus may fail to elicit a secondary immune response. A way round this problem is to develop alternative viral vectors to be used as booster vaccinations, an area which is being actively explored.

Recombinant technology has also been applied to bacterial infections and *Strep. equi* is an obvious candidate. It has been possible to insert genes responsible for the production of M protein of *Strep. equi* into avirulent strains of *Salmonella typhimurium* and *Escherichia coli*. The recombinant can then be administered by the oral route and elicit a local immune response in the extensive lymphoid tissue of the intestine. This local immunity is transferred to other similar sites including the lymphoid tissue of the upper respiratory tract to provide protection against invasion by *Strep. equi*. The production of secretory IgA antibodies by this method does not appear to be inhibited by the presence of circulating IgG antibodies.

Considerable effort is currently focused on means of preventing the various clinical manifestations of equine herpesvirus infection. Studies are concentrating on characterizing the immune response to EHV-1 and identifying the surface glycoproteins of the virus that elicit this response. The complete nucleotide sequence of genes which code for several of the major glycoprotein antigens has been established and others are in the process of being identified. Once these have been characterized it will be possible to chemically synthesize a series of peptides that resemble these genes. These could then be used to generate a source of highly specific antigens to induce protection against equine herpesvirus.

Traditionally antigen for inclusion in killed vaccines derived from whole virus particles was produced in eggs or tissue culture. By recombinant technology it is now possible to express viral proteins and peptides in a variety of yeast, insect and mammalian cells to produce antigens for inclusion in subunit vaccines. This method has already been used to produce influenza subunit vaccines containing only the haemagglutinin and neuraminidase glycoproteins. Studies are currently underway to insert genetic segments of African horse sickness virus into a harmless insect baculovirus which is then allowed to replicate in tissue culture. Antigen derived by this method could then be used to develop an inactivated subunit vaccine against the various serotypes of African horse sickness.

Further reading

Beran G W (1981) *Handbook series in zoonoses. Section B, viral zoonoses*, vol. 1. CRC Press, Boca Raton, FL.

Klein J (1982) *Immunology. The science of self-nonself discrimination.* John Wiley & Sons, New York.

Powell D G (1988) *Equine infectious diseases V. Proceedings of the fifth international conference.* University Press of Kentucky, Lexington.

Timoney J F, Gillespie J H, Scott F W, Barlough J E (1988) *Hagan and Bruner's microbiology and infectious diseases of domestic animals*, 8th edn. Cornell University Press, Ithaca.

Tizard I R (1987) *Veterinary immunology: An introduction*, 3rd edn. W B Saunders, Philadelphia.

Veterinary pharmaceuticals and biologicals (1988) Veterinary Medicine Publishing, Kansas.

9 FOAL MANAGEMENT, DISINFECTION AND HYGIENE
ROBERTA M. DWYER, DVM, MS

Summary
Intestinal disease
Respiratory disease
The balance of health
Role of management in disease prevention
Disinfection
Hygiene
Further reading
Appendix 9.1: Management schedule
Appendix 9.2: Disinfectant checklist

Summary

Providing the newborn foal with a clean environment in which to grow and develop is equally important as proper vaccination, adequate nutrition and regular deworming. Reducing the exposure of the foal to potential pathogenic agents by management practices, disinfection and daily hygiene is critical to infectious disease prevention and control. The management and disinfection measures discussed in this chapter have been field tested and proved to be effective in controlling and preventing outbreaks of disease on horse farms.

Equine preventive health evolves around several factors including vaccination, nutrition, deworming practices and hoof care, which are discussed in detail in other chapters of this book. However, in the midst of a disease outbreak caused by rotavirus, *Salmonella* or *Streptococcus*, none of the preventive measures mentioned will stop the spread of infection. This chapter discusses the practical aspects of foal management, stall disinfection and hygiene to control disease outbreaks of an infectious or contagious nature. All three require planning, are labour intensive and are hence relatively costly. Before discussing each approach in detail, an understanding of the diseases we are trying to prevent is necessary.

As soon as the foal is born, it is exposed to a host of infectious and contagious agents. Maternal colostral antibody is the primary source of defence against many but not all pathogens. Vaccines are available against several bacterial and viral agents which cause diseases in young foals including tetanus, botulism and influenza, as discussed in Chapter 8. The foal is protected providing the mare was vaccinated during the last month of gestation, and the foal received adequate transfer of passive immunity via the colostrum. However, diseases which are highly contagious may threaten entire groups of foals. Besides identifying the pathogens of risk to foals, their mode of transmission must also be understood. Viruses and bacteria are transmitted in several ways including ingestion, inhalation, contact and during pregnancy from the dam to the foetus (*in utero* infection). Transmission may also occur by indirect means, for instance when a pathogen is carried from one animal to another on hands and inanimate objects such as pitchforks, brooms, brushes, boots, etc. These indirect modes of transmission are important and should never be overlooked.

Several pathogens, including *Salmonella* spp., rotavirus, influenza and *Streptococcus* spp. have the potential to cause widespread outbreaks of gastrointestinal and respiratory disease. Others such as *Clostridium tetani* and *Cl. botulinum* are infectious but not contagious and generally cause only individual cases of disease. Being aware of their epidemiological features will help in understanding the need for isolation requirements to prevent their transmission. A list of the more common bacterial infections of foals is provided in Table 9.1.

Intestinal disease

Salmonella species have long been recognized as a common cause of diarrhoea among foals. There are many serotypes of *Salmonella* known to infect horses; several of the more common isolates recently reported in the USA include *S. typhimurium*, *S. agona*, *S. saint-paul*, and *S. ohio*. The source of these various serotypes may be an asymptomatic adult carrier shedding bacteria in its faeces, contaminated feed, birds and domestic or wild animals. Following ingestion, salmonellae invade the small intestine and cause an enteritis of variable severity, although foals may also develop an acute life-threatening septicaemia. Morbidity may be as high as 50% of foals on the farm. Of those animals which develop severe septicemia, half may die. To isolate salmonellae, faecal samples may need to be taken over several days before a positive is identified. Diarrhoeic animals cause extensive faecal contamination of the immediate environment. Apparently healthy foals may be asymptomatic intermittent shedders of salmonellae, but become sick and constant shedders under conditions of stress including transport, surgery, prolonged confinement and orthopaedic problems. The presence of undetected shedders and the lack of a proven

Table 9.1 Common bacterial infections of foals

Pathogen	Classification	Diseases	Mode of transmission
Salmonella spp.[1]	Gram-negative	Salmonellosis: septicaemia, diarrhoea	Ingestion, *in utero*, umbilical
Rhodococcus equi[1]	Gram-positive	*R. equi* pneumonia, rarely diarrhoea	Aerosol, ingestion
Streptococcus equi[1]	Gram-positive	Strangles	Aerosol/respiratory secretions
Streptococcus zooepidemicus[1]	Gram-positive	Septicaemia	*In utero*, umbilical, ingestion, inhalation
Escherichia coli	Gram-negative	Septicaemia	*In utero*, umbilical, ingestion, inhalation
Actinobacillus spp.	Gram-negative	Septicaemia	*In utero*, umbilical, ingestion, inhalation
Pseudomonas	Gram-negative	Septicaemia	*In utero*, umbilical, ingestion, inhalation
Klebsiella	Gram-negative	Septicaemia	*In utero*, umbilical, ingestion, inhalation
Enterobacter	Gram-negative	Septicaemia	*In utero*, umbilical, ingestion, inhalation
Clostridium botulinum	Gram-positive sporeforming	Shaker foal syndrome (botulism)	Ingestion
Clostridium tetani	Gram-positive sporeforming	Tetanus	Wound contamination
Clostridium perfringens	Gram-positive sporeforming	Acute haemorrhagic diarrhoea, shock, death	Ingestion

[1] Pathogens with potential for multiple cases on a farm.

vaccine make salmonellosis a potential threat to foals, especially those on farms with a high concentration of animals.

Following ingestion, rotavirus causes diarrhoea in foals of all ages, with young foals being more susceptible to severe life-threatening diarrhoea and dehydration. The virus invades the small intestine, causing enteritis and the shedding of very high concentrations of virus, as much as 10^7 particles/gram of faeces as shown in Figure 9.1. This causes extensive contamination of the environment, with other foals in the same barn being exposed by direct or indirect contact. The disease is highly contagious and spreads rapidly among groups of foals. Apparently healthy or asymptomatic foals may shed rotavirus during outbreaks and diarrhoeic foals shed virus several days prior to and up to 9 days after the diarrhoeic period. Morbidity may be 70% and while mortality

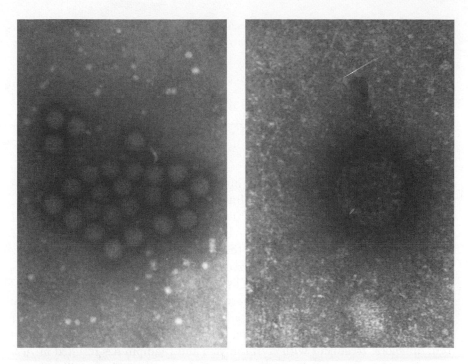

Figure 9.1 Electron microscopic photograph of rotavirus particles at × 135 000 (left) and a single particle magnified × 300 000 (right). This virus is resistant to many disinfectants and can remain viable in the environment for 9 months or more.

is low, foals less than 1 week of age are at the greatest risk of death. Rotavirus can survive for months in the environment and is resistant to many commonly used disinfectants. No equine rotavirus vaccine is currently available.

Other agents may also cause diarrhoea in foals. The protozoan parasite *Cryptosporidium* is known to cause severe diarrhoea in foals associated with failure of passive transfer (FPT), but its role in diarrhoeic immunocompetent foals is still under investigation. The coccidian parasite *Eimeria leuckarti* may be seen on faecal examinations, but is not thought to be a cause of foal diarrhoea. Severe infestations of small strongyles may cause foal diarrhoea, and this is encountered on farms with inadequate worming protocols. Parvovirus, known to cause intestinal infection of dogs, has been diagnosed as a cause of foal diarrhoea. Due to the very small size of the virus, electron microscopy, a procedure not readily available to practitioners, is required to make a diagnosis, therefore the extent of the problem remains undetermined. The anaerobic bacterium *Bacteroides fragilis* has been detected in the faeces of diarrhoeic foals, but the sophisticated culturing methods needed to identify toxigenic strains are not commonly performed. Other bacteria, including *Escherichia coli*, *Actinobacillus*, *Pseudomonas*, *Klebsiella*, *Enterobacter* and *Clostridium*

(Table 9.1), may be isolated from faecal samples obtained from sick foals, but are likely to be secondary invaders to a primary pathogen, most frequently rotavirus.

Respiratory disease

The respiratory viruses of influenza (influenza virus type A) and equine rhino-pneumonitis (EHV-1) cause similar clinical signs in the foal including anorexia, depression, serous nasal discharge, fever, cough, enlarged parapharyngeal lymph nodes and pneumonia. Both viruses are transmitted by inhalation of aerosolized virus, so close contact is the most common mode of transmission, although indirect contact may also contribute to their dissemination.

Rhodococcus equi, formerly known as *Corynebacterium equi*, is a Gram-negative bacterium which causes severe abscessing pneumonia among foals usually 2–4 months of age. Mortality of 50% has been reported. Initial documented outbreaks had upwards of 80% mortality among those affected, however current antibiotic treatment with erythromycin and rifampin has resulted in 70% recovery rates. Recovered animals may suffer a loss of athletic ability due to impaired pulmonary function. Transmission is by inhalation and/or ingestion of the organism present in soil and manure. No vaccine is available although the use of hyperimmune plasma to treat foals at risk has produced encouraging results.

Strangles is an infection of the submandibular and pharyngeal lymph nodes caused by the Gram-positive bacterium *Streptococcus equi*. Mucopurulent nasal discharge, ruptured abscesses, fever and anorexia are the signs of infection and can rapidly spread among horses of all ages. *S. equi* is transmitted by direct or indirect contact with the discharges from an infected animal. Horses have been shown to shed *S. equi* for several months after clinical recovery. Most outbreaks are thought to occur when an asymptomatic shedder is brought into a herd of susceptible animals. Although vaccines are available, their efficacy is in question, as discussed in Chapter 8.

The balance of health

The various viral and bacterial pathogens considered here are not the sole agents causing disease among foals, but rather ones that modern veterinary medicine is able to detect. No doubt many other agents which cause disease remain unidentified. Moreover, the shedding period of various pathogens is not known precisely, therefore it is necessary to guard against the threat of asymptomatic shedders. Many bacteria which cause septicaemia survive in the stable environment and clostridial spores are always present in faeces and dirt.

With asymptomatic shedding horses and a variety of agents present in the stable and pastures, why do so many foals remain healthy? Figure 9.2 illus-

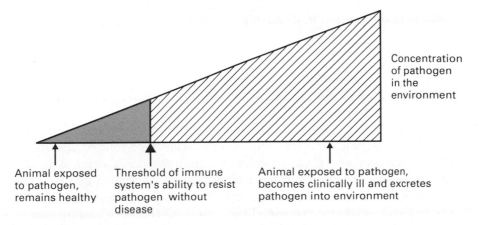

Concentration of pathogen in the environment

Animal exposed to pathogen, remains healthy

Threshold of immune system's ability to resist pathogen without disease

Animal exposed to pathogen, becomes clinically ill and excretes pathogen into environment

Positive Factors
Pre- and post-partum health care of dam (vaccination, deworming, nutrition)
Genetic predisposition
Adequate colostrum intake
Clean, disinfected, well-ventilated environment
Housing in same stall / paddock through weaning age

Negative Factors
Build–up of pathogens in environment due to poor disinfection techniques
Failure of passive transfer
Heavy parasitism, malnutrition
Stresses due to transportation, surgery, confinement, orthopaedic devices
Poor ventilation / draughty stalls
Overcrowding
Virulence of pathogen

Figure 9.2 Balance between health and disease.

trates the fine balance between health and disease in animals exposed to an infectious agent. The positive factors which bolster the foal's immune system to deal with various pathogens are listed. Once the immune system's threshold is exceeded, the balance tips in favour of the pathogen and the disease process commences. The negative factors favour the pathogen's ability to overwhelm the immune system. In the case of highly contagious diseases, large numbers of infectious agents are shed and the contaminated environment poses a threat to other foals by direct or indirect transmission. The foal with FPT has a compromised ability to handle even very low doses of infectious agents.

A key point to recognize from Figure 9.2 is that besides the routine preventive health measures of vaccination, parasite control and correct feeding, preventing the build-up of pathogens in the environment will help maintain the balance in favour of a healthy foal. The primary means of accomplishing this are management, disinfection and hygiene.

Role of management in disease prevention

Care of the newborn foal

Proper care of the newborn foal is essential for its future health and includes ensuring sufficient colostrum intake, care of the umbilical cord and prevention of retained meconium.

The foal is born without antibody protection, which is obtained by suckling the mare's first milk, or colostrum. Colostrum contains a concentrated source of immunoglobulins (Ig) or antibodies present in the mare's serum as a result of her exposure to natural infection and vaccination. The foal's intestine is able to absorb these antibodies only during the first 24 hours of life. Therefore, it is essential that foals begin to nurse within 2 hours of being born, and continue to suckle their dam at frequent intervals during this period. Studies have shown that the foal's ability to absorb Ig is greatest in the first 6 hours of life and rapidly decreases until 24 hours, when antibodies are no longer absorbed. In the case of weak foals, colostrum can be milked from the mare and bottle fed or administered by stomach tube.

Good quality colostrum should have a thick, sticky consistency; the higher the specific gravity, the greater the immunoglobulin concentration. The specific gravity of colostrum can be tested by using a colostrometer (Equine Colostrometer, Jorgenson Laboratories, Loveland, CO). Colostrum with a specific gravity of above 1.06 is associated with high levels of immuno-globulins.

Problems with passive transfer of antibodies may occur for several reasons: the mare may have run colostrum prior to parturition and not have sufficient amounts to give to the foal; the mare, especially a maiden mare, may have poor quality or insufficient colostrum; the foal may not have ingested enough colos-trum; or the foal may have some intestinal defect which prevents absorption of Ig. Foals which do not absorb adequate amounts in the first 24 hours have failure of passive transfer (FPT) and are susceptible to septicaemia, pneu-monia, diarrhoea and other infections.

Several different commercially available test kits can be used to determine the foal's level of immunoglobulins (specifically IgG) at 18–24 hours of age. Much discussion and debate has taken place over the appropriate level of IgG in the serum of foals. In a recent study involving 132 Standardbred foals on a farm in New York, it was found that serum IgG concentration was not related to the prevalence or severity of illness or to survival rate. Erring on the side of safety, foals should have minimum levels of 400 mg/dl of IgG at 18–24 hours of age. Foals which have less may require transfusions of plasma, an expensive and time-consuming procedure.

In order to provide a source of colostrum for foals when a mare dies or does not have an adequate supply, a colostrum bank should be established. Mares normally produce 1.5–2.0 litres of colostrum. A mare which has an uncomplicated delivery, and has colostrum with a specific gravity of greater than 1.06 is a good source. At least 250 ml of colostrum can be collected from a mare by milking the un-nursed teat after the foal first suckles. Colostrum should be frozen in plastic jars or bags (glass may break with freezing) at regular home freezer temperature and should be used within 18 months of storage.

Besides ensuring adequate intake of colostrum, other preventive health procedures need to be performed within the first few hours of the foal's life. Because of continual transfer of blood from mare to foal, the umbilical cord should not be manually broken. The cord naturally breaks when the dam gets to her feet after foaling. The umbilical stump, usually about 5 cm (2 in) long, is a pathway for bacteria to gain entrance to the body. To prevent this, it is important to dip the stump in a 2% iodine solution immediately after the cord breaks and twice a day for 2–3 days. This can be performed with the iodine in a small disposable paper cup held up to the ventral abdominal wall of the foal. Stronger concentrations of iodine should be avoided as they are too caustic to the skin and umbilicus. The area should be inspected daily for the presence of heat, swelling and dribbling of urine or blood. These signs indicate the presence of an abscess, hernia or a patent urachus, all of which require prompt veterinary attention.

Meconium is the first faeces passed by the foal after birth. This material is dark greenish to brown in colour and has a soft, tar-like consistency. Signs of meconium impaction are straining, restlessness, tail elevation and colic. To facilitate passage of meconium, a warmed enema using 150 ml of liquid paraffin or up to 1 litre of soapy water, or a human enema product may be given via a soft rubber tube. Care must always be taken to use soft tubing in the rectum as the rectal mucosa can be easily damaged. If the foal is still straining and uncomfortable after two enemas, veterinary intervention is required.

Healthy foals born without complications do not require administration of antibiotics. Routine injections of penicillin or penicillin/streptomycin are discouraged since most neonatal infections are caused by Gram-negative bacteria which are resistant to these drugs. A single administration of any antibiotic is inadequate to prevent or treat a bacterial infection and may cause development of antibiotic resistant strains of bacteria. Oral doses of vitamins, bacterial inoculum preparations or intestinal protectants should *not* be administered within the first 24 hours of age due to the ability of the small intestine to non-selectively absorb large proteins. Foal deaths have been reported following administration of vitamin preparations containing iron shortly after birth. Intestinal protectants and adsorbant products for treatment of diarrhoea, and any other orally dosed product should be given only by veterinary direction.

Foals born to mares which had not been vaccinated with tetanus toxoid 4–6 weeks prepartum should receive 1500 units of tetanus antitoxin by intramuscular injection. This protection usually lasts for 3 months, the time when routine vaccination for other diseases should be initiated.

Every farm has its own husbandry practices and history of disease problems. A broodmare farm with a closed herd and each mare having its own stall is very different from a boarding stable with mares and foals circulating through a limited number of stalls during the year. The recommendations which follow should be implemented where practical on an individual farm basis.

Horse movement

Any horse coming onto the farm, whether from a neighbouring stable or from another country, should be isolated for a minimum of 7–10 days prior to joining the resident herd. This will cover the incubation period of most respiratory viruses and stress-induced diarrhoeal diseases, but strangles remains a continuous threat. Isolating all new arrivals for a longer period may not be practical. A complete vaccination and health history should be obtained on every incoming horse and any additional vaccinations and medications should be administered during the isolation period.

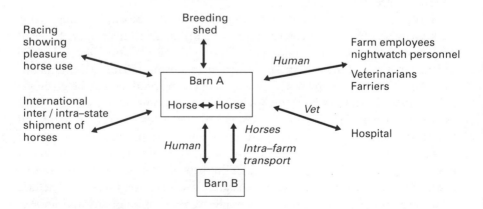

Figure 9.3 Potential sources of contamination on horse farms either by direct animal contact or fomite transmission.

Figure 9.3 indicates the enormous amount of human and equine traffic which goes through a single barn. Besides the increased horse traffic during the foaling season, veterinarians and other visitors may be a source of infectious disease agents. Much of this movement is an essential part of everyday farm operations, but show horses or racehorses should not be mixed into a barn or field of broodmares. The stall and paddock arrangements should be planned so that horse traffic to different areas of the farm is kept to the absolute minimum. The ideal situation would be to have a mare housed in the same stall/paddock area for the entire foaling season. Shuffling mares and foals from barn to barn is contraindicated. Although the practice of housing mares close to foaling in a special foaling unit economizes on labour, especially of nightwatch personnel, the potential for the build-up of pathogens in this area is very high. If individual stalls are adequate in size and construction, mares should be allowed to foal in their own stall. If use of central foaling stalls is necessary, it is essential that they be *thoroughly* cleaned and disinfected after each foaling.

Mares with similar foaling dates should be grouped together so that foals of similar age will be housed in the same barn and paddock. This helps not only in the control of infectious disease, but also in easing the stress of weaning. Likewise, horses of similar type should be grouped together: resident broodmares, yearlings, horses in training, and boarders or transient residents. This reduces the stresses of a changing 'pecking order' and limits the introduction and spread of diseases. Even on farms with no disease problems, farm employees, farriers and veterinarians should work with younger foals and their dams first, then weanlings, yearlings and finally adult horses. Although this may seem an overly strict and needless exercise, if animals have been grouped by age and use, it becomes a practical means of preventing the spread of disease agents from asymptomatic adult carriers to young foals.

Employee education

Prior to the foaling season, farm employees should be instructed about the disease prevention programme on the farm. All farm personnel need to understand the reasons why specific measures are being instituted and that their absolute co-operation is essential to the success of the programme. The management schedule in Appendix 9.1 at the end of the chapter should be given to each farm employee and displayed in a prominent place in the barn.

Procedures to be adopted during a disease outbreak

Besides treating individual animals, containment of a contagious disease outbreak is paramount. When the foal's immune system is overwhelmed by the large concentrations of pathogens, the disease process is initiated as illustrated in Figure 9.2. Animals which appear clinically normal may be in the incubative phase of sickness and shedding pathogens into the environment. When a foal is diagnosed as having a contagious disease, *all in-contact animals should be considered to have been exposed*. The practice of moving 'healthy' foals to other barns as a way of preventing them from becoming infected usually ensures further spread of the disease as these foals may already be infected.

How is it possible to prevent disease transmission from one animal to another within a barn? The provision of a separate barn with easily disinfected stalls for the sole purpose of isolating sick animals is the ideal solution. Sick animals shed large numbers of microorganisms, and so removing them from asymptomatic animals will limit contamination of the barn. Sick animals and the employees caring for them need to be isolated from other horses on the farm. Farm employees and night watchmen attending sick foals can effectively transmit disease to other foals if precautions are not taken.

Animals should be kept isolated even after recovery from clinical signs, the duration being dependent upon the shedding pattern of the pathogen, as discussed earlier. If a separate isolation facility is unavailable, a regime as illustrated in Figure 9.4 should be implemented. Assume that foals in stalls D,

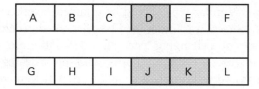

Figure 9.4 Twelve-stall barn with mares and foals.

J and K have developed a contagious disease. The movement of personnel into those stalls and that half of the barn should be kept to an absolute minimum and all traffic into and out of the barn restricted severely. Foals in adjoining stalls have to be considered exposed and at high risk of developing disease. Personnel going into and out of stalls D, J and K should take extreme precautions to limit the transmission of disease including the use of protective clothing, disposable boots and frequent hand washing.

Vehicles such as manure and hay wagons should move from the left of the barn to the right to prevent disease transmission. Veterinarians, farriers and other outside personnel should work first with healthy animals in other barns, followed by healthy animals in 'sick' barns and finally sick animals in isolation.

Manure disposal

Spreading manure on pastures is a common disposal practice on most farms. In the knowledge that rotavirus can survive for an extended period of time outside the host, and is transmitted by ingestion, manure collected during rotavirus diarrhoea outbreaks should *never* be spread on pastures. Rather, it should be composted in a manure pile that is inaccessible to horses and foals.

Disinfection

The primary objective of disinfection is to keep the level of pathogenic organisms in the environment to a level which will not cause disease. The types of surfaces which are to be disinfected strongly influence the effectiveness of the disinfectant. Foals are exposed to two different environments: pasture and a stall or man-made enclosure. As it is not possible nor desirable to disinfect pastures, this discussion will concentrate on the cleaning of stall or stable surfaces. Horse vans and trailers also need to be routinely disinfected, but they generally have similar surfaces as stalls.

No stall flooring is ideal when durability, economy, drainage, horse comfort and ease of cleaning are taken into consideration. The advantages and disadvantages of a variety of flooring materials are discussed in Chapter 5. Little information, however, is available regarding the suitability of flooring materials for disinfection procedures. To control infectious or contagious disease through disinfection, a solid floor is essential. A slope of 3° in the stall floor will assist drainage and not place a strain on the horse's legs. Concrete provides a hard surface which is easily cleaned, but unless the stall is deeply bedded it can cause leg problems and is slick when wet. Porous 'popcorn' asphalt has a rough surface so that horses will not slip when getting to their feet. This surface is composed of a large particle asphalt which is raked instead of rolled when installed. Rubber mats are resilient and easy on horses' legs but are expensive. Microorganisms may accumulate in the crevices between and under the mats, requiring that the mats are removed for cleaning. Packed clay is comfortable for horses to stand on for long periods of time, but may become uneven with extensive use. Clay, along with sand and soil, is very difficult if not impossible to adequately disinfect. If a disease outbreak occurs in a barn with soil flooring, the only way to 'clean' the stall floor is to remove the top 15–30 cm (6–12 in) and replace with fresh material.

Synthetic plastics and other man-made materials have recently become available, from interlocking synthetic 'bricks' to heavy duty plastic connecting squares under a sand bedding. These are durable, aesthetically pleasing and probably comfortable for the horse. As for disease prevention, however, the more crevices where dirt and microorganisms can accumulate, the more difficult the floor is to disinfect.

Besides floor construction, stall walls also become contaminated with organic matter, including faeces, urine, blood and various discharges. Most stall walls are constructed of concrete block or wood. Basic concrete blocks are porous and should be painted with a high quality enamel paint to facilitate cleaning, as seen in Figure 9.5. Unfinished wood is impossible to clean ad-

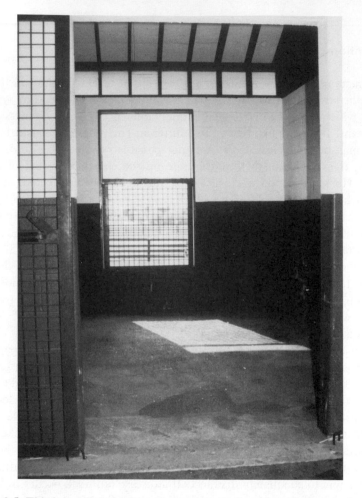

Figure 9.5 This is a well-designed stall constructed of roughened concrete floors and concrete block walls coated with epoxy paint. The metal mesh doors provide a bright, well-ventilated environment.

equately. One way to seal wood and facilitate thorough cleaning is to fill in knots and holes with plastic wood to eliminate spaces where organic matter and microorganisms may harbour. Then apply one or two coats of a quality marine varnish, or wood water sealant followed by a coat of polyurethane to seal the wood, allowing adequate cleaning of the resultant smooth surface.

Choice of disinfectant

The choice of disinfectant should be based on the following criteria: effectiveness at killing targeted pathogenic organisms; ability to work in a specific environment (horse stalls); activity in the presence of organic matter and hard water; safety for animals and people; and biodegradability.

Of the pathogens discussed, the primary targeted organisms are lipid-enveloped influenza and herpes viruses, rotavirus, Gram-positive and Gram-negative bacteria and spore-forming bacteria. Of the viruses which cause outbreaks of disease, rotavirus is the most resistant to disinfection. Because of its importance on broodmare farms, much of the discussion on the choice of disinfectants will concern the use of those which are effective against rotavirus. At this stage it is important to emphasize that no disinfectant is going to be 100% effective against every organism found in the environment.

An effective disinfectant for farm use should not be readily inactivated by organic matter. Organic matter provides a physical barrier to any chemical and also inactivates some compounds. Since no disinfectant will work on a dirty surface, the initial step in disinfecting stalls is to clean the walls and floors with a detergent. Detergents may consist of one or a combination of three different types: anionic, cationic or non-ionic. The choice of a specific disinfectant will determine which type of detergent is used in cleaning since certain disinfectants and detergents are incompatible. Anionic detergents can be found in the laundry cleaning section of stores. Most labels indicate whether the compound is biodegradable, and if it is anionic, cationic, non-ionic or a combination. In general, most powdered detergents are anionic, whereas liquid detergents, even if under the same tradename as their powdered counterparts, are combinations of anionic, cationic and non-ionic compounds. These combinations should not be utilized in cleaning stalls. Several commercial disinfectants are formulated with a detergent and may be used in the cleaning step as well as for disinfecting.

Water hardness can directly reduce the germicidal action of a disinfectant due to the presence of calcium and magnesium ions. The label should list the disinfectant's effectiveness in hard water. 'Hardness' is defined as the level of calcium carbonate ($CaCO_3$) in parts per million (ppm) found in a water sample. Look for label statements such as 'Germicidal testing shows this product is effective in the presence of 400 ppm $CaCO_3$ (as hard water)'. An inquiry to the local water department or water company will reveal the average level of hardness in tap water. Farms which have well or spring water should have the water tested for hardness in order to choose an appropriate disinfectant.

Disinfectants can be potentially harmful to people and animals. Abiding by the manufacturer's usage recommendations and using protective eye goggles and gloves can reduce the dangers associated with their use. A potential danger with long-term skin exposure to phenolic disinfectants is depigmentation of the skin; this is prevented by the use of protective clothing and rubber gloves. Compounds which have noxious fumes, or are extremely caustic are inappropriate for use by farm employees. The possibility exists of ingestion of disinfectants by small animals and pets and the reader is referred to an article by Coppack and colleagues included in the list of further reading.

With current awareness of environmental issues, the use of biodegradable products is important and should be taken into consideration when reading labels and choosing a commercial compound.

Classes of disinfectants

Textbooks, scientific articles and the mass of advertising literature on disinfectants provide a confusing list of organic chemical compounds and properties to consider. Most textbooks and articles describe the value of disinfection on surfaces in hospitals. Careful interpretation is necessary when reading information regarding the use of disinfectants in the stable. Useful references include *Disinfection in Veterinary and Farm Animal Practice*, *Disinfection Sterilization and Preservation*, and *Chemical Disinfection in Hospitals* (see Further Reading).

The types of disinfectants available for farm use include phenols, iodophores, quaternary ammonium compounds (QAC), hypochlorites and chlorhexidine. The activity of these disinfectants is summarized in Table 9.2.

Phenols

Phenolic compounds are derivatives of coal. Based on their chemical structure, many compounds may be formulated, each with potentially different germicidal actions. Phenols are effective against Gram-positive and Gram-negative bacteria (but not bacterial spores), yeasts and fungi. Lipid-enveloped viruses, including herpesvirus and influenza virus, are readily inactivated by o-phenylphenol, a common phenolic in commercial preparations. Tests of phenolic disinfectants on human rotavirus have shown a good range of activity against the virus. Disinfectants containing o-phenylphenol, o-benzyl chlorophenol and p-tertiary amyl phenol and sodium o-benzyl-p-chlorophenate were effective against rotavirus in the presence of organic matter. Of considerable practical significance is the use of detergents with phenolic compounds. Anionic detergents should be used, since cationic compounds are incompatible and non-ionic compounds inactivate the germicidal action of the phenols. If the detergent label does not indicate what type it is, call the manufacturer for information.

Several general principles need to be borne in mind when choosing a phenolic disinfectant. The active ingredient list should contain a combination of

Table 9.2 Germicidal activity of common disinfectants

	Rotavirus	Influenza	Herpes	Adenovirus	Gram-positive	Gram-negative	Bacterial sporicidal	Positive features	Negative features
Phenolics	+	+	+	+	+	+	–	Not readily inactivated in organic matter	Irritant, corrosive
Iodophores	+[1]	+	+	+	+	+	+	Used as a skin antiseptic	May cause skin sensitivity
Quaternary ammonium compounds (QACs)	–	+	+	+	+	–	–		Readily inactivated in organic matter
Hypochlorites (bleach)	–	+	+	+	+	+	+	Economical; commonly used as sanitizers in public buildings	Readily inactivated in organic matter
Chlorhexidine	–	–	–	–	+	+/–	–	Used for skin antiseptic	Readily inactivated in organic matter

[1] 10% povidone iodine.

the four chemicals listed above as active against rotavirus. Phenolic compounds have long chemical names, but can be recognized by the -phenol or -phenate at the end of the compound name. Each of the four phenolic compounds has various synonyms, arising from different nomenclature. (Note that o-phenylphenol is an entirely different compound than sodium o-phenylphenate.)

ortho-phenylphenol = o-phenylphenol = 2-phenylphenol

para-tertiary amyl phenol = p-tertiary amyl phenol = p-tert amyl phenol

ortho-benzyl chlorophenol = o-benzyl chlorophenol

sodium ortho-benzyl para-chlorophenate = Na o-benzyl p-chlorophenate

Note that sodium o-phenyl*phenate* is an entirely different compound from o-phenyl*phenol*.

Do not rely on buying a disinfectant based on brand name alone. Be sure to read the list of active ingredients. As an example, disinfectants under the name of Lysol® have formulations for the product packaged in the gallon size different from that packaged in the half gallon and pint size. Similarly, the phenolic disinfectant One Stroke Environ® (Calgon-Vestal Laboratories, St Louis, MO) may be confused with another disinfectant One Step-Environ 42®(Central Chemical Corp., Lexington, KY) which is a QAC. Because of this, the choice of disinfectant should be based on the list of active ingredients and not reference to a brand name. Under no circumstances should a disinfectant be mixed with other chemicals.

Because of their activity against various equine pathogens, the ability to disinfect in the presence of organic matter and their stability in solution, phenolic disinfectants are recommended for farm use.

Iodophores

Iodine by itself is bactericidal and sporicidal, but is irritating to the skin, is toxic and stains. A combination of iodine with a carrier produces a compound known as an iodophore, which increases solubility, improves wetting properties, aids the penetration of organic matter and is less toxic. When the carrier is polyvinylpyrrolidone, the solution is known as povidone iodine. Germicidal activity and ability to disinfect in the presence of organic matter are dependent upon the percent concentration of the iodine compound and an acidic pH (at least pH 4). The activity of iodophores is limited by excessive water hardness. It should be noted that due to the particular carrier or concentration, not all iodophores are equal in their ability to kill rotavirus. In one study an iodophore at 1:200 dilution did not inactivate rotavirus in the presence of organic matter, whereas a 10% concentration of povidone iodine solution was capable of killing the virus. Iodophores are not generally used for disinfecting stalls, but are commonly utilized as solutions and scrubs for skin antiseptics.

Quaternary ammonium compounds (QAC)

Quaternary ammonium compounds are classified as cationic surfactants and are the most numerous commercially available disinfectants. QACs can be recognized by the ending *-ammonium chloride* in their chemical name. Some disinfectants have just one QAC listed as an active ingredient (first generation products) while others have four different QACs listed (fourth generation products). QACs possess bactericidal activity against Gram-positive and Gram-negative organisms but are not sporicidal. Lipid-enveloped viruses are readily inactivated by this lipophilic compound. Even with the many different chemical formulations available, cationic surfactants are not able to inactivate rotavirus. The most important factor to be aware of with QACs is their inactivation in the presence of organic matter. Most QAC disinfectant labels state that the compound has been tested and proven effective in the presence of heavy organic matter (5% blood serum). Even so, they are *not* recommended for use in cleaning horse facilities because of their inactivation in the presence of organic matter.

Hypochlorites

Sodium hypochlorite, commonly known as bleach, has long been used as a disinfectant on horse farms both for stall cleaning and in footbath solutions. It is inexpensive, easy to obtain and leaves a fresh bleach odour associated with cleanliness. Hypochlorites have a wide bactericidal spectrum, are sporicidal, and are active against lipid-enveloped and non-enveloped viruses. Their germicidal activity is rapid but is dependent upon the concentration of available chlorine in solution. However, testing of hypochlorites against rotavirus has demonstrated that this virus is resistant to inactivation by bleach. Hypochlorites, like QACs, are readily inactivated in the presence of organic matter. They are unstable following long periods of storage and exposure to light and are incompatible with cationic detergents. Because of their rapid inactivation in the presence of faeces, urine, blood and discharges, as well as the inability to kill rotavirus, hypochlorites are not suitable as disinfecting agents on horse farms.

Chlorhexidine

The chlorhexidine group of compounds are commonly used as skin disinfectants or antiseptics. Their germicidal spectrum has greater activity against Gram-positive than Gram-negative bacteria, but they are not sporicidal. They are limited in activity against viruses and are inactivated by soap, anionic detergents and organic matter. Because of their low toxicity, they should be utilized as antiseptics and not as disinfectants for farm use.

Aldehydes

Glutaraldehyde is a compound which is very effective at killing bacterial microorganisms, spores and various viruses, including rotavirus, even in the presence of organic matter. Its germicidal action requires long periods of time, and most commercial preparations are for use in disinfecting surgical instruments and endoscopes, not for cleaning environmental surfaces. It is an irritant to eyes, skin and mucous membranes.

Formaldehyde is a potent germicidal agent, and is known as formalin when in aqueous solution. Although it is slow acting, this chemical will kill bacteria, viruses and spores even in the presence of organic matter. Swine and poultry units are commonly fumigated with formaldehyde, but because of the highly toxic nature of this compound, it is not used as a general disinfectant.

Pine oil

Pine oil has been used in horse barns for years, in part because of its fresh residual pine odour. Its ability to disinfect is dubious under farm conditions, and it should not be indiscriminately added to other disinfectants due to possible adverse chemical reactions.

Prospective buyers of disinfectants should critically evaluate the claims on any disinfectant label. Many of the commercially available disinfectants were developed for the human health industry: hospitals, nursing homes and clinics. The disinfectant label may define the compound as a multipurpose disinfectant cleaner for the hospital environment. However the hospital environment of stainless steel, linoleum and ceramic tiles is vastly different from the environment of a horse barn, even one that is meticulously clean. Other label statements which require critical analysis are claims of efficacy in the presence of 5% serum contamination; bearing in mind the contamination in a horse barn this is not impressive. Some labels state that the compound cleans and disinfects in one easy step. However, when dealing with horse stalls, cleaning and disinfecting cannot be completed in one step, as discussed later in this chapter. An ideal disinfectant for use on horse farms would be a compound labelled as bactericidal, virucidal, fungicidal, biodegradable, effective in the presence of 10% organic matter and 400 ppm hard water, and safe for responsible use around people and animals. A checklist to consider when choosing a disinfectant is included in Appendix 9.2 at the end of the chapter.

Disinfection of farm buildings

Stalls need to be disinfected after each mare has foaled, irrespective of whether a central foaling stall or individual stall was used. Disinfect gangways twice a week throughout the foaling season. If mares and foals need to be moved into a different stall, the stall should be disinfected prior to occupation. Stalls used for isolating incoming horses need to be disinfected after each use.

Disinfecting farm premises is a two-step process: physically cleaning the surfaces with a detergent followed by chemical disinfection. The cleaning step is clearly the most time consuming and labour intensive but is the most important, remembering that the best disinfectants cannot be expected to be effective in a heavily contaminated environment. Under farm conditions even though surfaces cannot be considered completely free from microorganisms, stall walls and floors must be visibly clean before the application of a disinfectant.

When cleaning and disinfecting an individual stall, the sequence of events should be as follows. All portable equipment must be removed from the stall including buckets, feed tubs, salt blocks, etc. Bedding must be removed and the floor thoroughly swept. Soak all surfaces with an anionic detergent/warm water solution for an hour to loosen dried faeces and organic matter. Stalls can then be cleaned in several ways. Dirt is removed manually with a stiff brush followed by washing down the surface. A nozzle attached to a hose provides added water pressure to remove dirt. Power steam washers (Figure 9.6), which deliver water at high temperatures (99 °C = 210 °F) and pressure (700–1000 pounds per square inch), represent a significant investment, approximately $US3000. Modern machines are equipped to deliver detergent and disinfectant solutions. Care must be taken when utilizing these high-pressure steam machines on painted surfaces, since their abrasiveness can remove paint. Wash down the stall with a pressure spray, starting at the top. Floors should be rinsed starting at the end opposite from where the water will eventually drain. Any stubbornly stained areas should be scrubbed again by hand with a stiff brush and detergent solution, and thoroughly rinsed. When all visible surfaces and corners are clean, allow to dry. According to manufacturer's instructions, dilute the disinfectant and pour into the pressure sprayer or a hand-held pressurized applicator which costs approximately $US50–70. Since phenol compounds are irritating, safety goggles and rubber gloves should be worn. Spray all wall and floor surfaces with particular attention to corners and crevices. After allowing the surfaces to dry apply a second coat of disinfectant to the stall. Surfaces should *not* be rinsed. Allowing the disinfectant to dry

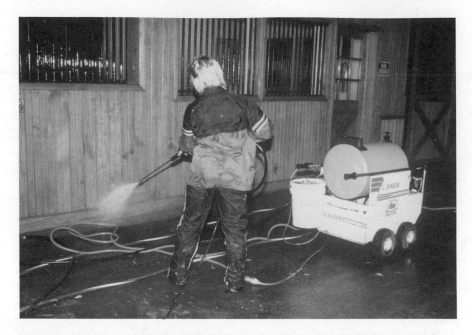

Figure 9.6 Steam cleaners are made to deliver high-pressure/high-temperature water with detergents and/or disinfectants. This allows for thorough cleaning of farm premises. Notice the weatherproof clothing of the worker.

increases the contact time and also the germicidal effectiveness. Drying time varies depending upon the temperature and relative humidity and may range from one to several hours, but can be hastened by using fans. Water and feed buckets should be cleaned with a detergent, rinsed with the disinfectant and then completely rinsed with water. Read the manufacturer's label regarding the use of the disinfectant on feeding/watering equipment. Brooms, rakes and shovels need to be disinfected; in cases of strangles, brushes, combs and other horse equipment used on affected horses also need to be cleaned and scrubbed with a detergent and soaked in a disinfectant solution for 10 minutes before being allowed to dry. Coveralls, clothing, towels and other cloth materials used on infected horses can be soaked in detergent to remove dirt and then soaked for 10 minutes in disinfectant solution before regular washing. Again, the disinfectant label should indicate if the compound is safe for use on fabrics.

Disinfection during a disease outbreak

Every endeavour should be made to keep stalls of sick animals as clean as possible. Pitchforks, shovels, brooms, rakes, feed/water buckets as well as combs, brushes and other equipment taken into the stall should be considered as contaminated. Equipment used for healthy foals should be kept separate from that used for sick foals. If this is not possible, equipment should be used first on and around healthy foals, then sick foals, followed by thorough cleaning and disinfection. Footwear is an effective means of transferring pathogens from stall to stall. Footbaths filled with phenolic disinfectants should be placed at every entrance to the barn and in the case of strangles and diseases causing diarrhoea, placed at every stall entrance, as shown in Figure 9.7. Footbath solutions need to be changed every day as the level of organic contamination is high following routine use.

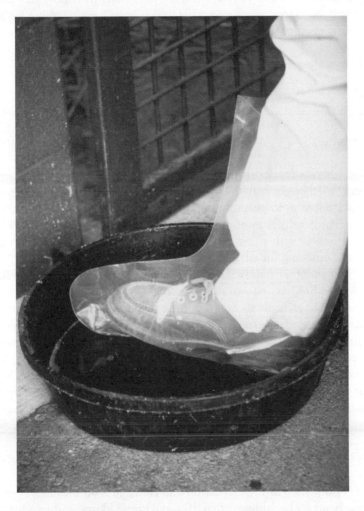

Figure 9.7 Footbaths with phenolic disinfectants should be used in the midst of disease outbreaks. A separate pair of plastic disposable footwear can be used for each stall to prevent transmission of diseases from foal to foal.

Special treatments

Cryptosporidium is an intracellular coccidian parasite which invades the small intestine to produce clinical or subclinical infections in many species of animals and humans. This organism is not species specific and therefore may pose a zoonotic threat. Since infective oocysts are shed in the faeces and the survival time in the environment is unknown, the choice of disinfectant is critical. The common disinfectants previously discussed are ineffective in killing oocysts. In disinfectant trials, only after an 18-hour exposure to 10% formol saline or 5% ammonia were the oocysts effectively killed. Fumigation with these compounds is dangerous and requires trained personnel to handle these noxious, toxic chemicals. Barns containing foals which have been diagnosed with cryptosporidiosis need to be cleaned by this method of fumigation.

Hygiene

The hard labour of stall disinfection may seem sufficient to prevent the spread of contagious disease, but daily hygiene practices especially when handling sick foals are just as important. Little has been reported regarding the role of antiseptic handwashing solutions in disease prevention on the farm. The preparation of hands with a 5-minute scrub, as performed by doctors prior to gloving and gowning for surgery, is hardly practical.

How important is handwashing, especially during a rotavirus diarrhoea outbreak? Studies have shown that rotavirus can remain infective on hands for several hours. Diarrhoeic faeces from foals infected with rotavirus contain high concentrations of the virus, and even after an hour's drying time, virus-contaminated human skin is still infectious to foals. Hands are therefore an effective means of disseminating rotavirus from one foal to another, stressing the importance of thorough hand washing.

What are the most effective handwashing solutions that are not inactivated by organic matter? In discussing this subject, active ingredients, not tradenames will be used because there are numerous products available with the same active ingredients. Tradenames change and product names vary from country to country, so reading the list of active ingredients on a product label is necessary.

A study published in 1983 by Sattar and colleagues on the efficacy of various antiseptic handwashes showed that 10% povidone iodine and two hexachlorophene handwashes inactivated rotavirus in the presence of organic matter. Hexachlorophene is absorbed through the skin and has potential neurotoxicity for humans. It has been removed from the general commercial market in the USA and is not recommended for human use. Chlorhexidine gluconate 4% and an iodophore compound of unspecified concentration did not significantly inactivate rotavirus. Other compounds including 1.5% chlorhexidine gluconate with 15.0% cetrimide and a QAC were inactivated in the presence of organic matter. Another study found that a product with active ingredients ethanol (78.2% w/w) and phenol (0.1% w/w) effectively decreased rotavirus contamination on hands after a one-minute scrub.

What information can be gained from these studies and applied on horse farms? Disposable gloves should be used *every* time a sick foal is handled. Employees, including nightwatch personnel, should be instructed to wash their hands thoroughly before handling very young foals and after handling sick foals. To further facilitate employee compliance, each barn should have accessible warm water and a clean washbasin, a pump dispenser for the liquid antiseptic, a hand brush, disposable paper towels and a waste container. A liquid handsoap should be available throughout the year. In the midst of a contagious disease outbreak, the routine use of a 10% povidone iodine scrub is recommended. In cases where people have a skin sensitivity to povidone iodine, a triclosan medicated soap could be used. Hand-scrub solutions may be obtained through most medical supply companies. Ethyl or isopropyl alcohol (60–70%)/emollient foam products (waterless hand antiseptics) which are rubbed on cleaned hands and allowed to dry are also recommended. Hand foams such as Derma Stat® (Minnetonka Medical, Chaska, MN) and Alcare® (Calgon-Vestal Laboratories, St Louis, MO) contain 62–65% ethyl alcohol and can be obtained through medical supply stores. Alcohols have rapid bactericidal and virucidal action at 60–70% concentrations. They do not penetrate organic matter, so hands should be washed prior to use. Since these compounds are flammable, care must be taken not to use around an open flame. Even though alcohols are effective germicides, they are not used in stall disinfection because of flammability, inactivity in the presence of organic matter and the cost of using large volumes of undiluted alcohols. QACs are not appropriate agents for handwashing due to their inactivity in the presence of organic matter and their inability to kill rotavirus. Even though no hand antiseptic is totally germicidal, the outcome is well worth the individual effort.

To prevent the spread of contagious diseases from foal to foal, disposable footwear should be used when working with sick foals. With cases of salmonellosis, rotavirus diarrhoea and strangles, disposable gowns or separate coveralls should be available.

Further reading

Ambrosiano N W, Harcourt M F (1989) *Complete plans for building horse barns big and small*. Breakthrough Publications, Ossining, New York, pp 48–50.

Ayliffe G A, Coates D, Hoffman P N (1984) *Chemical disinfection in hospitals*. Public Health Laboratory Service, London.

Baldwin J L, Cooper W L, Vanderwall D K, Erb H N (1991) Prevalence (treatment days) and severity of illness in hypogammaglobulinemic and normogammaglobulinemic foals. *Journal of the American Veterinary Medical Association*, **198**: 423–8.

Block S S (1983) *Disinfection, sterilization and preservation*. Lea & Febiger, Philadelphia, PA.

Claybough D L, Conboy H S, Roberts M C (1989) Comparison of four screening techniques for the diagnosis of equine neonatal hypogammaglobulinemia. *Journal of the American Veterinary Medical Association*, **194**: 1717–20.

Coppock R W, Mostrom M S, Lillie L E (1988) The toxicology of detergents, bleaches, antiseptics and disinfectants in small animals. *Veterinary and Human Toxicology*, **30**: 463–73.

Dwyer R M, Powell D G, Roberts W, Donahue M, Lyons E T, Osborne M, Woode G (1990) A study of the etiology and control of infectious diarrhea among foals in Central Kentucky. In: Royer M G (ed) *Proceedings of the 36th Annual Convention of the American Association of Equine Practitioners*, Lexington, pp 337–55.

Ellis D R (1990) Care of neonatal foals—normal and abnormal. *In Practice* **12**: 193–7.

Koterba A M, Drummond W H, Kosch P C (1990) *Equine clinical neonatology*. Lea & Febiger, Philadelphia, PA.

LeBlanc M M, McLaurin B I, Boswell R (1986) Relationships among serum immunoglobulin concentration in foals, colostral specific gravity and colostral immunoglobulin concentration. *Journal of the American Veterinary Medical Association*, **189**: 57–60.

Linton A H, Hugo W B, Russell A D (1987) *Disinfection in veterinary and farm animal practice*. Blackwell Scientific Publications, London.

Madigan J E (1991) *Manual of equine neonatal medicine*, 2nd edn. Live Oak Publishing, Woodland, CA.

Springthorpe V S, Grenier J L, Lloyd-Evans N, Sattar S A (1986) Chemical disinfection of human rotaviruses: efficacy of commercially-available products in suspension tests. *Journal of Hygiene (Camb)*, **97**: 139–61.

Appendix 9.1

Management schedule

I. Prior to foaling season

Institute an isolation protocol for any horses coming onto the farm.

Avoid use of central foaling stalls. If this is not possible, plan stall and paddock assignments for foaling mares to minimize the movement of horses during the year, but especially during the foaling season.

Completely clean and disinfect stalls and aisleways of barns prior to occupation by foaling mares.

Educate *all* farm personnel about isolation and disinfection procedures, the need for disinfecting premises and general hygiene, including handwashing. Brief all employees on techniques to be employed in the midst of an infectious disease outbreak.

Provide adequate handwashing facilities including hot water, handwashing solution (povidone iodine scrub or chlorhexidine scrub) in pump containers; hand/nail scrub brush, and disposable paper towels.

II. *During the foaling season*

After each foaling completely clean and disinfect the stall.

Water buckets and feed equipment within stalls should be completely cleaned and disinfected prior to use by another mare and foal.

At least once or twice a week, barn aisleways should be thoroughly swept and sprayed with disinfectant.

Wash hands prior to handling very young foals.

Have separate employees work with newborn foals or have employees handle youngest or most susceptible foals first and older foals last.

III. *During an outbreak*

If an unoccupied isolation barn is available, sick foals and mares should be moved as soon as clinical signs are evident; other mares and foals remain confined to their respective stalls and paddocks.

Employees working with foals in the isolation unit should not work around any other horses and could be assigned to other non-animal duties e.g. fence repair, painting, etc.

ABSOLUTELY NO MOVEMENT OF HORSES BETWEEN BARNS/PAD-DOCKS SHOULD TAKE PLACE. Consider all horses in a barn containing an animal with a contagious disease as having been exposed and potentially incubating the disease.

Limit the movement of farm employees and vehicles (e.g. tractors, feed wagons) between barns on the farm.

Enforce traffic control of veterinarians, farriers and other necessary personnel from unaffected barns of horses → unaffected animals within the 'sick' barn → sick foals → sick animals within an isolation facility.

Protective clothing (disposable gloves, footwear, and gowns/overalls) should be used by all personnel prior to handling any sick foal. Separate sets of protective clothing should be available at the entrance of *each* sick foal's stall.

Hands should be thoroughly washed before and after handling each sick foal.

A separate set of rakes, pitchforks and other stall cleaning equipment should be available for stalls of sick foals and be disinfected after use. Alternatively, stalls of healthy foals should be cleaned first, with equipment used on sick foal's stalls last, after which equipment is thoroughly cleaned and disinfected.

Consider setting up footbaths or providing disposable footwear for use in every stall, especially in the foaling barn and with stalls of foals less than 2 weeks of age.

Clean and disinfect towels, cloths and uniforms contaminated with infectious material (faeces, discharges, etc.) by first rinsing to remove gross filth, soaking for 10 minutes in a phenol disinfectant solution and then machine washing. Brushes, combs and other equipment can be washed, soaked and rinsed similarly. In the midst of an outbreak, these materials and equipment are very effective transmitters of pathogens and should not be overlooked in the overall disinfection protocol.

Appendix 9.2

Disinfectant Checklist

What class of disinfectant is the product: phenol, QAC, hypochlorite, iodophore, chlorhexidine, other?

What specific active ingredients are listed?

What is the concentration of the active ingredients?

Is a detergent incorporated in the compound?

Is the product advertising geared toward the human health industry or toward the agricultural/animal industry?

Is the product labelled for use in hard water? If so, at what level of water hardness (ppm)? What is the average hardness of the tap water used on the farm (check with local water utilities or have the water tested)?

Has the product been tested for germicidal activity in the presence of 10% organic matter?

Is the product biodegradable?

Does the product have a pleasant odour or are there dangers of noxious fumes?

Is the product a fungicide?

Is the product labelled for use on feed and water buckets or is it potentially toxic?

Can the disinfectant also be used to soak and clean clothing and other fabrics?

What safety precautions must be taken when using the product besides standard eye goggles and rubber gloves?

Is the compound stable with shelf storage, freezing/thawing, heat (as in outdoor storage during summer months), light exposure?

Is the compound flammable?

Is the compound safe for use on the porous and non-porous surfaces?

What is the recommended dilution of the compound per litre of water for disinfecting faecally contaminated surfaces?

How many litres of disinfectant solution can be made from one litre of undiluted disinfectant?

Example Disinfectant A
Dilution 4 ml per litre water
(1 litre of disinfectant = 1000 millilitres)

Therefore 1000 ml disinfectant $\dfrac{1 \text{ litre solution}}{4 \text{ ml disinfectant}}$ = 250 litres of disinfectant solution

Use this factor to calculate a cost comparison with an equivalent product.

What is the cost per litre? Is there a discount for buying in volume?

Is the manufacturing company reputable with knowledgeable sales representatives and technical service personnel?

10 CARE OF THE FOOT
STEPHEN G. JACKSON, PhD

Summary

The equine foot is a very complex structure which serves to absorb concussion during exercise and support the weight of the horse during activities requiring agility and soundness. The basic principles involved in the care of the foot as well as several of the more common diseases and abnormalities are discussed.

The often quoted adage 'no foot no horse' indicates the importance of the foot to the ultimate athletic ability of the horse. The equine foot is a sophisticated system of bones and tissues which provides an effective interface with the ground. This chapter will discuss the care of the foot and several of the more common diseases and abnormalities. Details regarding the anatomy of the foot and shoeing are covered only superficially and the reader is referred to the list of 'Further reading' at the end of the chapter for additional information.

Basic anatomy

Skeletal structures of the foot

Each foot contains two and a half bones, the coffin bone (distal or third phalanx), the navicular bone (distal sesamoid) and the distal end of the short pastern bone (second phalanx) as shown in Figure 10.1. The coffin bone, also referred to as the pedal bone, is completely contained within the hoof wall; in the forelimb it is rounder than in the hindlimb. The coffin bone gives the foot

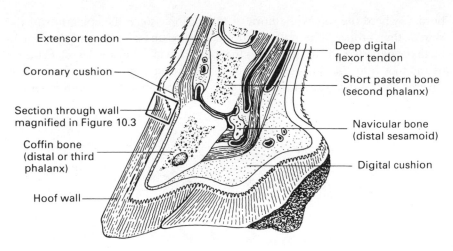

Extensor tendon

Coronary cushion

Section through wall magnified in Figure 10.3

Coffin bone (distal or third phalanx)

Hoof wall

Deep digital flexor tendon

Short pastern bone (second phalanx)

Navicular bone (distal sesamoid)

Digital cushion

Figure 10.1 Section through the foot.

its rigid structure and allows for attachment and protection of blood vessels and nerves that nourish the sensitive structures of the foot. The coffin bone is the point of attachment for the tendons that allow flexion and extension of the foot. The common digital extensor tendon in the forelimb and the long digital extensor tendon in the hindlimb are attached to the extensor process of the cranial edge of the coffin bone. The deep digital flexor tendon is attached to the semilunar crest of the coffin bone. Both the extensor and flexor tendons originate in muscles of the upper leg.

The navicular (distal sesamoid) bone sits behind the articulation of the coffin bone and short pastern bone which together form the distal interphalangeal or coffin joint. The navicular bone serves as a fulcrum for the deep digital flexor tendon as it passes behind and under the navicular bone prior to its attachment to the coffin bone. The navicular bone is subject to injury and wear and the development of navicular diseases, which will be discussed later.

The lower end of the short pastern bone is rounded to form condyles that articulate with corresponding concave depressions of the coffin bone. The rounded ends of the short pastern bone which articulate with the coffin bone allow lateral adjustment of the foot to compensate for uneven terrain.

Structure of the hoof

The hoof is the epidermal keratinized structure that surrounds the lower part of the foot; it is derived from the coronary corium or dermis that lies at the junction of the skin and hoof wall. The hoof wall is the portion seen when the horse is in the standing position and extends from the ground to the coronary border, where the soft white horn of the periople joins the epidermis of the skin at the coronet. The wall is reflected to the under surface of the foot to form the bars, which are two ridges that converge to delineate the solar surface of the foot into the sole and the frog as shown in Figure 10.2. The wall is covered by a waxy substance secreted by the periople that controls loss of

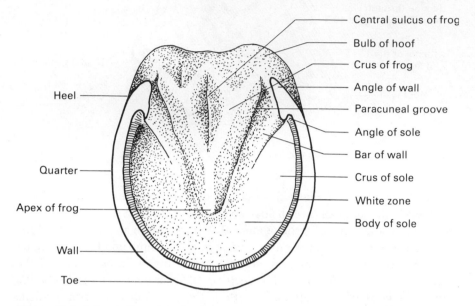

Figure 10.2 Solar surface of the hoof.

moisture from the hoof. The insensitive stratum medium forms the bulk of the wall and exhibits parallel ridges and depressions that extend from the base to the coronary band, which lies at the junction of the hoof and the skin. The deeper inner portion of the wall is referred to as the laminar corium and is formed by approximately 600 primary epidermal laminae, each of which gives off a hundred or so secondary laminae as shown in Figure 10.3. These interlock with corresponding vascular primary dermal laminae of the laminar corium that blends into the periosteum of the coffin bone. The coffin bone is actually suspended within the hoof by the interlocking of the dermal and epidermal laminae.

The hoof wall is thickest at the toe, thinner at the quarters and widens again at the heels. The sole makes up the greater portion of the ground surface of the foot. The hardened tissue of the sole is produced by the underlying corium which is an extension of the laminar corium covering the coffin bone. The white zone or line is the linear junction formed by the periphery of the sole with laminae of the hoof wall. It is thickest at the toe and thinnest at the heel and is readily apparent after the foot has been trimmed and rasped. As the

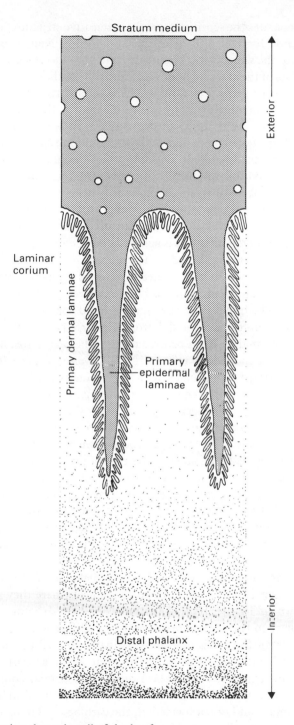

Figure 10.3 Section through wall of the hoof.

white zone separates the sensitive from the insensitive structures of the hoof it is used as a guide for nail placement during shoeing. Nails should be driven peripherally to the white zone. The white zone serves to absorb shock between the movements of the sole and hoof wall. The cells of the sole become cornified and harden as they grow providing its characteristic rigidity. Growth of solar tissue is at approximately the same rate as the hoof wall; however, wear of the sole is more rapid due to its softer consistency—it is composed of one-third water. One of the more common mistakes in trimming and shoeing horses is to remove excessive sole material. The sole is not designed as a weight-bearing structure and is concave to protect it from constant ground contact. The foot should be encouraged to retain its natural concavity when shod and direct contact of the sole and shoe should be minimized. The concavity of the sole serves not only to protect the underlying sensitive structures but also to increase traction. The sole of the hind foot is generally more concave than the front foot.

The frog is a triangular shaped structure that covers a portion of the coffin bone and the digital cushion. The healthy frog is a pliable, spongy structure containing 50% water and unlike other structures of the foot contains fat-secreting cells. The frog should have some ground contact in order to function properly. The pointed area of the frog is referred to as the apex and the depression in the middle is the central sulcus. The raised area near the heel at the widest area of the frog is referred to as the crus (Figure 10.2). The rear portion of the frog is continuous with the coronary cushion allowing more efficient shock absorption. The healthy frog maintains the consistency of a rubber eraser due to the fat-secreting cells and is shed about twice a year if left untrimmed. It is generally pared away during normal trimming, and shedding may not be noticeable. The frog is a good barometer of the health of the foot and becomes atrophied and small in the case of over-paring, contracted heels and if affected by thrush. Besides protecting the coffin bone, the frog is an integral part of the shock-absorbing mechanism of the foot and aids in traction. It has frequently been referred to as the heart of the foot and has been credited with improving blood circulation in the foot, acting as a hydraulic pump. The frog should not be over-pared as this prevents it from maintaining width in the heel.

Two cartilages attach to the lateral and medial side of the coffin bone just beneath the dermal laminae and extend to the heel where they are covered by skin as shown in Figure 10.4. They are wing-like structures made of soft hyaline cartilage in the young horse, and fibrocartilage in the older horse. The uppermost part of the cartilages can be palpated toward the heel of the foot. Because of their attachment to the coffin bone and rear portion of the hoof wall, they allow expansion of the heel during the ground contact phase of a stride and reduce concussion to the coffin bone and hoof wall. Due to age, concussion, injury and or conformation, the cartilages often ossify in the older horse. When the cartilages become ossified, the condition is referred to as

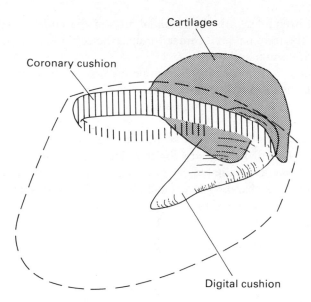

Figure 10.4 Diagrammatic representation of the cartilages and coronary and digital cushions.

sidebone. Although not a severe fault, sidebone does increase the concussive forces to which the foot is subjected and may lead to more wear and tear on the foot.

The digital cushion is part of the shock-absorbing, elastic structure 'sling' of the foot and is located deep to the frog. The digital cushion is a meshwork of collagenous and elastic fibres, deposits of fat and tough fibrocartilage. The base of the cushion bulges to form the bulbs of the heel and is continuous with the coronary cushion. The coronary cushion lies deep to the proliferative cells of the hoof wall. It is attached to the main extensor tendon and covers the extensor process of the coffin bone in the front of the foot and attaches to the lateral cartilages near the quarters of the foot. The function of the coronary cushion is protection of the extensor process and shock absorption.

Blood supply to the foot

The foot receives arterial blood from medial and lateral digital arteries which descend in each limb and are palpable over the proximal sesamoid bones at the fetlock and over the latero-palmar aspect of the first phalanx. The strength of the digital pulses are used to determine inflammation or active disease within the foot. Both digital arteries give off numerous branches in the area of the short pastern bone to supply blood to various structures of the foot. Each digital artery enters an opening in the bone (solar foramen) and joins with the other digital artery to form the terminal arch of the coffin bone. Branches arising from the terminal arch course through the coffin bone to supply blood to the laminar corium and sole.

Three venous networks or plexuses drain the vascular beds of the foot—the dorsal plexus in the laminar corium, the coronary plexus in the coronary corium and the palmar plexus consisting of venous channels from the coria of the frog, sole, digital cushion and the inner surfaces of the cartilages of the coffin bone. At the proximal edge of the cartilages the venous plexuses converge to join the medial and lateral digital veins. Besides the plexuses, venous return in the foot is facilitated by deep veins within the coffin bone and beneath the coronary band. A functional blood perfusion system in the foot is critical to the maintenance of the health of the foot.

Mechanics and maintenance of a healthy foot

Hoof growth

The hoof wall grows evenly from the coronary border at the rate of 6–9.5 mm (¼–⅜ in) per month so the youngest portion of the wall is at the heel. Since most horses have a 7.5–10 cm (3–4 in) toe this means it will grow a 'new foot' once a year. The rate of growth varies from horse to horse and several factors alone and in combination significantly affect the growth and integrity of the hoof wall. A sound solid hoof wall that grows at a reasonable rate and holds a shoe well is as much a function of breeding as any other single factor. Sound footed horses tend to produce horses with good feet. Beyond breeding, growth and integrity of the hoof wall are affected by nutrition, exercise, environment, moisture and overall general health. Horses on a good plane of nutrition tend to show accelerated hoof growth when compared to horses on a deficient plane. The water-soluble vitamin biotin and the sulphur-bearing amino acid methionine are particularly involved in promoting the production of a healthy hoof wall. Any factor that promotes circulation of blood in the foot and moisture retention impacts positively on hoof growth. Dry, hot weather and hard terrain appear to decrease hoof growth or it may be that under these conditions wear simply outstrips growth. Retaining elasticity, moisture and circulation in the foot will result in accelerated hoof growth and should be the goals of a foot-care programme, especially when horses are kept shod or under intensive training. There is a considerable difference of opinion among veterinarians and farriers with respect to the efficacy of hoof dressings applied topically. These products do no real harm and if they result in greater hoof moisture and pliability they may be of some benefit. It is worthy of note that those who are conscientious enough to go through a daily regimen of dressing the hoof are probably doing other procedures which are also necessary for correct hoof health.

Sanitation and daily care

Regular observation and cleaning of the feet will do much to ensure the foot remains healthy and free from disease. Daily cleaning of the feet may be impractical for large groups of horses turned out to pasture and receiving minimal individual care and is less important than for stabled horses. Stabled horses in work should have their feet picked daily as most are shod causing manure and bedding to become packed under the feet. Thrush and other bacterial diseases of the feet can be eliminated if the horse is kept on a routine hoof hygiene programme. Other diseases of the foot such as abscesses can be identified early and their severity minimized if the feet are cleaned and inspected daily. Cleaning of the feet ensures that the handler gives the horse at least one thorough examination daily. Teaching the horse to stand quietly while the feet are picked is a good discipline in preparation for the farrier who comes to trim or shoe the horse. Feet should be cleaned with a blunt instrument, preferably a hoof pick, to ensure the foot is not damaged. The feet should be cleaned from heel to toe rather than starting at the toe and working toward the heel. This will prevent damage to the foot if the horse has thrush or if it puts the foot down while being cleaned. All debris should be removed from around the frog and the foot examined for signs of puncture wounds, abscesses or gravels.

Routine trimming—balancing the foot

Although the inside (medial) hoof wall is steeper than the outside (lateral) hoof wall, the hoof wall should appear symmetrical from side to side and from the coronary band to the ground surface. When held the balanced foot should be flat and level. If a line is drawn down the middle of the pastern it should bisect the foot into equal parts and a line drawn across the foot should be perpendicular to the line drawn through the middle of the pastern bones. The hoof wall should be thick enough to bear weight and not wear excessively when unshod. Thin walls in foals or older horses may collapse in the quarters and exert pressure on the adjacent laminar corium and coffin bone. In the normal unshod hoof, the toe becomes worn at the point of breakover, which should occur at the centre of the toe. The concave sole should be thick enough to protect the sensitive structures of the foot, yet be free of excess horn. The frog should be broad and well developed and clear the ground except at the angle of the wall. The angle of the toe with the ground reflects the angle of the coffin bone and pastern and should be similar to the angle of the shoulder. The angle of the forefoot will vary with the overall conformation of the horse from 45 to 60°. The narrower, more pointed hind foot reflects the shape of the coffin bone. The angle of the toe in the hind foot is generally steeper than that of the front foot and varies from 55 to 60°.

From the front or rear all limbs should appear straight, with a line drawn from the point of the shoulder or point of the hip bisecting the fore and hind limbs as shown in Figure 10.5. Deviation is an indication of an angular deformity. If the joint and toe do not rest in proper alignment then a rotational limb deviation exists.

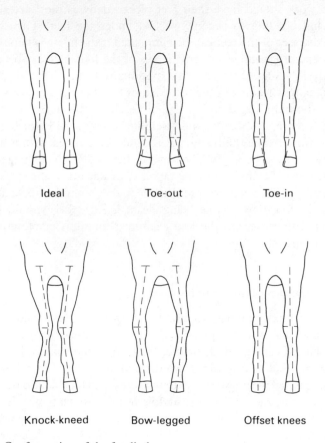

Figure 10.5 Conformation of the forelimb.

Trimming the foot should result in a balanced foot, one which is shaped to maximize function and long-term soundness. It gives the opportunity to remove excess growth and alter the growth pattern of the external hoof wall to produce a sounder foot. Trimming should be performed only as frequently as necessary and may vary widely between individuals, season and geographical locations. The time between trimmings has by convention been set at every 4–6 weeks but should be done only when needed. *Over-trimming may have a negative impact on the growth and development of the normal foot, especially in young horses.* The reasons for trimming are to remove excess growth prior to its breaking off, to remove flares and other hoof abnormalities, to change the angle of the hoof and prevent uneven wear.

The tools necessary are a hoof knife, a rasp and a set of hoof nippers. Before trimming, the foot should be examined for balance and point of breakover. The foot should be cleaned with a hoof pick or the blunt side of the hoof knife. After removal of debris the hoof knife should be used to pare away the excess sole from the bottom of the foot and trim the frog and bars of the foot. Care should be taken to thoroughly clean out the commissures (or paracuneal groove as illustrated in Figure 10.2) of the foot and any tissue that may trap debris and provide a site for the development of thrush. After paring the sole to a shiny consistency, which is characteristic of healthy sole tissue, the nippers should be used to remove excess hoof wall. The nippers should be held and used perpendicular to the ground surface of the foot. After the nippers, a rasp should level the foot and round the edges of the wall to prevent sand cracks.

Pathological conditions of the foot

Thrush

Thrush is an infection associated with poor sanitation and neglect caused by a variety of anaerobic bacteria. It is characterized by a foul smell and a sticky black exudate from affected areas of the foot causing tissue necrosis and sloughing. The frog and commissures of the foot are the most commonly affected and in severe cases the frog and underlying tissues may completely lose their functional integrity. The condition occurs more frequently in stabled horses and among horses that are infrequently trimmed. Thrush is found most commonly in the central sulcus of the frog and in the commissures, although any part of the foot may be affected. The hind feet are more prone than the front feet and horses with contracted heels and very concave feet are susceptible, especially if the frogs are not pared when the feet are trimmed or shod. Prevention of thrush requires regular trimming and cleaning of the feet, taking special care to pare away tissues in the central sulcus or commissures that may trap debris. Good hygiene in the stall, removal of soiled and damp bedding and maintaining good ventilation will prevent the occurrence of thrush. Treatment is relatively straightforward in mild cases, but is very demanding in severe cases where the sole is undermined. The first step in the elimination of thrush is removal of all necrotic tissue. As the causative organisms are primarily anaerobic, exposure of the tissue to the atmosphere is beneficial. After thorough trimming, the area should be treated with a bactericidal cleanser and antiseptic. Frequently used remedies include but are not limited to Clorox® bleach (The Clorox Company, Oakland, CA), iodine, caustic powder, or any strong antiseptic. A more severe and seldom used treatment is chemical cautery using iodine crystals and turpentine. Prevention is a much better option than cure in the case of thrush.

Quittor

Quittor involves necrosis of the cartilages of the coffin bone. The initial cause may be a bruise, laceration or puncture wound close to the coronet and is characterized by a chronic, purulent, foul-smelling discharge. Multiple drainage tracts may be evident and should be probed to determine their depth and number. Without intervention, quittor will not resolve due to poor drainage in the affected area. Horses may be sporadically lame as the wound cyclically bursts, partially heals and seals over allowing pressure to build within the foot. Treatment involves establishing effective drainage, removal of necrotic tissue and treatment with antiseptics. Partial hoof-wall resection in some cases is necessary to obtain adequate drainage and allow permanent resolution.

Gravels and abscesses

Gravels are most frequently caused by a nail driven into the white zone of the foot or by a stone bruise or puncture wound. The causes of gravel may also result in a sub-solar abscess and so these conditions will be discussed together. In a severe case there is a palpable digital pulse, heat and noticeable lameness. If an abscess is located using a hoof tester or by paring the sole, aggressive treatment is required to find the black spot or line where the abscess is located. Horses that are severely lame will be nearly sound once the pus is drained and pressure on the foot removed. The following is a step-wise procedure for the treatment of abscesses in the sole of the foot.

1. Locate the abscess using a hoof tester or hoof knife.
2. Explore the area with the knife and try to locate the origin of the abscess. If the abscess is too deep or if one is not readily found, it may be prudent to apply a poultice to soften the sole and draw the abscess.
3. After the abscess is allowed to drain, it is important to pare away all the

affected, necrotic tissue. Any necrotic tissue left is a source of re-infection.

4. Following removal of necrotic tissue the lesion should be protected with a bandage and treated with furacin or other antibacterial ointment for several days.

5. Following treatment, caustic powder should be applied to harden viable tissue and allow remaining necrotic tissue to slough off. During the time caustic powder is used the lesion should be bandaged.

6. After healing has occurred, the horse should be shod with a pad to protect the sensitive area. At this point the horse may be put back into work.

Corns

Corns occur as a result of haemorrhage or bruising of the sole of the foot. They may be present as a circular dry bruise or a moist suppurating area that is extremely sensitive and resembles a gravel. Corns are generally the result of improper shoeing, infrequent re-setting of shoes or bad conformation of the foot. Sometimes farriers will turn the branches of the shoe in the area of the heel to prevent a horse from reaching with the hind foot and removing a front shoe. Whilst this is an effective technique for protecting the heel of the shoe, if it impinges on the sole, a corn may develop. Another mistake that produces corns is setting the shoe too tight in the heel so that pressure from the shoe is exerted on the sole rather than the wall. Corns will occur if the heels of the foot are too low, either from improper trimming or faulty conformation. Infrequent shoeing, allowing the foot to grow out over the shoe will also result in pressure on the sole and the appearance of corns. Corns are not a severe problem and are easily treated by removing pressure from the sole. Making the sole concave in the area of the corn to reduce contact with the shoe will effectively eliminate the problem in the majority of cases. Occasionally it may be necessary to apply a wide web shoe, a rim pad or in cases when there is an open wound, a full pad. A bar shoe, 'eased', or taken out of contact at the site of the corn may be used to treat severe cases.

Seedy toe

Seedy toe, also referred to as white line disease, is characterized by separation of the laminae of the wall and sole, usually at the toe. The wall in the affected area sounds hollow when rapped with a hammer and generally there is a dished appearance to the foot. The cause is not known though faulty foot conformation will predispose to the development of seedy toe. It is often seen in flat-footed horses and infrequently trimmed or shod horses. An effective way to treat seedy toe is to re-establish the normal angle of the hoof. The defective wall should be trimmed away and the diseased part of the hoof wall and sole removed. Occasionally a rim shoe or a rocker toe shoe may be necessary to decrease pressure on the defective wall.

Cracks

Sandcracks and toe cracks are the result of improper or infrequent trimming and are frequently seen among horses with flared feet and thin hoof walls. They are vertical cracks in the hoof wall that affect the surface of the wall or extend completely through the hoof wall. The former are primarily cosmetic and may be due to very dry conditions or not rounding the edges of the wall in unshod horses. The latter are more serious and may affect the functional integrity of the foot. Deep cracks such as quarter cracks are caused by improper trimming, not getting the foot level prior to shoeing, not trimming unshod horses and excessive pressure being exerted on the hoof wall. Horizontal cracks generally appear following a gravel or injury in the area of the coronet. It is important to stabilize or immobilize the crack allowing the foot to grow out normally. In shod horses it is important to take the wall out of contact with the shoe in the area of the crack. For quarter cracks, clips may be drawn on either side of the crack to keep it from spreading. Severe cracks may have a plate placed across and screwed into the hoof wall on either side of the crack. Surface cracks can be prevented from extending up the foot by rasping a groove or burning a hole in the top of the crack. If these methods are used, the depth of the groove should be as deep as the crack or half the thickness of the hoof wall.

Buttress foot

Buttress foot is characterized by a swelling just above the coronary band in the region of the extensor process of the coffin bone. It is caused by fracture of the extensor process of the coffin bone, or by low ringbone. Other conditions that give rise to buttress foot are abscesses or injury to the coronary band resulting in damage to cells responsible for generation of the hoof wall. Treatment includes balancing the foot and using a rolled or rocker toe shoe to reduce pressure. Pads and silicone may also alleviate pressure and reduce the extent of lameness.

Brittle feet

One of the more frustrating conditions is brittle feet. Brittle feet are prone to quarter and toe cracks and do not support a nail. Frequently brittle feet occur in conjunction with white line disease, badly flared or flat feet. The methods previously described for treating these problems may be utilized but it is important to restore normal hoof angle and concavity of the foot. When flares exist, there is a great deal of force exerted on the hoof wall which causes the wall to break away. In cases of brittle feet it is advantageous to provide extra biotin in the diet. Biotin intake should be set at a minimum of 30 mg/day until the foot starts to respond, with subsequently a maintenance level of 20 mg/day. The use of a biotin supplement containing methionine, a sulphur-bearing amino acid, is also warranted as sulphur-bearing amino acids (methionine, cystine, cysteine) are responsible for the sulphydryl bonds providing the cross-links in hoof-wall protein. Wide web shoes and thin shanked nails should be used on horses with brittle feet. Driving nails outside the white line causes the wall to break to a greater extent than when nails are driven in the outer half of the white line. The more wall that is used in attaching the shoe the less pressure is exerted on any given nail. Also of value is hand punching of shoes when horses are re-shod, allowing nails to be positioned in different areas of the foot at each shoeing. The weight of shoes for horses with brittle feet should be only as heavy as is necessary to prevent the shoe from bending. It is also a good practice to use shoes with clips drawn to reduce the pressure on the nails. Rim shoes may be used in severe cases to hold the shoe in place or glue-on shoes may be utilized if there is inadequate hoof wall. After the foot has grown out and sound hoof material is available on the ground surface, glue-on shoes may be replaced with conventional shoes. Frequent resetting, before the shoes become loose, will do much to ensure that a sound hoof wall is maintained.

Club foot

Club foot is characterized by a very steep hoof angle at the toe, a pastern–hoof axis that is broken forward, dishing of the feet and excessive growth at the heel. The condition may be congenital or develop after foaling and there is a strong genetic predisposition. Club foot may also be caused by lameness when the horse does not use the leg or only uses the toe causing excessive wear to the toe and inadequate wear on the heel. It is seen in foals with acquired forelimb contracture, fractured coffin bones and when the ground is very hard and dry and the baby feet break off prematurely. Elimination of the condition occurs infrequently, especially in congenital cases. The foot should be trimmed such that the heel is gradually lowered and an extended toe shoe or a shoe that fits full at the toe applied to encourage growth at the toe. If the affected horse is allowed to go unshod, the toe will continue to wear more than the heel, resulting in a foot that continues to appear clubby. In some instances there may be some rotation of the coffin bone, which can be seen radiographically. Although many club-footed horses compete very well, it is a fault that diminishes the horse's value.

Flat feet

Flat-footed horses do not have the normal concave sole and are more likely to develop sole abscesses. Flat feet are seen in horses that have a tendency for flared feet and seedy toe. An attempt should be made to restore or create the normal concave sole, and flat-footed horses should be shod with a bevelled shoe to ensure weight-bearing is on the hoof wall rather than the sole. Rim pads or full pads may be used to protect the foot if the horse is to be used on rocky or uneven terrain.

Contracted heels

Contracted heels are narrower at the bulbs of the heel than normal. Frequently the frog is atrophied due to lack of ground contact and the bars of the foot are thicker and more pronounced than horses with adequate width in the heels. Horses with contracted heels are prone to thrush and navicular disease. Although contracted heels seem to predispose a horse to navicular disease, in many cases they may be as much a result as a cause. Treatment includes restoring normal moisture to the foot, trimming out the bars to allow the foot to spread, restoring normal frog pressure, and providing a slippered heel shoe. It may speed treatment to weaken the wall in the area of the heel to allow the foot to spread. A bar shoe may be used to increase weight-bearing in the area of the heel.

Sloping or underslung heels

Underslung heels may result from a congenital defect or from improper trimming or shoeing and are seen most often with a long toe-low heel conformation typical of some racehorses. The base of support is moved farther forward than it should be and the pressure on the deep digital flexor tendon is consequently increased. Leaving too much toe and consistently taking off too much heel leads to the condition. Treatment includes taking off more toe, not trimming the heel, shoeing with a wedge pad to raise the heels, and fitting the shoes full in the heel to increase support. As the pastern–hoof axis is often broken backward, re-establishment of the proper angle is important.

Navicular disease

Navicular disease is characterized by degenerative changes in the distal sesamoid or navicular bone. Navicular disease, though over-diagnosed as a cause of lameness, is responsible for roughly a third of all chronic forelimb lameness. Prior to diagnosing navicular disease other causes of lameness should be ruled out. Especially common as causes of lameness similar to navicular disease are bruised heels, sheared heels, unbalanced heels and abscesses.

Navicular disease is characterized by chronic forelimb lameness, pointing of the toe, attempts to bear weight on the toe rather than on the heels (probably the reason why navicular disease horses exhibit contracted heels), and changes in gait including stumbling and a short choppy stride. Horses in the initial stages of the syndrome frequently lose the lameness after warming up and respond to phenylbutazone or aspirin therapy. As the disease progresses, lameness is more pronounced and the gait becomes more characteristic of the navicular horse.

Treatment should begin with balancing the foot and establishing the normal axis of the hoof and pastern. The use of wedge pads or full pads may alleviate pain and allow the horse to go sound. Often, if changes in the navicular bone are slight, shoeing may result in cessation of the signs. In more severe cases, the heel of the foot should be raised using a wedge shoe or pad and the toe should be rolled, allowing for the foot to break over more easily and exert less pressure on the deep digital flexor tendon. A bar shoe will provide added support and stability to the heel area as well as protecting the frog from trauma. The use of bar shoes appears particularly effective in treating horses with a low heel, long toe conformation which is characteristic of many race-horses. A method of treatment which has recently received attention is the use of an egg-bar shoe. The egg-bar is rounded in the palmar area of the foot making it easier to move the horse's base of support backwards, consequently reducing the stress on the deep digital flexor tendon. Egg-bar shoes are par-ticularly effective in treating horses with sheared or underslung heels.

Besides shoeing therapy, navicular disease has been treated with varying degrees of success by medication. Medication should only follow the advice of a veterinarian who has examined the animal and includes non-steroidal anti-inflammatory drugs such as phenylbutazone, sodium hyaluronate, polysul-phated glycosaminoglycan, warfarin (an anticoagulant), isoxsuprine and corti-costeroids.

Horses with navicular disease appear to benefit from limited exercise. The positive effects of exercise are derived from increased blood perfusion to the foot. Other options for treatment include acupuncture and palmar digital neurectomy.

Laminitis

Laminitis or founder is one of the more severe disease states involving the foot. By definition laminitis is an inflammation of the laminar structures of the foot and varies significantly in degrees of severity. Although the predisposing causes are varied, the basic pathology involves interruption of laminar blood flow followed by necrosis of the interdigitation between the dermal and epidermal laminae. This inflammation and damage to the laminar bed results in loss of functional integrity of the support structure of the foot. It is the degree to which function is compromised that determines the severity of a case of laminitis.

The incidence of laminitis is highest in ponies, lower in geldings and least in stallions and mares. Seasonal variation of the disease is seen: with early growth of pasture in the spring, overweight horses especially ponies on pasture are susceptible. Laminitis is caused by a number of different factors acting alone or in combination. The classical one and one that has been investigated in greatest detail is excessive intake of carbohydrate in the diet. Abnormal amounts of carbohydrate in the diet overwhelm the digestive capacity of the horse causing increased quantities of readily fermentable starch to enter the hind gut. Rapid fermentation results in the formation of lactic acid, causing the caecal pH to fall dramatically. The acid pH results in lysis of caecal bacteria with the release of bacterial endotoxins that are absorbed through the gut mucosa into the circulation. The endotoxins are thought to be the triggering mechanism for vasoactive mediators resulting in damage to the laminae due to loss of the blood supply. However, the exact chain of events remains obscure. Toxaemia secondary to retained placenta and acute gastrointestinal disease such as Potomac horse fever may also cause laminitis.

Traumatic laminitis can occur when overweight horses are exercised on a hard surface. Laminitis may also develop in a forelimb which has to bear excessive weight during the recuperative phase when the other forelimb is recovering from a fracture. Drug-induced laminitis has been observed following the administration of certain corticosteroids and following excessive consumption of cold water after exercise.

Laminitis in the acute form should be treated as an emergency requiring immediate attention. Although the front feet are most commonly affected all four feet may be involved. Lameness develops rapidly and animals shift their weight from one foot to another. The stance of a horse with acute laminitis is quite typical. The horse will rock back on the heels of the front feet taking more weight onto the hindlimbs by shifting them forward under the body. This stance is exaggerated when the horse is made to walk or turn in a circle. Horses in severe pain will remain recumbent. There is excessive warmth in the hoof area and an exaggerated digital pulse. Hoof testers when applied to the sole will evoke a pain response. Radiographic examination will reveal whether rotation of the coffin bone has occurred. When exacerbation of the disease occurs and no improvement is seen following therapy the condition should be considered refractory and carries an unfavourable prognosis. The chronic form of laminitis causes recurrent lameness aggravated by recent foot trimming and exercise on a hard surface. The chronic form follows the acute or refractory form in which rotation of the coffin bone has occurred. Damage to the laminae results in abnormal hoof growth observed as rings around the hoof wall. A flattened or convex sole (dropped sole) and abnormally long toe will develop if trimming is not regularly undertaken. Horses with chronic laminitis usually move with a two-phase placement of the feet—heel toe, heel toe—best observed when the horse is trotting. There is increased sensitivity of the sole to the hoof tester and a greater tendency of the hoof wall to crack and for development of abscesses beneath the sole.

As the blood supply to the laminae is disrupted, tissue necrosis occurs causing a separation of the dermal from the epidermal laminae. Laminar separation results in two major anatomical derangements, rotation of the third phalanx and a condition referred to as sinking. In cases where rotation occurs the laminae on the dorsal aspect of the foot separate allowing the coffin bone to rotate downward. The degree of rotation is the major criterion for assessing the severity and therefore the prognosis for recovery. In cases referred to as sinkers, the laminae around the total circumference of the foot become detached causing the coffin bone to slide downward. Both rotation and sinking of the coffin bone further occlude the blood supply by causing tearing and compression of the blood vessels. As the cascade of events continues and rotation and/or sinking proceeds, further necrosis of the foot occurs. The coffin bone may eventually penetrate the sole and the entire foot may slough off. Improper or inadequate treatment during the acute or chronic phase will reduce the chance of the horse's recovery and it is critical that treatment of laminitis-affected horses begins as soon as any signs are noticed.

If the cause of the acute laminitis is known, therapy should be instituted to reduce the severity of the metabolic disturbance. Mineral oil should be given by nasogastric tube to coat the gut mucosa so reducing the uptake of endotoxins and increasing the rate of passage of digesta. Intravenous fluids can be given to correct electrolyte and fluid imbalances and antibiotics administered if septicaemia is present. Although exercise causes vasodilation and an increase in blood flow, it should be avoided in the acute stages as further mechanical damage may occur. The administration of phenylbutazone and antihistamines to reduce pain and inflammation is generally recommended. Laminitic horses should be fed only grass hay during the acute phase and if the horse is overweight it should be placed on a reduced diet thereafter. A case of acute laminitis may take several days or weeks to respond. A variety of medications to treat the acute and refractory forms have been used with a variable degree of success. They include dimethyl sulphoxide (DMSO), acepromazine, acetyl salicylate (aspirin), flunixin meglumine (banamine), heparin, isoxsuprine and warfarin.

As regards shoeing of the laminitic horse, stabilization of the coffin bone and reduction of pressure on the pedal vasculature are of primary concern. Support of the frog is critical, which is best achieved by applying a heart-bar shoe following advice from the attending veterinarian.

Further reading

Butler K D (1974) *The principles of horseshoeing*. Doug Butler Publishing, Maryville, MO.

Greely R C (1970) *The art and science of horseshoeing*. J B Lippincott, Philadelphia.

Rooney J R (1969) *Biomechanics of lameness in horses*. Williams & Wilkins, Baltimore.

Stashak T S (1987) *Adam's lameness in horses*, 4th edn. Lea & Febiger, Philadelphia.

Stick J A (1987) Foot diseases. In Robinson N E (ed) *Current therapy in equine medicine*, 2nd ed. W B Saunders, Philadelphia, pp 255–90.

Yovich J Y (1989) *The equine foot*. The Veterinary Clinics of North America, Equine Practice. W B Saunders, Philadelphia.

GLOSSARY

acid–base balance   a state of equilibrium in the buffering system of blood.

amyloidosis   an abnormal condition characterized by deposition of a waxy translucent substance consisting of protein and polysaccharide in tissues, particularly the liver.

anaerobic   living in the absence of free oxygen.

anaphylactoid   resembling anaphylaxis.

anaphylaxis   a hypersensitivity reaction following an injection of antigen.

aneurysm   a permanent abnormal blood-filled dilation of a blood vessel resulting from disease of the vessel wall.

anionic   composed of negatively charged particles.

anorexia   loss of appetite.

anthelmintic   a drug that expels and destroys parasitic worms of the intestine.

antibodies   serum proteins which are produced by the immune system following contact with antigen. They bind specifically to the antigen which induced their formation.

antigen   a protein or carbohydrate substance capable of stimulating an immune response.

antiseptic   a substance which inhibits the growth and development of microorganisms but does not necessarily kill them; usually in reference to use on skin or living tissue.

antiserum   serum from an animal containing specific antibodies produced by repeated immunization.

antitoxin   antibody that is capable of neutralizing a specific toxin.

artificial vagina   a device for collecting semen from the stallion.

atrophy   decrease in size or wasting away of a part of the body or tissue.

bacterin   a suspension of killed or attenuated bacteria for use as a vaccine.

bactericidal   the ability to kill bacteria.

bacteriostatic   inhibiting the growth or multiplication of bacteria.

barren mare   a mare that has been mated but is not pregnant.

biodegradable   capable of being broken down into innocuous products by the action of living cells.

bolus   a soft mass of chewed food.

caecum   the blind pouch in which the large intestine begins and into which the ileum opens from one side.

cationic   composed of positively charged particles.

cervix   the narrow lower or outer end of the uterus.

chorion   the highly vascular outer embryonic membrane that, with the allantois, forms the placenta.

clitoral sinuses   cavities in the clitoris—a small organ situated in the ventral part of the vulva.

coccidia   common name given to certain protozoan parasites.

coccidiostat   a chemical compound usually added to animal feeds to partially inhibit or delay the development of coccidiosis.

colic   acute abdominal pain of the intestine caused by spasm, obstruction or twisting.

complement   one of the serum enzyme systems whose functions include mediating inflammation, engulfing foreign antigens and damaging invading pathogens.

contagious   capable of being transmitted by contact.

copraphagy   the eating of faecal matter.

corium (dermis)   the sensitive vascular inner layer of the skin.

coronet   the junction between the skin and the hoof.

cribber   a horse with the vice of gnawing at solid objects.

crimp   mechanically breaking the outer coating of grains to improve their digestibility.

croup   the part of the top line of the horse that lies distal to the hip bones and in front of the tailhead.

cultivar   a plant originating and persisting under cultivation.

cytology   a branch of biology dealing with the structure, function, multiplication, pathology and life history of cells.

deamination   to remove the amino group from a compound.

disinfection   the act of killing pathogenic organisms.

diurnal   active during the daytime.

DNA (deoxyribonucleic acid)   a complex nucleic acid occurring in cell nuclei which is the molecular basis of heredity.

dystocia   a slow or difficult birth delivery.

embolus   an abnormal particle such as a blood clot circulating in the blood.

encephalitis   inflammation of the brain.

encephalomyelitis   inflammation of the brain and spinal cord.

endemic (or enzootic)   restricted or peculiar to a locality or region.

endometrial cups   tissue of foetal origin which invades the endometrium at 36 to 38 days of gestation producing pregnant mare's serum gonadotrophin (PMSG), which assists in the maintenance of pregnancy.

endometrial cyst   a closed sac having a distinct membrane which develops as a result of a blocked or dilated endometrial gland.

endometrium   the mucous membrane lining the uterus.

endophyte a parasite living inside another organism.

endotoxaemia the presence of endotoxins in the blood.

endotoxin a poisonous substance present in bacteria but separable from the cell only on its disintegration.

endotoxoid a toxoid derived from an endotoxin.

enterotoxaemia a condition resulting from absorption of toxin from the intestine.

eosinophil a leucocyte 'white blood cell' with cytoplasmic inclusions readily stained by eosin.

epidemic (or **epizootic**) affecting many individuals within the population at the same time.

epiphysitis inflammation of the end of a long bone.

flares lateral and medial horny outgrowths at the base of the hoof that are not weight-bearing, causing the foot to become asymmetrical.

flat plates horseshoes without toe grabs or heel calks.

footings an enlargement at the lower end of a foundation which helps to distribute the load.

fungicide an agent that kills fungi.

fungistat an agent that inhibits the growth of fungi without destroying them.

genome the total genetic material in a cell.

glycolysis the enzymatic breakdown of a carbohydrate (as glucose) with the production of pyruvic or lactic acid and energy.

glycoprotein a conjugated protein in which the non-protein group is a carbohydrate.

granulocytes (**polymorphs**) phagocytic cells distributed throughout the organs of the body whose function is to engulf antigenic and tissue particles.

haematoma a tumour or swelling containing blood.

haemoglobin an iron-containing protein pigment in red blood cells responsible for transporting oxygen from the lungs to the tissues of the body.

herbicide an agent used to destroy or inhibit plant growth.

herbivore a plant-eating animal.

homeostasis the maintenance of stable physiological conditions such as body temperature and pH of the blood.

hypercalcitoninism increased secretion of the hormone calcitonin from the thyroid, which lowers the level of calcium in plasma.

hyperimmune serum serum containing large quantities of a specific antibody.

hyperparathyroidism the presence of excess parathormone resulting in a disturbance of calcium metabolism.

hypodont describing teeth having high or deep crowns and short roots.

hypothalamus a part of the brain which releases a hormone to initiate secretion of hormones from the pituitary gland.

immunization the procedure of antigen administration to induce antibodies or produce protective immunity.

immunocompetent   capable of mounting a normal immune response.
immunoglobulin (Ig)   a synonym for antibody.
infectious   the invasion and multiplication of microorganisms in body tissues.
instar   a stage in the life of an insect between two successive moults.
interferon   any of a group of molecules which limit the spread of viral infection.

laminitis   inflammation of the laminae in the hoof of the horse.
leucocytes   any of the white or colourless nucleated blood cells that occur in mammals.
lymph node   small encapsulated organs in the lymphoid network containing aggregates of lymphocytes.
lymphocytes   cells which control the immune response.
lymphokines   substances other than antibodies produced by lymphocytes that act as chemical signals between the cells of the immune system.

macrophage   a large phagocytic cell.
maiden mare   a mare that has never been mated.
marsupial   an order of mammals including kangaroos which have a pouch on the abdomen of the female for carrying the young.
mast cells   cells that contain granules which when released mediate the inflammatory response.
monocytes   a type of leucocyte that migrates into tissues to become a macrophage.
morbidity   the incidence of disease in a population.
mortality   the number of deaths occurring in a population at a given time or place.
mycelium   the mass of filamentous hyphae that form the vegetative portion of a fungus.

neutrophils   the most abundant type of leucocyte in the blood that has phagocytic properties.
non-ionic   composed of neutral (non-charged) particles.
nucleotide   any of several compounds that are the basic structural units of RNA and DNA.

occlusal   describing the biting or grinding surface of the teeth.
oestradiol   a synthetic oestrogenic hormone.
oestrogen   a hormone which promotes oestrus and stimulates the development of secondary sexual characteristics.
oestrous cycle   the cycle of changes in the endocrine and reproductive systems of a female mammal from the beginning of one oestrus period to the beginning of the next.
oestrus   a regularly recurrent state of sexual excitability during which the female will accept the male and is capable of conceiving.
oocysts   the encysted form of a coccidian parasite which develops into the next generation.
opaline   resembling opal in appearance.
osmotic balance   the state which the concentrations of the components on either side of a living membrane reach equilibrium.
ossification   the process of bone formation.

ossify   to form or be transformed into bone.

osteochondrosis   a disease in which an ossification centre, especially in the epiphyses of long bones, undergoes degeneration followed by calcification.

osteomalacia   a disease characterized by softening of bones in the mature horse.

osteoporosis   a condition characterized by a decrease in bone mass as a result of disturbance of nutrition and mineral metabolism.

oviduct   a tube that carries ova from the ovary to the uterus.

palmar   relating to the undersurface of the forefoot.

parakeratosis   an abnormality of the horny layer of the skin.

pathogen   a causative agent of disease.

perinatal   occurring around the time of birth.

periople   the thin outer waxy layer of the hoof.

periosteum   the membrane of connective tissue that closely invests all bones except at the articular surface.

phagocytes   cells, including monocytes, macrophages and neutrophils, that have the ability to engulf foreign material and tissue debris.

phagocytosis   the process by which phagocyte cells engulf particles and microorganisms.

photosynthesis   the formation of carbohydrates from carbon dioxide and hydrogen by chlorophyll-containing plants exposed to light.

phytate   a salt or ester of phytic acid.

pineal gland   a small endocrine gland arising from the brain that may be a vestigial third eye.

pituitary gland   an endocrine organ of the brain which secretes several hormones influencing other endocrine glands controlling growth and development of smooth muscle, renal function and reproduction.

placenta   the vascular organ in mammals that unites the foetus to the maternal uterus and mediates metabolic exchange.

plasma cells (antibody-forming cells)   cells derived from B-lymphocytes devoted to the secretion of antibody.

platelets   constituents of blood that assist in clotting.

progesterone   a steroid hormone produced by the corpus luteum or produced synthetically.

progestogen   a collective name for progestational steroids.

prostaglandins   substances which have a variety of hormone–like actions including the control of smooth muscle.

pseudostem   the region of the plant above the ground but below the leafy portion.

purpura haemorrhagica   small haemorrhages in the skin and mucous membranes caused by a reduction in circulating blood platelets.

rhabdomyolysis   the destruction or degeneration of skeletal muscle.

rhizome   a horizontal plant stem that differs from a root in possessing buds, nodes and leaves.

rickets   a condition characterized by soft and deformed bones in the young, caused by a failure to assimilate and use calcium and phosphorus due to inadequate sunlight or vitamin D.

septicaemia   invasion of the bloodstream by virulent bacteria.

serotype a group of intimately related organisms distinguished by a common set of antigens.

serum sickness a hypersensitivity reaction occurring in individuals injected with foreign serum.

slot seeding a shallow channel cut in the ground in which seed is placed.

speculum an instrument for inserting into a body passage to facilitate visual inspection.

sporicidal able to kill spores.

steam rolled steam processing of grains by flattening or rolling to facilitate their digestibility.

stolon a horizontal branch from the base of a plant that produces new plants from buds at its tip.

subchondral situated beneath cartilage.

testosterone a male hormone produced by the testes or made synthetically which is responsible for inducing and maintaining male secondary sex characteristics.

thrombus a clot of blood formed within a blood vessel that remains attached to its place of origin.

thymus a primary lymphoid organ seeded by lymphoid cells from the bone marrow that produces T-lymphocytes.

thyroid a large endocrine gland situated at the anterior ventral part of the thorax which produces an iodine-containing hormone that has a profound effect on growth, development and metabolic rate.

toxoid a toxin of a pathogenic organism treated so as to destroy its toxicity but which is still capable of inducing antibody formation.

umbilical cord a cord that connects the foetus with the placenta and contains the umbilical arteries and veins.

ungulate hoofed mammals.

urachus a cord of fibrous tissue extending from the bladder to the umbilicus.

urticaria an allergic reaction causing raised swellings on the skin and mucous membrane.

vagina a canal in the female mammal that leads from the uterus to the external orifice.

vestibule the space between the labia and lips of the external female genitalia.

viraemia the presence of virus particles in the blood.

virucidal able to kill viruses.

vulva the external parts of the female genital organs.

windrow (swath) forage cut with a mower piled in a row prior to baling.

withers the ridge between the shoulder bones of a horse.

zoonosis any disease which is transmitted from animals to people.

INDEX